CONTEMPORARY CASE STUDIES IN CLINICAL MENTAL HEALTH FOR CHILDREN AND ADOLESCENTS

CONTEMPORARY CASE STUDIES IN CLINICAL MENTAL HEALTH FOR CHILDREN AND ADOLESCENTS

JENNIFER N. BAGGERLY
University of North Texas at Dallas

ATHENA A. DREWES
New York Association for Play Therapy

ROWMAN & LITTLEFIELD
Lanham • Boulder • New York • London

Acquisitions Editor: Lilith Dorko
Assistant Acquisitions Editor: Sarah Rinehart
Sales and Marketing Inquiries: textbooks@rowman.com

Published by Rowman & Littlefield
An imprint of The Rowman & Littlefield Publishing Group, Inc.
4501 Forbes Boulevard, Suite 200, Lanham, Maryland 20706
www.rowman.com

86-90 Paul Street, London EC2A 4NE

British Library Cataloguing in Publication Information Available

Library of Congress Cataloging-in-Publication Data
Names: Baggerly, Jennifer, editor. | Drewes, Athena A., 1948– editor.
Title: Contemporary case studies in clinical mental health for children and adolescents /
    Jennifer N. Baggerly, University of North Texas at Dallas, Athena A. Drewes, New York
    Association for Play Therapy.
Description: Lanham : Rowman & Littlefield, [2024] | Includes bibliographical references and
    index.
Identifiers: LCCN 2023038904 (print) | LCCN 2023038905 (ebook) | ISBN 9781538173626
    (hardback) | ISBN 9781538173633 (paperback) | ISBN 9781538173640 (epub)
Subjects: LCSH: Mental illness—Diagnosis. | Adolescent psychotherapy. | Psychology, Pathological.
Classification: LCC RJ503.5 .C66 2024 (print) | LCC RJ503.5 (ebook) | DDC
    616.89/140835—dc23/eng/20231031
LC record available at https://lccn.loc.gov/2023038904
LC ebook record available at https://lccn.loc.gov/2023038905

I, Jennifer Baggerly, dedicate this book to my father and stepmother, Dr. Leo Baggerly and Mrs. Carole Baggerly, for their lifetime of support and inspiration to me and my daughter, Katelyn Jean Baggerly.

I, Athena Drewes, dedicate this book to my husband, Dr. (Nelson) Keith Seibert, whose love and support make my life full of wonderful adventures.

Brief Contents

Contents

PART II: ADOLESCENTS

List of Figures, Tables, and Textboxes

Textboxes

Foreword

In early 2002, while in an internship, I saw my first child and adolescent clients. I was a second-year student completing a master's degree in community counseling. At that point, my training to work with child and adolescent clients consisted of two courses: introduction to play therapy and child and adolescent counseling. What I had to offer was funneled through knowledge gained, yet, I had little practical experience applying this knowledge. Running through my head were many theories, skills, and techniques and a lot of fear. The fear was centered on the fact that I was working with a vulnerable population who had little choice in their outcomes. Surrounding all the information I had learned was a statement that I had heard over and over: meet them where they are.

Though children and adolescents have always experienced difficulties, in the 20 years or so since my first clients, it seems that these difficulties are more frequent and pervasive. As we find ourselves following several years of an unexpected and overwhelming pandemic, we are more aware than ever of the mental health issues facing children and adolescents. Did the pandemic cause more mental health issues? Yes, but it did much more. The pandemic removed many of the avenues of support available to children and adolescents, leaving mental health issues an unencumbered path in which issues thrive.

While reflecting on my abilities 20 years ago and the pandemic, I could conclude that had I started practicing during the pandemic, I might have been underprepared. Then again, maybe not, because so much of what I learned through working with my first clients came from being present and attentive. It came from a hypothesis (diagnosis) and a conceptualization and was guided by a theoretical philosophy and a willingness to meet them where they were. So, whether in the room with them or connected through a teleconferencing platform, I believe that I would have relied on what had guided my facilitation in the past.

Now, after having been an educator for more than 15 years, I understand what helped me become a competent practitioner and educator. I learned that all clients are unique and present with varying circumstances, but our first few clients help us develop case conceptualization skills that can be applied to the next clients. Case conceptualizations are not easy. They take practice and experience. Our first case conceptualizations are akin to trial and error and hunches and are only guided by the facts we have collected. Through practice, we learn to look deeper.

I believe that had I had a text like *Contemporary Case Studies in Clinical Mental Health for Children and Adolescents*, my journey into case conceptualization and client work would have been easier. The text adds to our foundation in child and adolescent therapy as it is full of robust case examples covering numerous mental health issues. Across the child and adolescent cases, multiple theoretical approaches are described and linked to treatment goals and objectives. Adding to the practical nature of the text are realistic session descriptions providing readers with a glimpse into how sessions might progress. Throughout the 20 chapters, as one reads, I believe each reader will see themselves in the therapist's place. Seldom covered in most texts, but highlighted in this text, are the sections, in each chapter, on parent and/or teacher consultation.

Contemporary Case Studies in Clinical Mental Health for Children and Adolescents is not prescriptive, in that it does not attempt to assert that what is described is the only way to work with a child or adolescent experiencing a specific issue. The seasoned editors, Jennifer Baggerly and Athena Drewes, transparently state that the text is not intended to be a step-by-step manual. Rather, the extensive use of case illustrations along with questions for reflection make it possible for practitioners to extrapolate beneficial principles that can be applied to their clients.

As mental health practitioners, we are expected to conceptualize our clients to develop the best course of action to help remediate their issues. The case conceptualization process gives us a starting point to which we can connect empirically supported interventions. Through texts such as *Contemporary Case Studies in Clinical Mental Health for Children and Adolescents*, we're able to see the linking of case conceptualization to empirically supported intervention. We can see, through our clients' worldview and circumstances, how one's theoretical lens can be applied.

As a counselor educator, I found *Contemporary Case Studies in Clinical Mental Health for Children and Adolescents* to be an exceptional guide to help my counseling students conceptualize and treat culturally diverse children and adolescents. As a seasoned child and adolescent clinician, I found it to be a refreshing reminder about applying key therapeutic principles and evidence-based procedures with each unique client. I also found it to be a challenging call to consider expanding my clinical strategies. In summary, this text is valuable for beginning and experienced clinicians working with children and adolescents post-pandemic and beyond.

Edward (Franc) Hudspeth, PhD, NCC,
LPC-S, ACS, RPT-S, RPh
Program Coordinator, EdS in Counselor
Education-Play Therapy
University of Mississippi

Preface

Jennifer N. Baggerly and Athena A. Drewes

Inspiration

The inspiration for *Contemporary Case Studies in Clinical Mental Health for Children and Adolescents* came during the world's life-altering COVID-19 pandemic during 2020, referred to as "the year from hell" (Wikipedia). In January of 2020, I (JB) heard a medical professional say on television, "Life as you know it will change because of this coronavirus." I thought to myself, *well, that seems a little extreme*. I wish I were wrong, but as we now know, millions of lives were impacted for at least two years and some for even more.

Children's and adolescents' mental health plummeted. The pandemic triggered some children to experience anxiety, depression, abuse, and grief. Children who already had ADHD became more symptomatic during the COVID quarantine. Then the death of George Floyd ignited a social fire, in which some people protested for justice while others balked. Hate crimes and political extremist groups increased. This anger and tension in the community at large seemed to reflect anger and tension within families.

Early in the pandemic, many mental health professionals (MHP) experienced financial anxiety from not having as many clients and trying to figure out telehealth. Then the surge hit with parents, educators, and medical professionals inundating mental health professionals with referrals of children and adolescents desperate for relief. Indeed, mental health became the second wave of the COVID-19 crisis, cresting only after the medical outlook stabilized. It was all hands on deck. As a counselor educator, I (JB) was teaching classes, providing counseling to as many children and adolescents as possible, and supervising new professionals who were trying to keep up. One new counselor said to me, "I don't feel ready but so many children need me. I need more than weekly supervision because there are so many different problems that it seems I forgot how to counsel. I wish there was a book that gave me concrete examples of what to do and say and how to conceptualize treatment for lots of different children and adolescents."

Like many MHP, this new professional experienced the pressing urgency of numerous children struggling with contemporary challenges. Constant requests to serve more and more children resulted in some MHP feeling so overwhelmed that they worried that they had forgotten how to do things properly and forgot about self-care. A physical book with concrete examples as well as case conceptualization analysis was needed to remind us of all of the key theoretical concepts and strategies that lead to therapeutic change. We need to be reminded of how to counsel lots of different types of children and adolescents struggling with lots of different recent realities. We need contemporary case studies that reflect this changing world. We need *Contemporary Case Studies in Clinical Mental Health for Children and Adolescents*.

Book Chapter Authors

Along with Athena Drewes, we contacted experts in specific counseling approaches for specific presenting problems. We developed "the dream team" of passionate, seasoned therapists to share case studies of diverse children and adolescents including Caucasian, Black, Latinx, Asian, indigenous, LGBTQ, and neurodivergent. We divided the sections into children and adolescents with common presenting problems such as depression, anxiety, ADHD, divorce, domestic violence, sexual abuse, self-harm, eating disorders, and substance abuse. For children, theoretical approaches include Child-Centered Play Therapy (CCPT) and variants such as Trauma-Informed CCPT and Critical Race Theory with CCPT; Adlerian Play Therapy; Cognitive Behavioral Play Therapy; AutPlay; sand tray; Filial Therapy; and Child-Parent Relationship Therapy. For adolescents, theoretical approaches include Cognitive Behavior Therapy (CBT) with expressive arts, Mindfulness CBT, Trauma-Focused CBT, equine therapy, motivational interviewing, queer and liberatory approaches, and narrative therapy. In summary, our book is unique in describing how to treat numerous presenting problems with various theoretical approaches for uniquely diverse clients.

What the Book Is Not

This book is *not* a one-size-fits-all approach to counseling. We recognize that the intersectionality of gender, age, racial and ethnic identity, language, religion, family status, personality, presenting problems, and so forth impact the type of treatment approach for each client. We recognize that clients tend to have overlapping concerns beyond one diagnosis. We recognize that children and adolescents are people first and are more than just their problems. Some need a child-centered approach, others need a cognitive behavioral approach, others need an integrative approach. Yet most importantly, each needs an authentic relationship with a caring and trained mental health professional who provides genuineness, empathy, and unconditional positive regard.

This book is *not* a step-by-step approach for clients with a particular diagnosis. Not only do we see each child and adolescent as an individual who is very complex, but we see each MHP as very complex with various training and professional experiences. We honor MHPs' therapeutic judgment to prescriptively select a treatment approach for a particular client and encourage flexibility within the limits of MHP training. Some MHP are not trained in play therapy, beyond a day or two workshop, and should not state that they are providing play therapy. Likewise, others are not trained in equine therapy and should not provide it. Fortunately, we do provide resources where you can seek training.

What the Book Is

In this book, we offer a guide in how to conceptualize specific presenting problems and operationalize specific theoretical treatment strategies with a particular child or adolescent. We provide concrete illustrations through a sample transcript analysis. I (JB) learned this technique from the late great Nancy Boyd Webb. I realized it was important when one of my supervisees said, "Your suggested responses to my videos seem to come so easily to you. I wish there was a book that gave me examples of what to say in difficult cases." The therapeutic responses provided are examples of how to start or reminders of what is helpful.

This book does address controversial issues, especially Critical Race Theory (CRT), transgender youth, undocumented immigrants, and gun violence. The legislators in our states (Texas and Florida) have banned Critical Race Theory, which helps to conceptualize racism, from being taught in K–12 and have proposed legislation to ban CRT in higher education. The legislators in our states have also denied access to gender-affirming care for trans children; denied access to immigrants and rights to undocumented people; and protected access to semi-automatic guns. Yet, as mental health professionals, our clients face these issues, and we are called to provide ethical care for them. Our chapter authors are mental health experts who guide us in doing so.

Structure for Book Chapters

Our book chapter structures have several unique features that differ from other books.

Begin with Case Studies

We start with the case scenario to pique your interest and draw you into contemplation of a specific client's gender, age, race/ethnicity, culture, family context, and presenting problems. Starting with this holistic case study overview, which reflects actual case consultations, the reader gets to see how counselors make clinical decisions based on aspects of a particular client's needs and how it leads to tentative goals and then therapeutic approaches.

All case studies are composites, representing common characteristics and experiences of clients with specific diagnoses. Each case uses pseudonyms to protect the privacy of any client who may resemble the description.

Brief Overview of Issues and Treatment Approaches

Next, we provide a brief literature review to promote understanding of the complexity of presenting problems and cultural issues that may apply. Frequently, counselors brush past this and rely on past knowledge, which can lead to simplistic assumptions. Our up-to-date literature reviews bring to attention nuances and connections that even seasoned counselors may take for granted.

Descriptions of treatment approaches highlight key principles and procedures in a way that motivates commitment to them. Too frequently we lose the awe-inspiring holding and integration of theoretical tenets. Yet, these are the key to therapeutic success. Therefore, we encourage a fresh reading of the theoretical approach.

Treatment Goals and Objectives

Often treatment goals and objectives are written in an almost "cut and paste" obligatory manner. Prior to electronic records, many counselors kept treatment goals in the back of the file without regular review. This approach would be like driving from Florida to Washington state without looking at the GPS. You have a general direction but are bound to get lost and not know when you have reached your goal, resulting in inefficient progress toward agreed-upon goals. Regular review of treatment goals and objectives, with the client and family, helps to reinforce progress, strengthen collaboration, assess where treatment is in relationship to termination, and whether the approach needs to be adjusted. Reviews also help to ensure counselor accountability and that the treatment is in the best interest of the client.

Further, many counselors may feel at a loss as to what the treatment goals and objectives should be. This is partly because, in typical practice, counselors seldom discuss them with colleagues who hold a like theoretical perspective. Seeing how specific treatment goals and objectives for a specific client and situation are written will help clinicians create better treatment plans for their own cases.

Session Description and Transcript Analysis

To make session descriptions more personable and accessible, we had the authors use the first person, "I," to explain what they did. We wanted to approach the description as if a colleague asked, "What did you do with this client and how did it turn out?" The "I" approach is intended to be less academic and more friendly. After all, counselors are people, too. The "I" creates a vulnerability rather than a disconnected abstract idea of "the counselor."

Our session transcripts and analysis provide a glimpse into how a counselor implements theory, what she might say, and why she says it. This is the nuts-and-bolts approach. It is not a treatment manual of specific things you should or must say. Rather, it is an example of what session content can look like for this particular client in this particular context with this particular theory. Many times, you may think, *I say the same thing*, or *Oh, that is an interesting way to demonstrate that concept*, or *I would have said it differently*. All of these thoughts are fine. The transcript may confirm what you do or improve what you do. More importantly, the transcript analysis helps you to consider the "why" of what you do. I tell my counseling students, "I will stop your video at any random moment and ask you to provide a theoretical rationale for why you said what you did or did what you did." I always love seeing the look of panic on my students' faces when I say this because then I can help them realize they know or need to know the theoretical rationale. Then their faces turn to a look of contemplation and commitment to be the best counselor they can be in each session.

Ethical and Cultural Considerations

Ethics are so important that most state licensing boards and clinical associations require numerous hours in ethical training each renewal cycle. Our chapter authors remind us of both common and specific ethical considerations for each case study. They explain how they work toward aspirational ethics of evaluating their actions and ethical code to ensure that their clients receive services that exceed the expected standard of care, often through social justice advocacy.

For cultural considerations, our chapter authors discuss the client's intersectionality of gender, age, race, ethnicity, culture, religion, socioeconomic status, family context, school context, local community environment, broader societal events, political environment, and oppressive forces such as racism that they may have experienced. They provide guidance in honoring clients' culture through practical suggestions.

Parent and Teacher Consultation

Parent and teacher consultations are not often discussed in books. However, they are crucial for success because parents and teachers influence for better or worse the immediate environment of children and adolescents. MHP have wisdom to guide parents and teachers in new attitudes, skills, and directions to improve their children's lives. Our authors share their approach to enhance parents' and teachers' supports for children and adolescents.

Sample Case Notes

MHP seldom share case notes. Although MHP are required to write case notes after every session, these notes seem to be a mystery. What is amazing about our authors' case notes is that they are all different. Some use forms whereas others use SOAP (subjective, objective, assessment, plan) and others free write. It was validating to see that case notes can be so different and so on target.

Resources

Our chapter authors share their go-to resources for professional training, children, and parents. If you are new to a subject and don't know where to start, our chapter authors will point you in a helpful direction. If you are well versed in an approach, you may find something new.

Discussion Questions

Each chapter asks you specific questions to extend your thinking and learning, either on your own or in a group discussion. These questions are a helpful way to engage colleagues in professional development, for personal growth by journaling individually, and for use in academic settings to engage students in problem solving. Whichever way, we encourage you to think about and answer these questions.

Our Hope

Our hope for you, the reader, is to experience new learning and renewal as you work with contemporary issues and challenges with your clients. Honestly, we as editors have learned so much from each chapter author, which in turn has helped to improve our treatment approaches with some of our own clients. We believe you will find this volume clinically useful as well.

Acknowledgments

We also wish to thank the reviewers whose thoughtful comments and expertise guided our writing and revisions for the development of this book. As always, any errors and omissions are our own:

Carleton Brown, *University of Texas at El Paso*
Celeste Fiori, *University of Wyoming*
Kenisha Gordon, *Mississippi College*
Sueann Kenney-Noziska, *Play Therapy Corner*
Donna Kreskey, *California State University, Chico*
Craig LeCroy, *Arizona State University*
Misti Lindquist, *Azusa Pacific University*
Jack Peltz, *Daemen College*
Richard Ruth, *The George Washington University*
Sean Scanlan, *Chaminade University of Honolulu*
Anne Stewart, *James Madison University*
Hayley Stulmaker, *HLS Counseling PLLC*
Daniel Sweeney, *George Fox University*
Gabriel Young, *Pacific Oaks College*

PART I
Children

CHAPTER 1

Depression
Child-Centered Play Therapy with a Biracial Child
Peggy L. Ceballos and Marium Sadiq

Roberto is a 7-year-old biracial male (mom identifies as African American and father as Puerto Rican Latino) who was referred to counseling by the school. His parents are divorcing after 9 years of marriage and according to Roberto's parents, the divorce is causing a lot of problems between the two of them, which Roberto has witnessed. A more in-depth family history revealed that Roberto's mom has been diagnosed with major depressive disorder and currently takes medication for it. Roberto's teacher describes him as a child who is very "hyperactive" and extremely anxious. Recent incidents at school include Roberto crying uncontrollably when he could not perform an academic task, being very anxious in social situations, and tending to keep to himself in social situations. The teacher adds that Roberto is hyper and that she needs to call him out constantly for not following school rules. At home, Roberto is described as having angry outbursts. Roberto's parents also stated that Roberto tends to become anxious and that lately he has lost his appetite and refuses to eat during mealtimes. They have observed Roberto's anxiety coming up at times when he is afraid of a new situation or around new people. His mom explains he has always tended to want to do everything perfectly, and when he cannot accomplish a task, he feels very disappointed in himself. In general, his parents describe him as having a lot of negative self-thoughts such as "I am bad," "I cannot do things right," and "I am stupid." He has expressed to his mom feeling sad sometimes and wanting her and dad to get back together. The father stated that he thinks Roberto feels guilty about them separating and thinks it is his fault for misbehaving and for feeling sad. Roberto's parents clarified that they had noticed this sense of sadness and negative self-image in Roberto since he was about 4 years old.

Childhood Depression

According to the Centers for Disease Control and Prevention (CDC, 2023), approximately 2.7 million children, ages 3–17, were diagnosed with depression between 2016 and 2019. Symptoms of childhood depression can present in a variety of ways. Children experiencing depression may exhibit impairment across cognitive, affective, physiological, and social domains (Burgin & Ray, 2022;

Korczak, Madigan, & Colasanto, 2017). These symptoms can negatively impact children's level of functioning by impeding their school performance and impacting their ability to participate in interpersonal relationships (Garber, 2006).

Researchers associate childhood depression with exposure to early life stressors. LeMoult et al. (2020) conducted a meta-analysis and found that exposure to early life stressors such as physical abuse, emotional abuse, sexual abuse, the passing of a loved one, or domestic violence were linked to greater risk of being diagnosed with major depressive disorder before the age of 18 years. Other researchers have corroborated the significant link that exists between adverse childhood experiences and depression (Satinsky et al., 2021). In addition, family history of mental health problems such as depression (Maughan, Collishaw, & Stringaris, 2013; Mills & Baker, 2016) and lack of social support (Rueger, Malecki, Pyun, Aycock, & Coyle, 2016) are factors linked to childhood depression. It is important to note that childhood depression may leave the child prone to the development of other mental health conditions (Weisz et al., 2006; Avenevoli, Stolar, Li, Dierker, & Ries Merikangas, 2001).

According to Delaney and Smith (2012), the negative effects of early onset of depression continue into adulthood. When depression appears in childhood, there are more risks of developing comorbidity of mental health problems and major depressive disorder later in life (Zisook et al. 2007). This is concerning as statistics show that about 25% of children are diagnosed with major depressive disorder by adolescence (Abela & Hankin, 2008). Maughan et al. (2013) explained that depression in adolescents is preceded by anxiety, addictions, and disruptive behaviors. The authors concluded that a combination of environmental and genetic factors play a role in the development of depression during childhood, affecting more girls than boys. According to Maughan et al. (2013), diagnosing depression in childhood is difficult due to developmental concerns and how depression often presents itself in comorbidity with other disorders.

The criteria to diagnose depression center on symptoms of continued sadness, significant loss of interest in enjoyable activities, changes in appetite, fatigue or diminished physical activity, feeling a sense of worthlessness or guilt, inability to think concretely, and suicide ideation (American Psychiatric Association [APA], 2022). However, Allgaier et al. (2014) cautioned of the difficulties most mental health providers face when trying to diagnose depression during childhood. The authors explained several factors that contribute to this difficulty, including developmental factors that cause symptoms to present in an atypical manner, the presence of other disorders such as anxiety, and the struggle children face when trying to express verbally what is happening to them. According to Sánchez Rus, Solis, Rodriguez, & Suárez-Gómez (2021), because depressive symptoms in children may present as irritability, lack of attention, and hyperactivity, the diagnosis can be confused with ADHD. The authors also warned that both diagnoses can coexist, making it hard for mental health providers to determine the best treatment. Thus, Sánchez Rus et al. (2021) urged providers to closely monitor early diagnosis to lower chances for later complications.

When diagnosing depression, it is also important to have an in-depth understanding of the cultural background of the client. Research conducted in countries outside the United States have found that clients are more likely to show symptoms of depression through physical rather than psychological symptoms (Bibi, Masroor, & Iqbal, 2013; Mumford, Devereux, Maddy, & Johnston, 1991). In addition, studies have found that exposure to adverse childhood experiences (ACEs) such as living in unsafe, violent neighborhoods or lack of access to basic resources contribute to the onset of depression during childhood (Satinsky et al., 2021). Girls are more prompt to show depression symptoms than boys and to carry a major depressive diagnosis once they get to puberty (Maughan et al., 2013). These factors make it imperative for clinicians to properly consider cultural factors that may be affecting a child's depression symptoms. Thus, it is important to conduct a thorough family interview that includes attention to cultural factors such as how a family conceptualizes depression, understanding the client's intersectionality of identities (e.g., religion, language, disability, race/ethnicity) and the lived experiences these identities bring into the child's daily life (Strand & Bäärnhielm, 2022). Similarly, Bibi, Lin, Zhang, & Margraf (2020) remind clinicians to use culturally appropriate diagnostic measurements that account for cultural differences in symptomatology.

Child-Centered Play Therapy (CCPT)

Given Roberto's developmental stage and presenting problem, we believe that CCPT can be beneficial to help him deal with his presenting issues and symptoms of depression and ADHD. CCPT is a developmentally appropriate approach to therapy with children ages 3–10 (Landreth, 2012). CCPT was adapted from Carl Rogers's person-centered theory, and it expands on the nondirective tenants presented by Virginia Axline (1947). Landreth (2012) presents CCPT as an approach in which "play is the child's language" (p. 12). Within CCPT, the child attends therapy in a room with carefully curated toys so that the child can express their internal self through using these toys as their words. The therapist provides a culturally appropriate space in which the child experiences empathy, genuineness, and unconditional positive regard from the therapist. In addition, because in CCPT the therapist believes in the child's inner capacity for self-actualization, the therapist offers a structured yet nondirective space where the child is free to express himself freely (Landreth, 2012).

Responses used in play therapy, such as tracking, reflection of feelings, reflection of content, esteem building, reflection of meaning, facilitating decision making, facilitating creativity, facilitating relationship, and reflecting larger meanings (Ray, 2011), are used to communicate understanding and acceptance of the child (Landreth, 2012). These skills combined with the therapist's attitudinal conditions outlined by Carl Rogers (1957; i.e., genuineness, empathy, and unconditional positive regard) provide a psychologically safe environment for the child. Within the relationship, the child needs to experience the play therapist's attitudinal conditions to begin to integrate a more positive self-structure (Haas & Ray, 2020; Jayne & Ray, 2015).

CCPT with Childhood Depression

Lin and Bratton's (2015) meta-analysis found that CCPT showed a statistically significant effect on reducing symptoms for internalizing behavioral problems. This finding is corroborated by a meta-analysis conducted by Ray, Armstrong, Balkin, and Jayne (2015) that examined interventions conducted in school settings and found CCPT to be effective in reducing internalizing problems among other problem behaviors while increasing academic achievement. It is important to note that most studies used in these meta-analyses looked at internalizing behaviors in general, which include depression; however, these studies did not look at depression as a diagnosis by itself. To date, two studies have looked at CCPT and depression (Baggerly, 2004; Burgin & Ray, 2022). Baggerly (2004) conducted a nonrandomized study and concluded that homeless children improved in their symptomatology of depression after 12 sessions of CCPT as measured by the Children's Depression Inventory (Kovacs, 1978). In a more recent study, Burgin and Ray (2022) conducted a randomized clinical study with 71 children in five Title I schools. The experimental group received between 14 and 16 biweekly 30-minute individual CCPT sessions to be compared with the wait-list control group. Results showed a statistically significant improvement in depressive symptoms with a large effect size among children who participated in CCPT.

From a CCPT perspective, mental health problems arise when children start to form conditions of worth; external messages interfere with one's self-concept (Rogers, 1957). Conditions of worth create an ideal self as the child starts to live to external expectations. For example, in the case of Robert he may have created conditions of worth around having to be perfect to be worthy of being accepted, which has led to his negative self-image when he is not able to accomplish tasks. Conditions of worth create a dissonance between who Roberto truly is and who he internalizes he should be according to how he has experienced his world (Rogers, 1957). It is the tension created by this incongruence that has led him to the formation of psychological maladjustments. Thus, the healing process occurs when he can feel unconditionally accepted, which can lead him to reject previously internalized conditions of worth (Landreth, 2012). As he starts to achieve a sense of congruence between his two selves, he can decrease symptomatology (Landreth, 2012).

In CCPT, children can express their symptomatology of depression in a developmentally appropriate way as they are not required to verbalize their inner experience; instead, they use toys to play out their feelings and perceptions. The child-centered play therapist can provide a safe environment characterized by the core conditions (Landreth, 2012) using CCPT skills (Ray, 2011). This type of environment allows children to feel free to express themselves holistically (feelings, thoughts, behaviors) and to try new ways of being that allow them to experience more congruence with their real self. The child-centered play therapist believes in the child's self-actualizing force and therefore does not need to use activities or interventions (Landreth, 2012). Burgin and Ray (2022) stated that in CCPT the safe environment characterized by the core conditions and created by the application of CCPT skills "provide the child with the freedom to express their experiences of depression, naturally moving towards confronting their perceptions of inadequacy, and beginning to experience themselves as capable as they build coping skills, resulting in positive integrations to self-concept" (Ray, 2018).

Case Study Application

Roberto presents with signs of major depression disorder as specified by the DSM-V-TR (APA, 2022). He reports feeling negative about himself, withdrawn from social interactions in a way that is not expected at his age, and feeling sad. In addition, as expected in childhood depression, Roberto is expressing symptomatology that aligns with comorbidity of presenting issues (Burgin & Ray, 2022). The teacher describes him as hyperactive, which is characteristic of children experiencing depression (Sánchez Rus et al., 2021), and he is exhibiting anxiety and other behavioral problems such as anger outbursts also associated with the onset of depression in childhood (Allgaier et al., 2014).

From a child-centered theoretical approach, Roberto has been exposed to experiences that have created conditions of worth for him. These conditions of worth led him to experience incongruence between his true self and ideal self. For example, although his organismic experience is of a human being who learns through mistakes, he has learned through his interactions growing up that he is only worthy when he is perfect. This condition of worth led him to internalize negative messages about himself such as "I am not good at anything" and "I won't learn how to do things." This incongruence between his ideal self and true self creates feelings of sadness, anxiety, and anger, which externalize in behaviors such as hyperactivity, withdrawnness, anger outbursts, and crying uncontrollably.

Treatment Process

The CCPT treatment plan consisted of seeing Roberto once a week for 50 minutes. Prior to starting sessions, I (first author) completed an intake session with Roberto's parents to discuss presenting issues and administered the Children's Depression Inventory (Kovacs, 1978) with Roberto, which measures depressive symptoms in children over the age of 6. Roberto scored in the significant range for multiple subscales on the assessment. Based on the intake and assessment results, the parents and I collaborated to create the following therapeutic goals:

- increase Roberto's awareness of his own feelings and how he could express these feelings in socially acceptable ways,

- decrease the number of instances in which Roberto engaged in negative self-talk, and
- increase Roberto's ability to stay on task and follow directions in class and at home.

Throughout treatment, I conducted parent consultations every four weeks to assess for progress and changes in Roberto's disposition. I also conducted two teacher consultations to provide tools that would be helpful in supporting Roberto's educational success.

During sessions, I focused on providing the therapeutic conditions outlined by Axline & Carmichael (1947) for Roberto to feel safe enough to experience his true self in the playroom without fear of not being accepted. To this end, I provided Roberto with a level of unconditional acceptance, empathy, and congruence that he needed in the therapeutic relationship to feel safe to make mistakes and to express himself freely about his parents' divorce. The child-centered play therapist used the skills (reflection of feelings, tracking, reflection of meaning) to let Roberto know that I understood what he was expressing. In addition, I worked to return responsibility to Roberto to empower him and encourage him in social situations.

I used advanced skills such as setting limits to help Roberto develop an inner sense of self-control and learn alternative more appropriate ways to express feelings such as anger. In addition, due to his negative self-talk and beliefs about himself, I used skills such as encouragement to help him experience a new sense of self in the playroom. This new sense of self allowed him to perceive himself as someone who could try new tasks and value the process rather than the product. As Roberto was able to have these new experiences in the playroom, he was able to gain a new sense of self more aligned with his self-actualizing force and true self, thus reducing his need for symptomatology associated with depression. I saw these behaviors and skills play out over the next few sessions.

TABLE 1.1. ROBERTO: TRANSCRIPT/ANALYSIS

Transcript	Analysis
T: "Hello, Roberto, we are going to have our special playtime. In here, you can play with all the toys you want in many of the ways you want."	Introduction of the playroom and invitation to play with the toys. This informed the child that he gets to take the lead in the playroom.
R: "Can I play with that?"	Children often feel unsure and uneasy in a new situation. In addition, Roberto specifically tended to be anxious in new social situations.
T: "You're feeling nervous. You're not sure if you can play with what you want."	Reflection of feeling and meaning. Here, the therapist acknowledged Roberto's nerves.
R: "So, can I?"	Children are often unsure initially how to respond to reflections of feeling. Roberto was persistent in his questioning, still unsure of what he was allowed to do.
T: "Well, Roberto, in here that's something that you can decide."	I returned responsibility to Roberto. This both helped set the structure of play therapy and reminded Roberto that he was in charge of his own choices.
R: [Roberto quietly walks over to the dollhouse and removes half the family from the house. He begins arranging the figures in different positions.]	Roberto began playing with the toys. He remained hesitant around me, but he was drawn to the toys that allow him to express his reality.
T: "You're moving those around. It seems like you know where everybody goes."	I began tracking. This communicated interest and understanding to Roberto without imposing or leading the play.
R: [Roberto solemnly stares at the family and quietly responds to the therapist without making eye contact.] "Yeah."	While occupied with his play, Roberto expressed his sadness and experience through his voice, body language, and play.
T: "You feel sad [tone and body language should match the reflection]."	Reflection of feeling was used to bring Roberto's sadness to his awareness while continuing to provide a safe and supportive space to experience this sadness.
R: "Um, a little, but it's fine! Ooh, look, there are dinosaurs in here!"	It is not uncommon for children to appear uncomfortable with their difficult emotions. In addition, I began to see how Roberto's depressive symptoms appeared as difficulty staying on task.

TABLE 1.2. ROBERTO: TRANSCRIPT/ANALYSIS

Transcript	Analysis
R: [Roberto spends his eighth session hitting the bop bag with a sword. Meanwhile, he is shouting angrily at the bop bag.]	Roberto was much more comfortable in the counseling room and felt safe to express his anger to me.
T: "You are so mad! You want to show how angry you are."	I reflected Roberto's feelings and tracked what he is trying to do. I used a tone to communicate understanding and not judgment.
R: "DON'T SAY THAT! I DON'T WANT YOU TO TALK!" [Roberto hits the therapist on the leg with the sword.]	Roberto did not like his anger being seen as he had received the message that his anger was not allowed. This triggered his condition of worth that he must be "good" to be worthy.
T: "Roberto, I know you are very angry, but I am not for hitting. You can choose to hit the bop bag or you can choose to hit the dolls."	I used limit setting here to express to him that hitting people was not the appropriate way to express anger. By offering choices to express his feelings, I did not shut down his feelings but, rather, shared a way that he can express them.
R: [Roberto immediately shut down, embarrassed and concerned about his relationship with the therapist.] "I'm sorry; I didn't mean to hurt you. Please don't be mad; my teacher says I make bad choices."	Roberto was expressing his guilt. He began his negative self-talk.
T: "You're worried about how I feel about you. You were just trying to show me how mad you are."	I stayed with reflecting feelings here. It was not my goal to rescue the client but, rather, to express empathy and unconditional positive regard.
R: "Yeah." [Roberto begins to hit the bop bag again.]	Roberto felt understood by me and was able to continue his play.
T: "You chose to hit that instead. You knew just what to do!"	I used encouragement to reflect that Roberto was able to make choices on his own that helped him express his anger.

Ethical and Cultural Considerations

Ceballos et al. (2021) presented cultural considerations for the use of CCPT. These authors highlighted the need for play therapists to understand and apply the tenets of the theory within the cultural bounds of the client. For example, while self-actualization in individualistic cultures is understood as clients' taking decisions that promote independence, in collectivistic cultures, self-actualizing tendency can be viewed as an interdependence process. In the case of Roberto, both of his parents come from cultures known for being collectivistic (Sue & Sue, 2016). Taking this into account, I needed to understand that Roberto's self-actualization process may be understood within the context of what was in the best interest of the whole family and not only of him.

Ceballos, Post, and Rodríguez (2021) highlighted the need to account for the effects of oppressive factors on clients' self-actualizing force as oppression can play a role in children's ability to self-actualize. When working with Roberto, it was important to look at his experiences in school as a biracial child and whether these experiences had been negative or discriminatory, as exposure to discrimination could be an ongoing external stressor that negatively affected Roberto's self-actualizing force. In this case, engaging in advocacy actions on behalf of the client or with the client's parents was a way to intervene at the school. In addition, Cornelius-White (2016) cautioned about the importance of person-centered therapists acknowledging their intersectionality of identities in relation to their privileges. This awareness is critical to form genuine relationships with clients characterized by respect and empathy (Cornelius-White, 2016). While working with Roberto, it was important for me to engage in self-reflection about my own identity as an upper-middle-class Venezuelan woman who immigrated to the United States as a young adult and to consider any unconscious biases I may have.

Similarly, play therapists must be aware of how oppression affects the client's presenting problem and to what extent internalized oppression exists and contributes to the formation of conditions of worth. For example, in the case of Roberto, I had to conceptualize whether Roberto had internalized microaggressions about his racial identity or microaggressions he had witnessed his mother or father experience. If it was determined that he had internalized these messages received through his lived experiences with oppression, I had to conceptualize what, if any, conditions of worth Roberto had formed around these experiences. For example, later during the treatment, his father reported Roberto witnessed him experiencing discrimination for having an accent. This could have contributed to Roberto's sense of feeling that he was not good enough to belong in his school or with a group of friends.

Ethically, I had to be careful with confidentiality. Although Roberto was a minor and the parents had a legal right to access the therapeutic information, the play therapist had to consider Roberto's right to privacy and confidentiality (ACA, 2014). Thus, when talking to parents, I reported overall impressions and talked about emerging play therapy themes but never disclosed specific play behaviors or verbal disclosures that Roberto made unless it became necessary (e.g., disclosing wanting to harm himself). There is also an ethical obligation to attend to Roberto's cultural background (ACA, 2014) by delivering culturally responsive CCPT, which was done by following best practices provided in the literature (Ceballos et al., 2021). In addition, it was important for me to implement culturally and age-appropriate assessments with Roberto to ensure that results were valid and applicable to him. Finally, it was important for me to seek supervision and relevant information regarding the client's presenting issue (ACA, 2014). I made sure to have knowledge of depression in childhood and to seek peer supervision as needed throughout the case to maintain objectivity.

Parent and Teacher Consultations

I met with parents about once a month to discuss progress and with the teacher once at the beginning of treatment and once toward the middle of treatment (at about 12 sessions). When working with Roberto's parents and teachers, I had specific goals in mind that guided the consultation. First, I worked to help Roberto's parents and teacher differentiate between ADHD and depressive symptomatology. I did this by helping the parents and teachers notice the difference between Roberto's behaviors related to his inattention and behaviors related to his feelings of sadness. For example, through talking to his teacher, it was noted that Roberto tended to start talking about dinosaurs and become agitated when he no longer could sit in his sadness. When not looking for depression, it can be easy to mistake this type of behavior as a symptom of ADHD rather than depression.

In addition, I worked with Roberto's family and teachers to know how to respond to Roberto's feelings. Many of the skills used (reflection of feeling, returning responsibility, encouragement, and limit setting) were especially helpful to Roberto to create space for his feelings without perpetuating his conditions of worth (i.e., I must be happy to be worthy). Later during the treatment, Roberto's mother was able to participate in Child-Parent Relationship Therapy, which allowed her to gain a deeper understanding of these skills. I also provided psychoeducation about child development and childhood depression to increase the caregivers' empathy and ability to respond to Roberto in a more developmentally appropriate manner.

Conclusion

Throughout Roberto's time in therapy, he was able to make significant progress in identifying his feelings and noticing when they were coming up for him. Through his growth, he found ways to express his anger and sadness, which in turn reduced the angry outbursts that his teachers and parents reported. As he worked through these feelings, Roberto's parents and teacher also noticed a decrease in his anxiety and his willingness to participate more in social activities, although he still showed signs of anxiety when faced with new tasks and was shy when engaged with new people. I was able to effectively use CCPT with Roberto to create a space in which he was able to explore his feelings in a nonpunitive way and learn how to process and experience the symptoms of his depression. Through play therapy and my attitudinal conditions, Roberto felt accepted and was able to become more congruent without feeling further isolated. In addition to validating Roberto's feelings, I was able to validate his experience as a biracial child. Roberto's entire identity was considered in understanding him. Throughout therapy, I found out there had been experiences of bullying related to his and his parents' racial identity. I perceived these as factors contributing to his conditions of worth and perfectionistic themes. Through parent and teacher consultations, Roberto's parents and teachers increased insight into Roberto's experience, which in turn impacted their level of empathy for him. Overall, this case example shows ways that CCPT can be used in treating childhood depression.

Sample Case Notes

Session 1

Diagnosis/Presenting Problem: The child's parents brought the child to counseling to address angry outbursts, feelings of anxiety, and difficulty in school.
Intervention: Child-Centered Play Therapy
Description of Play: The child worked to explore the playroom and become familiar with the counselor. The client maintained a sad affect while playing with the dolls as evidenced by speaking low and body language. The client appeared uncomfortable with his sadness as evidenced by quickly changing the subject when the counselor brought attention to his feelings.
Assessment: The child engaged primarily in exploratory play while he familiarized himself with the playroom. It appeared important to the client that he was able to explore and be in charge of himself as evidenced by confirming that he was able to make his own choices in the playroom.

Session 8

Diagnosis/Presenting Problem: The child's parents brought the child to counseling to address angry outbursts, feelings of anxiety, and difficulty in school.
Intervention: Child-Centered Play Therapy
Limits Set: Counselor set limits to protect counselor safety and provided choices around how the client can express his anger.
Description of Play: The child worked to express his anger and, at the same time, to maintain his relationship with the counselor. The client demonstrated guilt when he was unsure of the appropriate way to express his anger as evidenced by negative self-talk.

Assessment: The child engaged in relationship and abandonment themes throughout the session as evidenced by wanting to repair his relationship with the therapist after the limit was set. The client experienced conditions of worth that made him believe that he had to control his emotions to be considered worthy.

Resources

For Professionals

Child-Centered Play Therapy Treatment Manual found in *Advanced Play Therapy: Essential Conditions, Knowledge, and Skills for Child Practice* by Dee C. Ray (2011).
Children's Depression Inventory Assessment by Maria Kovacs (1978).
Dibs in Search of Self: The Renowned, Deeply Moving Story of an Emotionally Lost Child Who Found His Way Back by Virginia Axline (1986).

For Children

A Terrible Thing Happened: A Story for Children Who Have Witnessed Violence or Trauma by Margaret M. Holmes (2000).
Was It the Chocolate Pudding?: A Story for Little Kids about Divorce by Sandra Levins & Bryan Langdo (2006).
When Sadness Is at Your Door by Eva Eland (2019).

For Parents

How to Talk So Teens Will Listen and Listen So Teens Will Talk by Adele Faber & Elaine Mazlish (2006).
The Whole-Brain Child: 12 Revolutionary Strategies to Nurture Your Child's Developing Mind by Daniel J. Siegel & Tina P. Bryson (2011).
Parents may also benefit from participating in a Child-Parent Relationship Therapy group to practice strategies that help them engage relationally with their child.

Discussion Questions

1. How do Roberto's experiences as a biracial child impact his conditions of worth?
2. How would you discuss Roberto's potential depression diagnosis with his parents and teachers?
3. What are different cultural views about depression that need to be considered. How would this knowledge be helpful in explaining Roberto's diagnosis to his family?
4. How did you see CCPT address Roberto's symptoms of depression? Please give specific examples.

5. Is there other information and/or resources that you believe would be helpful for parents and teachers to support Roberto?

References

Abela, J. R. Z., & Hankin, B. L. (2008). Cognitive vulnerability to depression in children and adolescents: A developmental psychopathology perspective. In J. R. Z. Abela & B. L. Hankin (Eds.), *Handbook of depression in children and adolescents* (pp. 35–78). Guilford Press.

Allgaier, A. K., Krick, K., Opitz, A., Saravo, B., Romanos, M., & Schulte-Körne, G. (2014). Improving early detection of childhood depression in mental health care: The children's depression screener (ChilD-S). *Psychiatry Research, 217*(3), 248–252. https://doi.org/10.1016/j.psychres.2014.03.037

American Counseling Association. (2014). *2014 ACA code of ethics.* https://www.counseling.org/docs/default-source/default-document-library/2014-code-of-ethics-finaladdress.pdf

American Psychiatric Association. (2022). *Diagnostic and statistical manual of mental disorders* (5th ed., text rev.). https://doi.org/10.1176/appi.books.9780890425787

Avenevoli, S., Stolar, M., Li, J., Dierker, L., & Ries Merikangas, K. (2001). Comorbidity of depression in children and adolescents: Models and evidence from a prospective high-risk family study. *Biological Psychiatry, 49*(12), 1071–1081. https://doi.org/10.1016/s0006-3223(01)01142-8

Axline, V. M. (1986). *Dibs in search of self.* Ballantine Books.

Axline, V. M., & Carmichael, L. (1947). *Play therapy: The inner dynamics of childhood.* Houghton Mifflin.

Baggerly, J. (2004). The effects of child-centered group play therapy on self-concept, depression, and anxiety of children who are homeless. *International Journal of Play Therapy, 13*(2), 31–51. https://doi-org.libproxy.library.unt.edu/10.1037/h0088889

Bibi, A., Lin, M., Zhang, X. C., & Margraf, J. (2020). Psychometric properties and measurement invariance of depression, anxiety and stress scales (DASS-21) across cultures. *International Journal of Psychology, 55*(6), 916–925. https://doi-org.libproxy.library.unt.edu/10.1002/ijop.12671

Bibi, A., Masroor, U., & Iqbal, N. (2013). Dysfunctional attitudes and demographic correlates of patients with conversion disorder; an exploratory study. *Journal of Pakistan Psychiatric Society, 10*(1), 25–29.

Burgin, E. E., & Ray, D. C. (2022). Child-centered play therapy and childhood depression: An effectiveness study in schools. *Journal of Child and Family Studies, 31*(1), 293–307. https://doi.org/10.1007/s10826-021-02198-6

Ceballos, P. L., Post, P., & Rodríguez, M. (2021). Practicing child-centered play therapy from a multicultural and social justice framework. In E. Gil & A. A. Drewes (Eds.), *Cultural issues in play therapy* (pp. 13–31). Guilford Press.

Centers for Disease Control and Prevention. (2023, March 8). *Data and statistics of children's mental health.* https://www.cdc.gov/childrensmentalhealth/data .html#print

Cornelius-White, J. (2016). *Person-centered approaches for counselors.* Sage Publications. https://doi.org/10.4135/9781506302621

Delaney, L., & Smith, J. P. (2012). Childhood health: Trends and consequences over the life course. *The Future of Children, 22*(1), 43–63. https://doi .org/10.1353/foc.2012.0003

Eland, E. (2019). *When sadness is at your door.* Random House Children's Books.

Faber, A., Mazlish, E., & Coe, K. A. (2016). *How to talk so teens will listen & listen so teens will talk.* Collins, an imprint of HarperCollins.

Garber, J. (2006). Depression in children and adolescents: Linking risk research and prevention. *American Journal of Preventive Medicine, 31*(6 Suppl 1), S104–S125. https://doi.org/10.1016/j.amepre.2006.07.007

Haas, S. C., & Ray, D. C. (2020). Child-centered play therapy with children affected by adverse childhood experiences: A single-case design. *International Journal of Play Therapy, 29*(4), 223–236. https://doi.org/10.1037/pla0000135

Holmes, M. M. (2000). *A terrible thing happened.* Magination Press.

Jayne, K. M., & Ray, D. C. (2015). Therapist-provided conditions in child-centered play therapy. *Journal of Humanistic Counseling, 54*(2), 86–103.

Korczak, D. J., Madigan, S., & Colasanto, M. (2017). Children's physical activity and depression: A meta-analysis. *Pediatrics, 139*(4), e20162266. https://doi .org/10.1542/peds.2016-2266

Kovacs, M. (1978). *Children's depression inventory (CDI)* [Database record]. APA PsycTests. https://doi.org/10.1037/t00788-000

Landreth, G. L. (2012). *Play therapy: The art of relationship* (3rd ed.). Routledge/ Taylor & Francis Group.

LeMoult, J., Humphreys, K. L., Tracy, A., Hoffmesiter, J., Ip, E., & Gotlib, I. H. (2020). Meta-analysis: Exposure to early life stress and risk for depression in childhood and adolescence. *Journal of the American Academy of Child & Adolescent Psychiatry, 59*(7), 942–855.

Levins, S., & Langdo, B. (2006). *Was it the chocolate pudding? A story for little kids about divorce.* Magination Press.

Lin, Y.-W., & Bratton, S. C. (2015). A meta-analytic review of child-centered play therapy approaches. *Journal of Counseling & Development, 93*, 45–58. https://doi.org/10.1002/j.1556-6676.2015.00180.x

Maughan, B., Collishaw, S., & Stringaris, A. (2013). Depression in childhood and adolescence. *Journal of the Canadian Academy of Child and Adolescent Psychiatry = Journal de l'Academie Canadienne de Psychiatrie de l'enfant et de l'adolescent, 22*(1), 35–40.

Mills, S. E. E., & Baker, L. D. (2016). Childhood depression. *InnovAiT, 9*(9), 524–530.

Mumford, D. B., Devereux, T. A., Maddy, P. J., & Johnston, J. V. (1991). Factors leading to the reporting of "functional" somatic symptoms by general practice attenders. *British Journal of General Practice: The Journal of the Royal College of General Practitioners, 41*(352), 454–458.

Ray, D. (2011). *Advanced play therapy: Essential conditions, knowledge, and skills for child practice* (1st ed.). Routledge. https://doi.org/10.4324/9780203837269

Ray, D. C. (2018, October). *Advanced play therapy.* Doctoral counseling course, Denton, TX.

Ray, D. C., Armstrong, S. A., Balkin, R. S., & Jayne, K. M. (2015). Child-centered play therapy in the schools: Review and meta-analysis. *Psychology in the Schools, 52*, 107–123. https://doi.org/10.1002/pits.21798

Rogers, C. R. (1957). The necessary and sufficient conditions of therapeutic personality change. *Journal of Consulting Psychology, 21*(2), 95–103. https://doi.org/10.1037/h0045357

Rueger, S. Y., Malecki, C. K., Pyun, Y., Aycock, C., & Coyle, S. (2016). A meta-analytic review of the association between perceived social support and depression in childhood and adolescence. *Psychological Bulletin, 142*(10), 1017–1067. https://doi.org/10.1037/bul0000058

Sánchez Rus, S. S., Solis, M. O., Rodriguez, L. S., & Suárez-Gómez, M. (2021). Depressive disorder in childhood: The importance of an early diagnosis for a functional recovery. Specific symptoms and treatment in an 8-years old patient with depression. *European Psychiatry, 64*(Suppl 1), S332. https://doi.org/10.1192/j.eurpsy.2021.891

Satinsky, E. N., Kakuhikire, B., Baguma, C., Rasmussen, J. D., Ashaba, S., Cooper-Vince, C. E., Perkins, J. M., Kiconco, A., Namara, E. B., Bangsberg, D. R., & Tsai, A. C. (2021). Adverse childhood experiences, adult depression, and suicidal ideation in rural Uganda: A cross-sectional, population-based study. *PLOS Medicine, 18*(5), e1003642. https://doi.org/10.1371/journal.pmed.1003642

Siegel, D. J., & Bryson, T. P. (2016). *The whole-brain child: 12 revolutionary strategies to nurture your child's developing mind.* Langara College.

Strand, M., & Bäärnhielm, S. (2022). Could the DSM-5 cultural formulation interview hold therapeutic potential? Suggestions for further exploration and adaptation within a framework of therapeutic assessment. *Culture, Medicine and Psychiatry, 46*(4), 846–863. https://doi.org/10.1007/s11013-021-09761-2

Sue, D. W., & Sue, D. (2016). *Counseling the culturally diverse: Theory and practice* (7th ed.). John Wiley & Sons.

Weisz, J. R., McCarty, C. A., & Valeri, S. M. (2006). Effects of psychotherapy for depression in children and adolescents: A meta-analysis. *Psychological Bulletin, 132*(1), 132–149. https://doi.org/10.1037/0033-2909.132.1.132

Zisook, S., Lesser, I., Stewart, J. W., Wisniewski, S. R., Balasubramani, G. K., Fava, M., Gilmer, W. S., Dresselhaus, T. R., Thase, M. E., Nierenberg, A. A., Trivedi, M. H., & Rush, A. J. (2007). Effect of age at onset on the course of major depressive disorder. *American Journal of Psychiatry, 164*(10), 1539–1546. https://doi.org/10.1176/appi.ajp.2007.06101757

CHAPTER 2

Adjustment Difficulties
Child-Centered Play Therapy and Critical Race Theory with a Biracial Child

Keith I. Raymond and Angela I. Sheely-Moore

Laenor "El" is an 8-year-old biracial, cis male who racially identifies as "pinkish." During the intake, El's Black American father, Daemon, and White mother, Laena, reported changes in El's demeanor since relocating to a new town the previous summer due to Laena's job promotion. Both parents expressed concerns about El's emotional and physical outbursts toward Laena when she attempts to discipline him when house rules are broken. Both parents noticed how El has withdrawn from expressing himself openly, with the exception of showing his anger and frustration. Both parents acknowledged that similar to their old neighborhood, their new town is predominantly White. However, with the recent move, they reported El having difficulty adjusting to their new home and community. Instead of meeting new friends, El prefers to stay home, gaming all day.

For this case study, consider the following questions:

1. How does history inform El's biracial identity development?
2. What is the rationale for using Child-Centered Play Therapy and Critical Race Theory with El?
3. What strengths, grounded in the Black American and other minoritized populations, can support El and his family?

Racial Identity Development in Children

It is essential to understand and support racial identity development for youth of color. In the case of El, we need to unpack how he navigates his biracial identity development to better understand his view of self, others, and the world (Gathier et al., 2014) within the context of a White-dominant culture in the United States. Before diving into El's world as a young biracial male, we need to understand the implications of the historical, legal racial classification of the "one drop rule" that continues to impact individuals of Black ancestry.

Black-categorization bias of bi- and multiracial people originated in 1702 with the "one drop rule" in the state of Virginia (Goodyer & Okitikpi, 2007; Roberts & Gelman, 2017). These authors explained how individuals with traces of African/Black ancestry were categorized as Black or more Black than White with the sole intention of distinguishing between and the division of Black and White people. Despite the US Census abandoning this policy in 2000, these authors indicated that White and monoracial people continue to maintain similar presumptions that bi- and multiracial people are more Black than White. Examining El's social and structural perspective of his biracial identity could serve as a catalyst to self-acceptance and pride in adopting a positive, healthy biracial identity. Hence, to prepare El for how US society will perceive him not as a young *biracial* male, but as a young *Black* male, El's father sought out a Black American play therapist (the first author of this book chapter) to provide representation and to increase El's comfort with his biracial identity status.

Although El's father encourages El to embrace his Black heritage, developing a firm biracial identity is a process in which El would need additional space to explore his Whiteness. Researchers (Gathier et al., 2014; Morrison & Bordere, 2001) proposed developmental stages for biracial children, which in some ways parallel the historical "one drop rule" by centering Whiteness as a critical aspect of this model. The first proposed stage occurs by the age of 2 when children begin to notice racial differences. During the second stage, which happens by the age of 3, children begin to recognize their own racial identity in a concrete manner, categorize people by race, and communicate a racial preference. For the third stage, children at the age of 4 start to recognize the social effects of skin color, show a pro-White bias, or feel a sense of pressure to choose between their biracial or multiracial identities. During stage four, 5-year-old children develop more favorable stereotypes of the dominant White racial group and more unfavorable stereotypes of marginalized racial groups. The remaining two stages involve children understanding the depth of racial identity, including being bi- or multiracial.

Although the aforementioned biracial identity development reflects a linear process with corresponding age ranges, El appears to fall within the second and third stages. Various internal and external factors (e.g., individual perception, personality, ethnicity, gender, family, society, political climate, and racist events such as George Floyd's murder) influence biracial children's identity development (Morrison & Bordere, 2001). For example, El's father identifies his son as Black, whereas his mother wants El to self-identify in a way that also honors her White ancestry. Many biracial children may struggle to form their racial identities due to feeling the need to compromise (Morrison & Bordere, 2001). Based on what El witnesses in his family unit and his surrounding White community, he chooses to label himself as "pinkish," possibly in hopes of finding a middle ground.

Clearly, El is processing his physical and social features associated with race, including his skin tone and his transition to a new home and community (Morrison & Bordere, 2001). As play therapists, it is essential to address El's racial identity while mitigating the potential conflict of choosing between his racial identities based on influences from his parents, the environment, and other social factors. El can form a strong biracial identity and choose how he self-identifies by providing a safe space to explore his identity through play.

Child-Centered Play Therapy

Given El's developmental level and environmental factors shared by his parents related to El's struggle in adjusting into his new and predominantly White community, Child-Centered Play Therapy (Axline, 1981; Landreth, 2012) and Critical Race Theory (Delgado & Stefancic, 2017) would benefit El for a few reasons. First, the innate propensity for self-understanding and self-acceptance is the cornerstone of the child-centered framework. Trusting in El's inner capacity to set his own pace to explore himself, others, and the world will not only enhance his self-esteem, but will also affirm his own personhood—including how he self-identifies racially. Promoting self-agency for El will also set the tone for him to process emotional and physical outbursts in a socially constructive and acceptable manner. Providing toys that can be used in "aggressive" ways (while keeping El, myself, and the toys clear of intentional physical harm) will enhance El's capacity to engage in self-control and, ultimately, self-responsibility for his actions. Last, race can be taxing and at times traumatic for persons of color who experience power over, lack of privileges, and oppression on a daily basis. Within the context of therapy, it is critical for play therapists to understand that play is *culturally contextualized* (Sheely-Moore, Ceballos, Lin, & Ogawa, 2020). To ignore the issue of race and racism would communicate disconnection and invalidation to El's experience as a biracial youth living in a predominantly White community.

Child-Centered Play Therapy (CCPT; Axline, 1981; Landreth, 2012) is based on the premise that children have the *innate* capacity to move in a forward, constructive manner. In essence, the core of human nature is good. My role as El's therapist using a CCPT framework is to promote his natural tendency to develop in a positive, healthy manner by communicating three key ways of being: unconditional positive regard, genuineness, and empathy (Landreth, 2012). Ultimately, my goal with El is to provide toys and other materials to give him a platform to communicate his perception of the world and how the world sees him. Doing so will enhance El's capacity to express a wide range of thoughts, feelings, and behaviors—while accepting all parts of himself, as I continuously demonstrate my acceptance of him.

Critical Race Theory

According to DiAngelo (2021) and Kendi (2019), racially colorblind ideology leads to support for racist policies and procedures. Play therapists practicing from a colorblind framework may thereby engage in and perpetuate racist practices. This colorblind framework can be reflected in counseling research that highlighted the negative impact of racism on Black, Brown, and indigenous clients through their underuse of mental health services when compared to their White counterparts (Kilmer et al., 2019) and experienced racial microaggressions in counseling (Sue et al., 2007).

Although play has been described as the universal language for all children (Landreth, 2012), the nuances of play remain culturally contextualized. Hence, it is important to include a theory that centers on the social and institutional embeddedness of race and the impact of race on disenfranchised members of society. Hence, it behooves play therapists to challenge and disrupt colorblind ideologies by acknowledging the impact of race and racism. Critical Race Theory (CRT) provides the grounding to engage in such actions. There are five main tenets of CRT, all of which centralize White people and their sociopolitical power to maintain this supremacy over others for their benefit (Delgado & Stefancic, 2017). Using a CRT framework, my role with El is to invite the conversation of race into the playroom by validating El's experience of racism, racial microaggressions, and racist events such as George Floyd's murder. Narrative storytelling (Trahan & Lemberger, 2014), one of CRT's tenets, honors the experiences shared by people of color. Within the US society, embedded in White privilege and power, the history of people of color is ignored and misrepresented—with minimal perspectives taken outside of a White person's lens (Delgado & Stefancic, 2017). Providing space for El to explore and articulate his experience of a biracial male living in a predominantly White community can affirm his experiences as real and not imagined or taken out of context. My goal with El is to affirm his biracial identity with equal value and worthiness for both racial backgrounds.

Case Study Application

Understanding El within a historical context of being Black in America, along with a nascent biracial identity developmental model and theoretical underpinnings for CCPT and CRT, we can return to El and explore how these concepts and tenets come to fruition in therapy. From a CCPT perspective, I conceptualize El as capable of uncovering and resolving challenges that he has faced, both past and present, within a therapeutic relationship that is based on the three core conditions (Axline, 1981; Landreth, 2012). Infusing a CRT lens within my work with El will provide opportunities to broach and unpack race and racism in an open, validating, and healing manner.

Session 1

The goals for my first session with El were twofold: to build rapport with El and to empower El by having him decide if he wants to continue play therapy sessions with me. After I introduced him to the playroom, El began to explore the area by pointing, hitting, and eventually punching the bop bag with more force when he learned that no video games were available in the playroom. He then proceeded to share his plan to draw a picture.

TABLE 2.1. **EL: SESSION 1**

Transcript	Analysis
El: [Starts to look through crayons available in the box] "Ugh . . . [sigh]."	El appeared frustrated while looking in the crayon box.
T: "You are looking really hard for something you can't find."	I communicated understanding of El's search for a specific crayon.
El: "I can't find the crayon that looks like me [makes grunting noise]."	El was clearly upset for not locating a particular shade of his skin tone.
T: "You are frustrated that you can't find the color that matches your skin color."	I validated El's emotions and communicated acceptance by exploring and acknowledging his racial identity in a developmentally appropriate manner.
El: "Which crayon do I use?"	El looked to an external locus of control to decide which crayon matched his skin color rather than depending upon himself to develop his self-concept.
T: "You can decide which color crayon to use."	I encouraged El to take the lead by trusting himself to form his own racial identity.
El: "I don't want to use these crayons. These crayons don't look like me."	El began to explore his racial identification instead of relying on me to determine his racial identity.
T: "You put a lot of thought into deciding you don't want to use these crayons because they don't match your skin."	I highlighted the strength it took for El to recognize that the selection of crayons did not match his skin color.
El: [Gets up from the table, walks over to the bop bag and punches it hard.]	El demonstrated a play disruption here when his feelings were challenging to process.

Treatment Goals

Upon receiving parental confirmation that El wanted to continue with therapy, we agreed to the following treatment plan: (1) reduce emotional and physical outbursts and aggressive behaviors and (2) increase the ability to communicate feelings more assertively and constructively. The treatment objectives were as follows:

1. Identify and express thoughts and feelings associated with emotional and physical outbursts.
2. Explore and create meaning for El's racial identity and develop a positive self-concept.
3. Conduct parent consultations to discuss treatment goals, progress, and recommendations.

During this same parent consultation, I shared the multicultural theme that emerged from his play. I knew El's play was interrupted because he could not locate a crayon that matched his skin tone. Therefore, I asked his parents for recommendations on toys that would be racially and ethnically appropriate to include in his play while avoiding making assumptions on my behalf.

Session 2

My objective for the second session was to incorporate additional toys and materials his parents suggested to better represent El's world. I also wanted El to take the lead by providing him opportunities to explore his biracial identity, which he did by beginning the second session excitedly locating a marker that represented his skin tone.

El experienced a significant breakthrough toward the end of the second session as he courageously recounted his painful experiences with covert racism and racial discrimination at school. El disclosed that his classmates made derogatory racial remarks about his skin tone and implied that his mother could not be his mother because she was White. From a CRT lens, it was my responsibility to dismantle the colorblind rhetoric that maintains racism and White supremacy in America. At that moment, I made it a priority to honor our racial identities and

TABLE 2.2. EL: SESSION 2

Transcript	Analysis
El: [Starts dancing and singing in the chair as he draws himself]	El's self-esteem increased when he identified the marker that resembled his skin color.
T: "You are working really hard drawing yourself."	I highlighted El's effort in creating a self-portrait.
El: [Looks at me several times] "You are darker than me, so I am going to use this marker."	El explored various shades of brown and black before selecting a marker that best matched my skin tone.
T: "You noticed the differences in our skin color and want to make sure you pick the right color."	I broached and highlighted El's observations about our differences in skin tone.
El: [Pause and slight smile] "You look like my favorite cousin."	El's comfort level seemed to have increased as this time was the first where he self-disclosed.
T: "I remind you of your cousin who is Black, just like me."	Often therapists avoid discussing race to avoid offending clients. However, I found it essential to share my Black racial identity to enhance our relationship and to increase El's comfort level to discuss race.
El: [Pause] "Yeah, but I don't see him anymore or anyone that looks like you."	Positive racial representation for youth of color can help ensure that they are validated, heard, and understood.
T: "You seem sad that you don't get to see your cousin or Black people often."	El expressed sadness for the first time, so it was important that I acknowledged his feelings.
El: "Yeah." [gets up from the table, walks over to the bop bag, and starts punching it]	El demonstrated play disruption as he expressed sadness about his disconnection with his cousin and other people of color.

empower El to narrate his own story to form his own racial identity. I facilitated this by fostering a space for El to engage in counter-storytelling through his drawings in opposition to the prevalent White dominant narratives told and upheld in El's occupied environments. I facilitated El's counter-stories by encouraging and empowering him to help him feel comfortable and confident in using his voice to share his counter-stories to combat racist and discriminatory narratives and to construct narratives that defined his experiences and worldview. I employed minimal tracking and paraphrasing responses to allow him to take the lead in telling his story. By leaning forward, matching my tone and attitude to his effect, and reflecting on El's feelings, I conveyed that I was with him, heard him, understood him, and acknowledged that his story mattered.

In the following sessions, El experienced intense emotions due to conflicting issues related to his biracial identity and experiences of racial prejudice, which required ordering a new bop bag to continue processing his feelings in a healthy manner. During the working stage of El's therapeutic process, he remained in stage three of the biracial identity development model. Specifically, El understood that he did not have the same privileges as his White peers. El began to articulate observed racial differences between himself and others, to express feelings of anger toward his mother, and to share how he often felt betrayed by his mom for scheduling play dates with the White parents of the students who made racist comments about him. Eventually, El demonstrated anxiety themes within his play as he attempted to determine his racial identity. In subsequent sessions the theme of anxiety dissipated with El's increased comfort when he began to share additional instances of racial prejudice within his social environments, which prompted me to schedule frequent phone calls with his parents.

Ethical and Cultural Considerations

Counselors are ethically bound to provide culturally and developmentally appropriate treatment to their clients. Hence, it is critical to examine my own cultural knowledge, biases, attitudes, and beliefs (Holcomb-McCoy, 2009) to avoid perpetuating colorblind ideology and racial microaggressions. The implementation of CCPT and CRT served to empower El by deconstructing race on his own terms and in his own time frame. Using these strength-based theoretical frameworks also prevented me from labeling El as defiant or misdiagnosing his exhibited emotions as having anger problems before understanding his worldview. With El's minor legal status, it was also imperative to engage his parents on a consistent basis while maintaining confidentiality and fidelity with El. Maintaining transparency with El's caregivers regarding what can and cannot be shared about El's session promoted agency within El to take the sessions where he needed them to go while keeping his parents informed on as-needed basis.

Parent Consultations

With El's presenting issue centered on race, including discrimination, I conducted regularly scheduled parent consultations to gain more insight into El's home, neighborhood, and school environment that seemed to impact El's daily functioning and views about himself. During these consultations I also had to consider the cultural impact of race on El's parents by exploring their family dynamics and cultural values (Holcomb-McCoy, 2009). Daemon and Laena had different views about how to parent their child racially and ethnically. Although they both identify El as Black, Laena did not want to disregard her White ancestry and was unsure how to share her thoughts related to this issue with the family.

Based on El's needs, I encouraged his parents to have conversations with El about their own cultural background, to share information about Black and biracial identity, and to encourage El to explore his racial identity freely. Using a CRT perspective, I discussed with his parents the potential benefits of imparting cultural knowledge and fostering a community that reflects both of his cultural identities by adopting a cultural relativistic paradigm (i.e., a person's behaviors, attitudes, beliefs, values, practices, and worldviews understood in light of their own culture and not judged by the standards of the White dominant group relative to the US societal context) to dismantle the universalistic paradigm that devalues people of color, such as El, and his position in predominantly White spaces.

Conclusion

El made significant progress in processing his racial identity issues and his experiences of racism, discrimination, and racial microaggressions. Prior to termination, El was able to communicate his thoughts, feelings, and experiences effectively without getting easily angered as evidenced by a decrease in aggressive play and the elimination of emotional and physical outbursts toward his mom. At the end of therapy, El reached the final stages of the biracial identity development model by gaining awareness of his biracial heritage and understanding that he can be both Black and White *and* still identify as a Black male. As a result, El developed a sense of pride in his biracial identity and gained self-confidence.

As a culturally competent therapist, I am aware that CCPT is a framework based on Eurocentric thought. Based on El's complex issues of racial identity, racism, racial microaggressions, and oppression, I knew I could not solely draw from a White ideological approach that would unjustly reflect and devalue his racial identity and discriminatory experiences. Integrating CRT, a social justice framework, alongside CCPT served to deconstruct Western colonist beliefs that negatively impacted El's daily life and impeded his racial identity development. Using both CCPT and CRT allowed me to help dismantle systems of White dominance and oppression experienced in El's occupied environments while demonstrating empathic understanding, genuineness, and acceptance. As a therapist, I learned the importance of cultivating an inclusive and nurturing environment where youth from different racial and ethnic backgrounds can freely form and learn to embrace their racial identities on their own.

Sample Case Notes

Session 1

Subjective: Client expressed frustration when he could not locate a crayon that matched his skin tone. Client stated, "I don't want to use any of these crayons" before hitting the bop bag.

Objective: Client's general appearance and dress were appropriate. Client's behavior shifted from calm to aggressive, releasing built-up tension. Throughout the session, client's mood fluctuated from happy, frustrated, and angry with congruent affect. Client spoke minimally but talked clearly at an average rate and volume.

Assessment: From a CCPT perspective, El demonstrated difficulty making decisions independently due to relying on others to develop his self-concept. El tended to communicate his thoughts and feelings by punching the bop bag rather than verbally articulating his experience.

Plan: Client will continue with weekly counseling sessions. Counselor will incorporate additional culturally and developmentally appropriate toys and materials in the playroom.

Session 2

Subjective: Client stated his feelings about the therapist: "I really like playing with you." Client explored self-racial identity and in relation to others when he stated, "You are darker than me, so I am going to use this marker" and "You look like my favorite cousin."

Objective: Client's speech was energetic while he drew a self-portrait and maintained direct eye contact with the therapist while selecting a marker. Client's eye contact decreased when he inquired about race and racial experiences. Client articulated his feelings verbally, nonverbally, and physically. Client's mood was a mixture of happy, angry, and sad with congruent affect.

Assessment: From a CCPT perspective, El was vulnerable when describing his disconnection with people of color and his experience of racial discrimination at school. The therapeutic connection deepened as the therapist demonstrated the three core conditions of CCPT. El felt more at ease disclosing personal information along with his feelings. From a CRT perspective, El was provided the opportunity to explore his own racial identity and dismantle White ideologies that did not accurately reflect his biracial identity.

Plan: Client will continue with weekly counseling sessions. The therapist will schedule a parent consultation to discuss possible strategies for broaching topics about racial identity.

Resources

For Mental Health Professionals

Atkin, A. L., & Yoo, H. C. (2019). Familial Racial-Ethnic Socialization of Multi-racial American Youth: A Systematic Review of the Literature with MultiCrit. *Developmental Review, 53,* 1–28.

For Children

Beauvais, G., & Jones, S. A. (2015). *I Am Mixed.* Stranger Comics.

Tyler, M., & Csicsko, D. L. (2005). *The Skin You Live In.* Chicago Children's Museum.

For Caregivers

The Conscious Kid. (2023). *The Conscious Kid: Definitions of Words and Phrases That Can Be Helpful to Understand When Discussing Race and Identity.* https://www.theconsciouskid.org/racial-literacy-key-terms

Parents. (2023). *Six Things to Stop Saying to Kids of Different Races and Ethnic Groups.* https://www.parents.com/parenting/better-parenting/things-to-stop -saying-to-kids-of-different-races-and-ethnic-groups/

Discussion Questions

1. Describe key considerations of El's biracial experience and how it relates to the historical structuring of race in America.
2. How did using CCPT and CRT in tandem work to help meet El's treatment goals? Provide examples.
3. As a therapist, what are some strategies that you would embody to avoid the perpetuation of a colorblind ideology and racial microaggressions when working with El and his family?

References

Axline, V. (1981). *Play therapy.* Ballantine Books.

Delgado, R., & Stefancic, J. (2017). *Critical race theory: An introduction* (3rd ed.). New York University Press.

DiAngelo, R. (2021). *Nice racism: How progressive White people perpetuate racial harm.* Beacon Press.

Gaither, S. E., Chen, E. E., Corriveau, K. H., Harris, P. L., Ambady, N., & Sommers, S. R. (2014). Monoracial and biracial children: Effects of racial identity saliency on social learning and social preferences. *Child Development, 85*(6), 2299–2316.

Goodyer, A., & Okitikpi, T. (2007). ". . . But . . . But I am Brown." The ascribed categories of identity: Children and young people of mixed parentage. *Child Care in Practice, 13*(2), 83–94.

Holcomb-McCoy, C. C. (2009). *Cultural considerations in parent consultation.* American Counseling Association.

Kendi, I. X. (2019). *How to be an antiracist.* One World.

Kilmer, E. D., Villarreal, C., Janis, B. M., Callahan, J. L., Ruggero, C. J., Kilmer, J. N., Love, P. K., & Cox, R. J. (2019). Differential early termination is tied to client race/ethnicity status. *Practice Innovations, 4*(2), 88–98. https://doi.org/10.1037/pri0000085

King, K., & Summers, L. (2020). Predictors of broaching: Multicultural competence, racial color blindness, and interpersonal communication. *Counselor Education & Supervision, 59*(1), 216–230. https://doi.org/10.1002.ceas.12185

Landreth, G. (2012). *Play therapy: The art of the relationship* (3rd ed.). Brunner-Routledge.

Morrison, J. W., & Bordere, T. (2001). Supporting biracial children's identity development. *Childhood Education, 77*(3), 134–138.

Ray, D. C. (2011). *Advanced play therapy: Essential conditions, knowledge, and skills for child practice.* Routledge/Taylor & Francis Group.

Roberts, S. O., & Gelman, S. A. (2017). Multiracial children's and adults' categorizations of multiracial individuals. *Journal of Cognition and Development, 18*(1), 1–15.

Sheely-Moore, A., Ceballos, P., Lin, Y. W., & Ogawa, Y. (2020). Culturally responsive child parent relationship therapy. In Landreth, G., & Bratton, S. (Eds.), *Child parent relationship therapy* (2nd ed.), 431–443. Routledge.

Sue, D. W., Capodilupo, C. M., Torino, G. C., Bucceri, J. M., Holder, A. M. B., Nadal, K. L., & Esquilin, M. (2007). Racial microaggressions in everyday life: Implications for clinical practice. *American Psychologist, 62*(4), 271–286.

Trahan, D., & Lemberger, M. (2014). Critical race theory as a decisional framework for the ethical counseling of African American clients. *Counseling and Values, 59*(1), 112–124. https://doi.org/10.1002/j.2161-007X.2014.00045.x

CHAPTER 3

Domestic Violence
Trauma-Informed Child-Centered Play Therapy with a White Child
Jennifer N. Baggerly

Carla is a White 5-year-old girl living with her mother and 3-year-old brother in a small apartment after her mother left her father due to domestic violence. Her mother, Sara, presents as anxious and timid. Sara quietly explained that Carla witnessed her father, Tim, yelling and slapping her (Sara) on a weekly basis for more than a year during the COVID-19 pandemic. Prior to this domestic violence, Tim lost his job due to pandemic layoffs and began drinking excessively. Sara escaped with her children and moved in with her parents until she was able to find an apartment. Sara obtained a restraining order so that her husband is not allowed near their new home. Sara is concerned that Carla has become very hyper and bossy toward her but cries excessively when Sara leaves her with anyone other than her grandparents.

For this case study, consider:

1. What is the physiological, emotional, and behavioral impact of domestic violence on Carla? How did the COVID-19 pandemic complicate these matters?
2. What is the rationale for using Trauma-Informed Child-Centered Play Therapy with Carla? Which strategies in each TI CCPT stage seemed to help Carla?
3. What unique ethical guidelines need to be considered? What does Carla's mother need to help Carla?

Impact of Domestic Violence on Young Children

The Centers for Disease Control and Prevention (n.d.) defines domestic violence, also known as intimate partner violence (IPV), as a current or former partner's physical violence such as hitting, kicking, or other types of physical force; sexual violence of forcing a partner to take part in a sex act; stalking or repeated unwanted contact that causes fear; and psychological aggression of verbal and nonverbal communication with the intent to harm mentally or emotionally.

Surveillance data shows that more than 10 million women and men experience IPV each year (Breiding, Basile, Smith, Black, & Mahendra, 2015).

Numerous studies reveal the short- and long-term impact of domestic violence on young children such as pervasive feelings of fear, powerlessness, and sadness (Noble, Moore, & McArthur, 2020); anxiety and depression (Chen & Lee, 2021); posttraumatic symptoms (Paul, 2019); disruptive behavior (Juan, Washington, & Kurlychek, 2020); and physical and psychological barriers to learning (Lloyd, 2018). This impact of domestic violence on young children is often revealed in their play during play therapy sessions (Tyndall-Lind, 2010; Weinreb & Groves, 2007). Kot & Tyndall-Lind (2005) found children exposed to IPV had play themes of aggression, killing, death, and escape. For example, they described a boy who engaged in aggressive play of shooting, hitting, and killing a Bobo blow-up doll until he collapsed in exhaustion. Another girl used scary animals (i.e., spiders, snakes, alligator, and other wild animals) to reenact the escape from her home after a violent episode.

Impact of COVID-19 Pandemic on Young Children

The World Health Organization (2020) and other studies (Cappa & Jijon, 2021) reported that IPV increased during the COVID-19 pandemic. Kelly and Morgan (2020) reported a 25% increase in calls to the domestic abuse hotline in the United Kingdom. This increased violence was triggered by financial stress from losing jobs, isolation due to quarantine, frequent volatile interactions because work and school were no longer an escape, and fewer checks and balances from outside family members, friends, and teachers (Ragavan, Garcia, Berger, & Miller, 2020). Parental burnout and child maltreatment also increased during the pandemic (Griffith, 2020; Russell, Hutchison, Tambling, Tomkunas, & Horton, 2020). Donagh (2020) stated, "The impact of COVID-19 has meant children and young people experiencing abuse have gone from being unnoticed to invisible" (p. 388).

Young children such as Carla who witnessed IPV during COVID-19 desperately needed treatment interventions (Donagh, 2020). Because Carla's developmental level at 5 years old limits her cognitive ability to understand abstract concepts, she needed a developmentally appropriate treatment intervention that allows for movement. Play therapy allows young children to express their experiences, feelings, and perceptions through their natural language of play (Landreth, 2012). When working with children who witnessed IPV, the play therapy needs to be trauma informed and promote coping strategies (Gil, 2017).

Trauma-Informed Child-Centered Play Therapy

Trauma-Informed Child-Centered Play Therapy (TI CCPT) (Baggerly, 2013) is a comprehensive treatment approach that combines knowledge of trauma and trauma-specific strategies with Landreth's (2012) Child-Centered Play Therapy.

The format of TI CCPT is 30 minutes of CCPT as described by Landreth (2012) followed by 15 to 20 minutes of psychoeducation based on neurophysiology and core components of children's trauma interventions (National Children's Traumatic Stress Network, n.d.). TI CCPT follows three fundamental stages of trauma recovery, identified in Judith Herman's (1992) seminal work: (1) establishing safety, (2) restorative retelling of the trauma story, and (3) restoring the connection between survivors and their community.

In stage one, safety in the setting is established by creating a warm and inviting playroom with toys from each category as described by Landreth (2012). Safety in the relationship is developed through implementing Axline's eight principles. In the second part of the session, safety is facilitated through play-based psychoeducation. Play therapists educate children and parents on basic neurophysiology through illustrations such as Daniel Siegel's hand model of the brain, found on YouTube. Then play therapists use playful games and children's books to teach physiological regulation strategies including deep breathing, progressive muscle relaxation, playful exercises, and mindful movements. Next, they help children develop a safety plan of where to hide and who to call for help. Finally, they teach positive cognitive strategies such as positive self-talk (e.g., "I am smart, and I am strong"), looking for clues that a place is safe, and thinking of the most likely thing that will happen rather than the worst thing that could happen. Resources for other coping strategies can be found in COVID-19 Interventions (O'Conner & Picard, 2021) accessible on the APT website; *Caroline Conquers Her Corona Fears* (Camelford et al., 2020); First Aid Arts (FirstAidArts.org, 2020); and Helping Children with Traumatic Separation or Traumatic Grief Related to COVID-19 (NCTSN, 2020).

In stage two, when children reenact their trauma experience during their non-directed play, play therapists facilitate understanding and enlarge the meaning. For example, "you like to be the one with the power to decide if I am stuck here or if I can go free" and "you know how scary it can be when there is no escape from danger." During psychoeducation, play therapists read children's books explaining trauma and domestic violence. Then they can guide children in making a book about their own experience. For example, "The happy things I remember about my family are when . . . ," "A scary thing that happened in my family was when . . . ," and "A hopeful thing about my future is . . ." Play therapists use other creative approaches such as puppet shows, sand tray, and art to facilitate a restorative retelling of children's trauma stories.

In stage three, play therapists help restore connection between children and their families, peers, and community members by reflecting or proposing effective interpersonal skills during nondirective play. For example, if the child is reenacting a scene of her dad yelling at her, then the play therapist could say, "The daddy doll yelled at the girl doll, who felt scared. The girl doll may be wishing daddy would just calmly say, 'Please pick up your toys.'" During psychoeducation, play therapists teach effective interpersonal skills such as "I" messages; compromising, encouraging words; and safe responses to harsh words. Children learn to say to angry siblings or peers, "I know you are angry. You look like you need time to calm down. I'll go do something else for now." In addition, play therapists invite parents who are safe and can regulate their own emotions into play sessions. Play therapists facilitate positive parent-child connections through strategies such as "I love you rituals" (Bailey, 2000), Theraplay activities (Booth & Jernberg, 2009), or Child-Parent Relationship Therapy (Landreth & Bratton, 2019).

Implementing TI CCPT with children who have experienced IPV during COVID-19 provides a safe space for children to develop an accurate emotional understanding of their experiences. Children can adjust their self-concept from "this is my fault, and I am helpless" to "even in scary situations, I am strong, and I know ways to help myself be safe and calm." Although it is difficult to witness the harsh impact of IPV in the pandemic, play therapists can take self-compassion breaks (Neff, n.d.) throughout the week and find inspiration in children's resilience.

Case Study Application

With this deeper understanding of the impact of domestic violence, the COVID-19 pandemic, and TI CCPT, we can now apply them to Carla. From a TI CCPT perspective, I conceptualize Carla as experiencing incongruence between her ideal self as a safe and emotionally regulated girl and her current self as experiencing trauma symptoms (e.g., permanent alert) with a desperate need to control to regain a sense of safety. Carla has inaccurately symbolized her experience as "the world is always unsafe so I must control people." She has denied to her awareness that her mother is growing stronger and is able to protect her. My treatment goals and objectives for Carla are as follows:

Treatment Goal: Decrease trauma symptoms of hypervigilance, separation anxiety, and controlling "bossy" behavior and increase effective emotional and behavioral regulation.

Objectives:

1. Express her feelings, experiences, and perceptions through play to gain an emotional understanding, mastery, and self-empowerment.
2. Identify and connect physiology, emotions, perceptions, and behavior related to trauma.
3. Develop effective safety and coping skills.

Session Overview

In the first play therapy session, Carla was intrigued enough about the playroom that she set aside her anxiety to investigate the toys. As in a typical first session, she explored all the toys, playing with them for a few minutes and then going on to the next toy. After 30 minutes of CCPT, I read *Don't Pop Your Cork on*

Mondays: Children's Anti-Stress Book (Moser, 1988) to help Carla develop basic calming strategies of deep breathing, progressive muscle relaxation, and so forth. By the third play session, Carla began to play out her feelings and perceptions related to IPV and COVID-19.

As shown in the Session 3 transcript below, Carla's play themes were aggression, power/control, nurturing, and protection. Through her play, she developed an emotional understanding of the danger she experienced and a sense of hope that she would be protected.

In the next sessions, I continued TI CCPT and stage one of psychoeducation for safety planning and anxiety management. Then I began stage two of restorative retelling of her trauma narrative by introducing books such as *A Terrible Thing Happened* (Holmes, 2000) and *The Strongest Thing: When Home Feels Hard* (Adelman, 2022). I facilitated a sand tray for Carla to show how she perceived the time living with dad. She depicted dad as "the Beast" from the Disney Movie *Beauty and the Beast*; her mom as "Belle," who was imprisoned by "the Beast"; her brother as a dog; and herself as a lioness. When asked what is different since they moved, Carla said, "The Beast is in a cage." Later she added that she hopes the Beast turns back into a prince.

TABLE 3.1. **CARLA: SESSION 3**

Transcript	Analysis
C: "Close your eyes." [Child put toy spiders on my shoulders.] "There are bugs all over you, and they are trying to crawl up your nose."	This appeared to be her concrete explanation of COVID-19, which is sometimes explained as a "bug" to children.
T: "Something strange and scary is happening to me."	Reflection of feeling and enlarging the meaning.
C: [Child used a rope to tie me to my chair], saying, "You can't escape these bugs. Now I have you trapped, and no one is going to come over to see." [She used a toy knife to pretend to stab me.]	This appeared to be her perception of danger within her family with limited protection due to the quarantine. Note: The child looped the rope loosely. Otherwise, I would have set a limit via "I know you would like to tie the rope behind me, but the rope is not for tying in the back. You can choose to tie it in the front."
T: "It is super scary because there is danger all around me, and I can't seem to escape."	Reflection of feeling and enlarging the meaning.
C: "No you can't escape. I won't let you," she said in a taunting voice with a smile.	Play theme was power and control, possibly representing her perception of dad controlling mom.
T: "You enjoy keeping me trapped. I feel powerless and need someone to help me."	Reflection of the power dynamic she is playing out. In my assigned role as "victim," I voice my need for help.
C: "No one will help you." [Walks around me] "But since you have bugs all over you, I will take you to the doctor because they bit you."	Child creates an escape to get help from the doctor. Medical personnel were often the only professionals a child would see during COVID. Because many children call me "Dr. Jennifer," she may see me as a rescuer.
T: "I feel relieved that I can get help from the doctor who can help take care of me and protect me."	Reflection of feeling and enlarging the meaning.

TABLE 3.2. **CARLA: SESSION 10**

Transcript	Analysis
C: "I'm the cop now, and I'm going to arrest you for being bad."	Play theme was still control but was serving a social purpose of being a helper.
T: "You are an important and powerful cop, and you know how to stop me from being bad."	Facilitated understanding of her strengths as an important and powerful person who no longer is out of control, watching bad things, but has the power to protect herself.
C: "Yes. Now, stay in there (behind the puppet stand) for 100 years. I'm going to make dinner. I get pizza, strawberries, and ice cream. You only get bread."	She created a safe space for her by jailing "the bad," which could represent IPV and/or her own misbehavior. She has enough power to nurture herself and show compassion to "the bad" by at least giving bread.
T: "You are making a safe place for yourself by making sure I won't get out for a really long time. You know how to get good things to eat for yourself. You're giving me bread, even though I've been bad."	Reflection of her agency in self-protection to the point of no longer being in constant state of alert but calm and confident enough to nurture herself while showing compassion.
C: "Now pretend to escape from jail." [Therapist pretends to sneak away] "Hey, I see you! Get back here. You're not going to trick me. Back in jail," she said with authority.	Establishes control over the fear of danger from tricky people. Demonstrates self-protection.
T: "You are strong and in charge even when I try to trick you. You have the power to protect yourself."	Encourages her confidence to protect herself.

By session 10, Carla had integrated a sense of safety and self-empowerment so that she could transform her role from being perpetrator to being the police.

In later play sessions, Carla was able to balance her need for control with cooperation as she engaged me in creative activities such as painting a rainbow forest. During stage three, I facilitated playful engagement between Carla and her mother, who had become much more confident and enjoyed Carla with smiles and laughs.

Ethical and Cultural Considerations

Ethical considerations in Carla's case began with her ongoing safety. Sara, her mother, had already obtained a restraining order so the father would not come to their new home. However, as is the case with many people, Carla's mother would occasionally visit her husband after being sweet-talked. Although I kept the information confidential, I still had a duty to protect Carla. I recommended that Sara not take Carla on these visits as they could turn violent. I followed the ethical principle of autonomy in respecting Sara's right to make her own decisions regarding her relationship.

Another ethical consideration was the likelihood of being subpoenaed for criminal charges against the father or custody battles. At the initial intake session, I reviewed our office policies that court appearances are charged at twice the usual session hourly fee. I clarified that I can only report what I directly witness, and I will not state an opinion on custody. I am careful not to overinterpret Carla's play in my documentation or possible testimony. For example, I can *not* say that Carla's play proves violence by the father or that he is a dangerous person. I can say, "In my professional opinion, Carla is processing perceptions of danger and feelings of fear." I can share assessment results from the Trauma Symptom Checklist for Children that indicate she is in the clinical range for trauma symptoms. I can also say that Carla needs to be in an environment in which she perceives safety and has consistently calm parenting.

A cultural consideration for Carla was related to her parents' religious belief that the husband is the head of the household, and the wife must submit to him. Because this belief is different from mine, I bracketed my beliefs and respected their freedom of choice. During a parent consultation, I briefly explained that spiritual faith often grows through different stages. Many adults are at a conventional stage of conforming to traditional beliefs while other adults grow into a more individual, reflective stage of analyzing their own values and becoming more flexible in some beliefs (Fowler, 1995). I asked Sara what changes, if any, she had noticed in her faith over the past few years. This prompted a discussion of how her faith grew to a different stage than her husband's. As a result, Sara felt proud of her growth and less judgmental toward her husband.

Parent Consultations

Given these ethical issues, it was crucial for me to have regular parent consultations with Carla's mom. Prior to seeing Carla, I conducted a parent consultation with Sara, her mother. Using Daniel Siegel's hand model of the brain, I explained strategies to calm the lower regions of Carla's brain through deep breathing, rocking, and soft voice rather than trying to reason with her prefrontal cortex, which was "offline" during her anxious times. To reinforce these concepts, I asked Sara to watch a parenting video by Tina Payne Bryson, *10 Brain-Based Strategies: Help Children Handle Their Emotions* and to read Siegel and Payne Bryson's (2016) *No-Drama Discipline*. These two resources helped Sara calm her own anxieties so she could provide co-regulation to help Carla calm down. After each play therapy session, I spent a few minutes informing Sara about what Carla had learned in psychoeducation so that Sara could encourage, not demand, the new skill at home.

To demonstrate my due diligence in my communication with Carla's dad, I emailed Tim to introduce myself and invited him to schedule a parent consultation with me. After a few weeks, he scheduled an online parent consultation. I reviewed with Tim the same information as with Carla's mother. Much of the session was spent with Tim explaining that there was a lot of misunderstanding, Sara had blown things out of proportion, and Carla was much better off with the family back together. I reflected his feelings and perceptions while also presenting him with facts. "You're very frustrated because, from your perspective, this was a misunderstanding. You just want things back the way they were. [Brief pause] And Sara sees it very differently; the judge granted a restraining order; and we all need to help Carla be less scared. This will be a much slower process than what you want, but the most important concern is Carla being calmer and confident. I know you want that for Carla. For now, I encourage you to focus on reading and viewing the resources I gave you."

Conclusion

Carla made remarkable progress over 20 sessions of TI CCPT. She transformed from being a perpetrator who put bugs on me while I was tied up to a calm, confident, and cooperative child. Her mother also became more confident, gave her choices, and set limits as needed. Her father chose not to engage with me past the parent consultation but continued to pressure Sara to reunite. Fortunately, Sara chose a calmer life for herself and Carla.

Sample Case Notes

Session 3

Subjective: Child expressed feelings of satisfaction, confidence, meanness, and projected fear and distrust.
Objective: During CCPT, child put toy spiders on Play Therapist's (PT) shoulders and said, "There are bugs all over you"; "You can't escape these bugs; you're trapped." Child used rope to pretend to tie PT to chair and pretended to stab me. During psychoeducation, the counselor read *Listening to My Body* (Garcia, 2017) to help the child understand physiological sensations, feelings, needs, and calming strategies.
Assessment: From a TI CCPT perspective, child is experiencing incongruence between her ideal self as a safe and emotionally regulated girl and her current self as experiencing fear with a desperate need to control to regain a sense of safety. Carla has inaccurately symbolized her experience as "the world is always unsafe so I must control people." Play themes were power and control, nurturing, and protection. She is developing an emotional understanding of the danger she experienced and a sense of hope that she will be protected.
Plan: Continue TI CCPT and psychoeducation book of *I Am Stronger Than Anxiety* (Cole, 2021) for stage one of establishing safety.

Session 10

Subjective: Child expressed feelings of confidence, determination, satisfaction, and annoyance.
Objective: Child put on police vest, held handcuffs and gun. She said, "I'm the cop now, and I'm going to arrest you for being bad." She used the kitchen food to make herself dinner and give the prisoner bread. Child caught prisoner from breaking out of jail and said, "You're not going to trick me."

Assessment: From a TI CCPT perspective, child is making progress as indicated by shifting her role from perpetrator to police. She is aware of safety strategies such as protecting herself from being tricked. She is integrating a helper and nurturer identity into her self-concept. Through this self-empowerment, she is mastering her trauma experience.

Plan: Continue TI CCPT and facilitate sand tray for stage two of restorative retelling of trauma narrative.

Resources

For Professionals

Mindful Self-Compassion Breaks (audio) as described by Kristin Neff at https://self-compassion.org/category/exercises/#exercises.

Posttraumatic Play in Children: What Clinicians Need to Know by Eliana Gil (2017).

For Children

A Terrible Thing Happened: A Story for Children Who Have Witnessed Violence or Trauma by Margaret Holmes (2000).

Don't Pop Your Cork on Mondays!: The Children's Anti-Stress Book by Adolph Moser (1988).

I Am Stronger Than Anxiety: Children's Book about Overcoming Worries, Stress and Fear by Elizabeth Cole (2021)

Listening to My Body by Gabi Garcia (2017)

The Strongest Thing: When Home Feels Hard by Hallee Adelman (2022).

For Parents

NCTSN, "Helping Children with Traumatic Separation or Traumatic Grief Related to COVID-19" (2020). https://www.nctsn.org/resources/helping-children-with-traumatic-separation-or-traumatic-grief-related-to-covid-19

No-Drama Discipline: The Whole Brain Way to Calm the Chaos and Nurture Your Child's Developing Mind by Daniel Siegel and Tina Payne Bryson (2016).

Recover and Rebuild: Moving on from Partner Abuse. Domestic Violence Workbook by Stacie Freudenberg (2020).

Discussion Questions

1. How did IPV and COVID-19 uniquely impact Carla's feelings, experiences, perceptions, and behavior?
2. How did TI CCPT facilitate the achievement of Carla's treatment goals? Give specific examples.

3. As a therapist, what beliefs, biases, and/or emotions would you need to bracket to effectively work with Carla and her family?
4. What steps would you take to manage ethical and legal issues related to Carla's case and family? How would you respond if you received a subpoena for a custody dispute?

References

Adelman, H. (2022). *The strongest thing: When home feels hard.* Albert Whitman & Company.

Baggerly, J. (2013). *Trauma informed child centered play therapy* [video]. Microtraining Associates and Alexander Street Press.

Baggerly, J. (2021, April 9). *Play therapy heroes for the coronavirus pandemic and national crises.* Texas Association for Play Therapy Conference. Virtual.

Bailey, B. (2000). *I love you rituals.* Harper.

Booth, P. B., & Jernberg, A. M. (2009). *Theraplay: Helping parents and children build better relationships through attachment-based play.* Jossey-Bass.

Breiding, M. J., Basile, K. C., Smith, S. G., Black, M. C., & Mahendra, R. (2015). *Intimate partner violence surveillance: Uniform definitions and recommended data elements.* Centers for Disease Control and Prevention. https://www.cdc.gov/violenceprevention/pdf/ipv/intimatepartnerviolence.pdf

Brown, S. M., Doom, J. R., Lechuga-Peña, S., Watamura, S. E., & Koppels, T. (2020). Stress and parenting during the global COVID-19 pandemic. *Child Abuse & Neglect, 110,* 104699. https://doi.org/10.1016/j.chiabu.2020104699

Camelford, K., Vaughn, K., & Dugan, E. (2020). *Caroline conquers her Corona fears.* LSU Health Sciences Center.

Cappa, C., & Jijon, I. (2021). COVID-19 and violence against children: A review of early studies. *Child Abuse & Neglect, 116* (Part 2). https://doi.org/10.1016/j.chiabu.2021.105053

Centers for Disease Control and Prevention. (n.d.). *What is intimate partner violence?* https://www.cdc.gov/violenceprevention/intimatepartnerviolence/index.html

Chen, W., & Lee, Y. (2021). Mother's exposure to domestic and community violence and its association with child's behavioral outcomes. *Journal of Community Psychology, 49,* 2623–2638. https://doi.org/10.1002/jcop.22508

Donagh, B. (2020). From unnoticed to invisible: The impact of COVID-19 on children and young people experiencing domestic violence and abuse. *Child Abuse Review, 29*(4), 387–391. https://doi.org/10.1002/car.2649

First Aid Arts (2020). *First Aid Arts Mini Toolkit: Tools for Mental & Emotional First Aid.* Seattle, WA. Available at https://www.firstaidarts.org/minitoolkit

Fowler, J. W. (1995). *Stages of faith: The psychology of human development and the quest for meaning.* HarperCollins.

Gil, E. (2017). *Posttraumatic play in children: What clinicians need to know.* Guilford Press.

Griffith, A. K. (2020). Parental burnout and child maltreatment during the COVID-19 pandemic. *Journal of Family Violence, 37,* 725–731. https://doi.org/10.1007/s10896-020-00172-2

Herman, J. (1992). *Trauma and recovery: The aftermath of violence—From domestic abuse to political terror.* Basic Books.

Juan, S.-C., Washington, H. M., & Kurlychek, M. C. (2020). Breaking the intergenerational cycle: Partner violence, child–parent attachment, and children's aggressive behaviors. *Journal of Interpersonal Violence, 35*(5–6), 1158–1181. https://doi.org/10.1177/0886260517692996

Kelly, J. & Morgan, T. (2020, April 6). Coronavirus: Domestic abuse calls up 25% since lockdown, charity says. *BBC News.* https://www.bbc.co.uk/news/uk-52157620

Kot, S., & Tyndall-Lind, A. (2005). Intensive play therapy with child witnesses of domestic violence. In L. A. Reddy, T. M. Files-Hall, & C. E. Schaefer (Eds.), *Empirically based play interventions for children* (pp. 31–49). American Psychological Association. https://doi.org/10.1037/11086-003

Landreth, G. (2012). *Child centered play therapy: The art of the relationship.* Routledge.

Landreth, G. L., & Bratton, S. C. (2019). *Child-parent relationship therapy (CPRT): An evidence-based 10-session filial therapy model* (2nd ed.). Routledge.

Lloyd, M. (2018). Domestic violence and education: Examining the impact of domestic violence on young children, children, and young people and the potential role of schools. *Frontiers in Psychology, 9.* https://doi.org/10.3389/fpsyg.2018.02094

National Children's Traumatic Stress Network. (n.d.). *Core components of interventions.* https://www.nctsn.org/treatments-and-practices/trauma-treatments/overview

Noble, C. D., Moore, T., & McArthur, M. (2020). Children's experiences and needs in relation to domestic and family violence: Findings from a meta-synthesis. *Child & Family Social Work, 25*(1), 182–191. https://doi.org/10.1111/cfs.12645

O'Conner, K., & Picard, S. (2021). *COVID-19 interventions.* Association for Play Therapy.

Paul, O. (2019). Perceptions of family relationships and post-traumatic stress symptoms of children exposed to domestic violence. *Journal of Family Violence, 34*(4), 331–343. https://doi.org/10.1007/s10896-018-00033-z

Ragavan, M. I., Garcia, R., Berger, R. P., & Miller, E. (2020). Supporting intimate partner violence survivors and their children during the COVID-19 pandemic. *Pediatrics, 146*(3). https://doi.org/10.1542/peds.2020-1276

Russell, B. S., Hutchison, M., Tambling, R., Tomkunas, A. J., & Horton, A. L. (2020). Initial challenges of caregiving during COVID-19: Caregiver burden, mental health, and the parent–child relationship. *Child Psychiatry & Human Development, 51*(5), 671–682. https://doi.org/10.1007/s10578-020-01037-x

Siegel, D., & Payne Bryson, T. (2016). *No-drama discipline: The whole-brain way to calm the chaos and nurture your child's developing mind.* Mind Your Brain.

Tyndall-Lind, A. (2010). Intensive sibling group play therapy with child witnesses of domestic violence. In J. N. Baggerly, D. C. Ray, & S. C. Bratton (Eds.), *Child-centered play therapy research: The evidence base for effective practice* (pp. 69–83). John Wiley & Sons.

Weinreb, M., & Groves, B. M. (2007). Child exposure to parental violence: Case of Amanda, age 4. In N. B. Webb (Ed.), *Play therapy with children in crisis: Individual, group, and family treatment* (3rd ed., pp. 73–90). Guilford Press.

World Health Organization. (2020, March 26). *COVID-19 and violence against women: What the health sector/system can do.* https://www.who.int/repro ductivehealth/publications/emergencies/COVID-19-VAW-full-text.pdf

CHAPTER 4

Disruptive Behavior after January 6 Washington, DC, Uprising
Cognitive Behavior Play Therapy with a White Child

Athena A. Drewes

Jake, a White 6-year-old boy in elementary school, who repeatedly witnessed the January 6 Washington, DC, uprising on television with his parents, started acting out at home and school. His parents, who were in favor of the uprising and very vocal about it while watching daily televised live reports and repeated showing of the events, used negative discipline on Jake's disruptive behaviors through harsh name calling, yelling, and periodic swats on Jake's bottom. Although Jake, his parents, and his older brother and sister did not directly have anyone they knew attend or die in the uprising, Jake began to experience nightmares, had anger management problems, became more oppositional at home, and had major behavioral problems in school. More specifically, his impulsivity resulted in rarely attempting his academic assignments, frequent disagreements with peers, whining and tattling on peers, temper tantrums and name-calling when he did not get his way on the playground, aggressive behavior by pushing and shoving peers, and pacing in class. Jake's parents noted increased negative behaviors at home that included physical aggression with siblings and neighborhood children, and frequent breaking of household rules. Jake was referred to the school psychologist for assessment and counseling.

For this case study, consider the following questions:

1. What were the main factors that contributed to Jake's disruptive behavior? Is Jake only responding to his environment, or is there an underlying diagnosis?
2. What is the rationale for using Cognitive Behavior Play Therapy with Jake? What specific strategies seemed to be helpful with Jake?

3. How would you manage your political views if they are different from the parents' views? Describe ethical considerations and consultation strategies you would use when working with the parents.

Disruptive Behaviors in Children

Disruptive or externalizing behaviors are an increasing concern in school-age children, with kindergarten teachers rating approximately 20% of students experiencing elevated behaviors (Murray, 2015). Externalizing behaviors are those characterized by aggressive, disruptive, oppositional, noncompliant, or antisocial behaviors (Murray, 2015). They include behaviors related to impulsivity and hyperactivity.

Various factors can trigger the emergence of disruptive behavior symptoms in children. Disruptive behaviors can be triggered by genetic/biological factors; emotional factors that include temperamental personality, frustration, fear, overstimulation, need for attention, or anxiety; family factors such as stress caused by parenting, parental marital dysfunction, or sibling conflicts; community environmental factors such as exposure to violence; and school environment factors (Afdal, Zikra, Sakmawati, Syapitri, & Fikeri, 2022). Further disruptive behavior can be triggered by physiological factors that include poor nutrition, hunger, fatigue, disease, and allergies as well as socioeconomic factors such as food insecurity or homelessness (Afdal et al., 2022). Fortunately, Hirshfeld-Becker and Bierderman (2002) found younger children to be more plastic in terms of behavior and their neurodevelopment. This plasticity continues throughout the lifetime, and brains can be rewired at any age (Siegel & Bryson, 2012); consequently, treatment interventions can have a positive impact. Considering Jake's disruptive behavior, I will focus on a few of these triggering factors, mainly ADHD, exposure to media violence, and family factors.

Attention-Deficit/Hyperactivity Disorder (ADHD)

Attention-Deficit/Hyperactivity Disorder (ADHD) is a complex neurodevelopmental disorder that is the most frequently diagnosed emotional/behavioral health disorder in children referred to school and mental health professionals. The prevalence in 2020 was 9.3% of children receiving an ADHD diagnosis (NSCH, 2021). This translates into 5.64 million children between the ages of 3 and 17 years. This prevalence has shown an increase over time. It is estimated that 5–10% of all school-age children have the disorder, resulting in approximately two to three children with ADHD in an average classroom (Kasiati, Naruvita, Harti, Yulia, & Yunitsari, 2022). Of children diagnosed with ADHD, 64%, or two in three children, suffer from at least one other psychiatric disorder, and 52% have comorbid behavioral or conduct problems (NSCH, 2021).

ADHD is associated with abnormalities in cognitive, psychomotor, and affective aspects and characterized by impulsive and hyperactive behavior. Factors that cause ADHD include heredity/genetic factors, brain damage during fetal development/after birth, smoking/alcohol during pregnancy, and babies born with low body weight resulting in delays in the prefrontal cortex. Neurological correlates of aggression in childhood, often comorbid with ADHD, were associated with smaller amygdala volume and decreased cortical thickness in the brain (Thijssen et al., 2015).

ADHD manifests in poor executive deficits in planning, attention, organization, monitoring, and self-control. Common behaviors seen include always being on the move, tapping fingers, shaking feet, pushing other children for no apparent reason, talking incessantly, and fidgeting. These children also find it difficult to concentrate on tasks with low task completion in a reasonable amount of time, show difficulty doing assignments at school or at home, difficulty listening, daydreaming, not having a lot of patience, often making noise, interrupting others, and difficulty calming down (Kasiati et al., 2022). Parents of children with ADHD often complain about disobedience, defiance, and rebelliousness with aggression at home (Jafari, Mohammadi, Khanbani, Farid, & Chiti, 2011).

As a result of these behaviors, many children with ADHD exhibit severe and chronic academic symptoms in school. Prevalence rates indicate that children with ADHD experience specific learning disabilities (SLD), which affects about 31% of the ADHD population across studies (Reddy, 2010). A child's high rate of externalizing behaviors can have a deleterious impact on classmates, teachers, and parents. Children's ADHD impulsivity can result in disagreements with peers, temper tantrums when the child does not get her way, aggressive behavior, whining, and tattling on peers.

Impact of Viewing Media Violence

The effect of violence in the media, especially television, on children is a well-known subject of research (Anderson et al., 2003; Husemann, Moise-Titus, Podolski, & Eron, 2003). Findings have demonstrated that exposure to high levels of violence in the media, television and computer or video games can lead to higher levels and increased probability of aggression in children. Because of their inability to distinguish fantasy from reality, preschool children and young schoolchildren, especially, are more likely to imitate the violence and aggression they see on television. As they watch more television, they become increasingly likely to resort to hostile and aggressive ways to solve problems (Berk, 2003). Seeing violence and aggression on television may spark hostile and aggressive thoughts and behavior in aggressive as well as nonaggressive children. Seeing violence can also make children more tolerant of aggression in others and in their environment. Research further shows that children will imitate what is seen on television or demonstrated by adults, even as young as the age of three (Calvert, 2006), and they become desensitized to its impact on others (Browne & Hamilton Giachritsis, 2005).

Family Setting

The family setting in which a child is raised plays an important role and can explain why some children are more aggressive than others. Research has shown that parents who are rejecting, use physical punishment in an inconsistent and erratic manner, and permit their children to express aggressive impulses are likely to raise aggressive and hostile children (Patterson, 2002). By ignoring their child's aggressive behavior, they are legitimizing it and failing to teach the child how to control their aggressive behaviors. Patterson compared families of aggressive children to families of the same socioeconomic status and size without aggressive children and found aggressive children often live in a setting where approval and affection are not expressed and where family members are constantly in conflict (e.g., arguing, threatening, fighting, and annoying each other). Patterson contended that these coercive homes with negative reinforcement maintain these coercive interactions.

Cognitive Behavioral Play Therapy

Cognitive Behavioral Play Therapy (CBPT) is a helpful treatment option for children with disruptive and aggressive behaviors as well as ADHD (Drewes, 2009). Cognitive behavioral play therapy interventions help ADHD children develop self-control and problem-solving skills by examining and correcting the thoughts that lead to actions. They can be used in both individual and group formats for treating a broad range of behaviors including impulsivity, social skills deficits, intrusiveness of thoughts, and anger management.

Cognitive behavioral therapy (CBT) (Beck, 1976) is a structured, goal-oriented therapy with a focus on deficits or distortions in thinking that interfere with appropriate social skills and behavior. CBT also increases the ability to express feelings, increases adaptive and realistic assessment of relationships, increases positive self-talk, and increases appropriate use of problem-solving skills. CBT is based on the work of theorists Ellis (1971), Beck (1976), and Bandura (1977). Behavioral therapy uses the concepts of antecedents, reinforcers, contingencies, and social learning therapy; cognitive therapy helps children learn to change their own behavior, change cognitions, and become part of their own treatment. The therapist and child develop goals for treatment. The therapist selects play materials and activities that will facilitate meeting the therapy goals. Modeling, role-playing, and behavioral techniques are used, mainly with children ages 10 and over who have abstraction skills.

Cognitive Behavioral Play Therapy (CBPT) (Drewes, 2009) is a theoretical framework based on cognitive behavioral principles and integrates these principles in a developmentally appropriate manner within a play therapy paradigm using empirically demonstrated techniques such as modeling and role-playing (Knell, 2009). It is usually used with children 10 and under who are concrete thinkers but can be used with older children and even teens. Play activities and verbal and non-verbal forms of communication are used to resolve problems. CBPT has several stages and components including forming a therapeutic relationship/alliance, identifying the problem of the child (through formal and informal assessments and observation), creating an individually tailored collaborative treatment plan (with child and parent), as well as teaching coping skills, social skills, and regulatory skills to increase behavioral tolerance and competence. In some cases, psychopharmacological therapy (medication) is added to help in regulating behavioral dysregulation and diminished attention/concentration (Perryman, 2016). Interventions might include use of games, bibliotherapy, role-playing, storytelling, modeling, desensitization, shaping, and positive reinforcement, as well as confronting any irrational beliefs that may be contributing to the child's difficulties (Knell, 2009; Perryman, 2016).

Play therapy with Cognitive Behavioral Therapy (CBPT) is effective for increasing the attention of children with ADHD, lessening impulsivity, and increasing self-control. Even on a short-term basis, positive gains are reported in building self-esteem, on-task behavior, self-control, channeling aggression appropriately, expression of anger through play, and practicing patience and problem solving (Jafari et al., 2011; Lochman, Powell, Boxmeyer, & Jimenez-Camargo, 2011; Murray, 2015; Sukhodolsky, Kassimnove, & Gorman, 2004). In their single case study, Chen and Chang (2014) found that CBPT had immediate and maintenance effects on increasing appropriate talking and playing with others and decreasing interrupting and loud responding. Agus, Bali, and Maula (2022) found that the use of role-playing in the classroom with the teacher had positive effects in increasing vocabulary, focus, peer interaction, and social relatedness in hyperactive schoolchildren.

School-Based Cognitive Behavioral Play Therapy

Schools are increasingly looked at as a viable service delivery system for primary mental health services, especially due to the prevalence of mental health issues involving anger management (Rones & Hoagwood, 2009). Play therapy is needed in the school setting to provide more developmentally appropriate interventions at an early age (Perryman, 2016). CBPT within schools is a time-efficient approach, with most behavioral interventions taking about 30 days (Perryman, 2016).

CBPT Techniques

Play therapy techniques such as role-playing, feelings identification, problem solving, developing social skills, and learning coping strategies are used. The parent component involves stress management, establishing rules and expectations, appropriate discipline to avoid punishing, improving parent-child relationship, giving effective instructions to children, academic support, family problem solving, family communication, family cohesion, and long-term planning.

During role-play, children can imitate or pretend to be someone by using objects around them and practice appropriate behavioral responses. This approach supports and enhances child development by promoting acquisition of cognitive, social, emotional, and language knowledge and skills (Viranda & Istiningtyas, 2019). By playing a role, children increase their ability to deal with experiences and interactions with friends and their social environment, develop empathy, add new feelings vocabulary, and anticipate future situations (Agus et al., 2022). Role-playing uses the therapeutic powers of play through accelerating knowledge acquisition, improving skills and attitudes, increasing self-confidence, and improving communication.

Additional techniques are chosen to cover six different modalities: affective, behavioral, cognitive, developmental, educational, and social. These activities may include storytelling, turtle technique, self-calming techniques, substituting behaviors when angry, and catharsis.

Case Study Application

As described above, CBPT will be a helpful treatment for Jake to treat his disruptive behavior, which seems to be triggered by ADHD, viewing violence on media, and his family environment. I began with a classroom observation of Jake, created a behavioral log to establish a baseline and monitoring mechanism, administered a formal assessment using the *Child Behavior Checklist* (Achenbach & Rescorla, 2001) completed by his teacher and parent, and conducted a play session with Jake. Based on this holistic information, I formulated a play-based treatment plan with Jake and his parents.

We agreed that the goals of treatment were to build self-esteem, teach on-task behavior, teach self-control, channel aggression appropriately, allow expression of anger through play, practice patience, and help problem solve through play. We also agreed that homework would be assigned after each counseling session for Jake to rehearse and practice his calming and coping skills at home and in the community. Finally, I taught his parents play skills and encouraged each parent to conduct special play sessions with Jake daily. I also taught his parents age-appropriate discipline techniques to counter harsh physical punishment.

Treatment Goals: Decrease disruptive and aggressive behaviors in school and increase affective and behavioral regulation, problem-solving skills, on-task academic behavior, and positive peer interactions.

Objectives were as follows:

1. Jake will learn the value of cooperating and supporting peers in the classroom through an increase in empathy skills.
2. Jake will decrease tattling on peers to zero per week.
3. Jake will gain experience in social problem solving so that tantrums and oppositional behavior incidents will be reduced to zero per week.
4. Jake will be able to modulate shifting between active and calm state and use his coping and calming skills at least once per day.
5. Jake will show an increased focus on academic tasks by remaining on task and completing assignments daily.

6. Parents will report a decrease in disruptive and negative behaviors at home to a minimum of once per week.

CBPT Strategies

I scheduled to see Jake for weekly 30-minute individual CBPT sessions for 8 weeks at his school. Throughout the sessions, I conducted numerous play-based activities such as feelings identification and expression (e.g., what is behind the anger; catharsis in expressing anger); self-calming techniques (e.g., the turtle technique, deep breathing); role-play (using puppets), a feelings thermometer and drawing and using clay.

Session 1

In the first play therapy session, the goal was to help Jake feel comfortable in the therapy room, know what the sessions would be like, and review the reason Jake was in counseling and his treatment goals. I read the bibliotherapy book *A Child's First Book about Play Therapy*. Jake engaged in child-directed play for 15 minutes, during which time he reenacted the uprising by having his characters scream and yell at the "grown-up" figures, bang and hit the block door and wall he created, push in to get the "grown-ups," and build up and smash down block buildings. This playtime gave Jake an opportunity to reenact the disaster, have

TABLE 4.1.   **JAKE: SESSION 1**

Transcript	Analysis
J: [Uses male doll to knock on the door he created] Yells, "Let me in. I'm going to stop you from doing that stuff!"	Jake reenacts what he saw on television of people pushing into the US Capitol. He does not understand what was being stopped, but he understood the anger.
T: "That guy is super angry and trying to force others to stop what he doesn't like."	Reflection of anger, force, and content.
J: "Yeah, me and my buddies are going to take over, and no one can stop us."	Jake observed the power of a group mob that loses self-control, defusing responsibility onto the group.
T: "They want to all be the boss but have lost self-control."	Highlights the responsibility of self-control.
J: "Well, watch this!" [Knocks down the wall he built]	Jake is proud of his power. He wants to be seen as a powerful boy, perhaps to feel safe.
T: "You want to show me how powerful you are, even if it means someone or something might get hurt."	Brings to Jake's awareness that misused power has consequences, and to introduce empathy.
J: "Well, I don't want to hurt anyone. I just want to show them my friends and I are in charge."	Jake adjusts his intentions. He starts to become aware that his underlying desire is to belong with strong people.
T: "You know it is important not to hurt others. What you really want is to be part of a group that is strong. There are lots of different ways to do that without causing destruction."	Reflected his value of not hurting others and his desire to belong. Provided some psychoeducation that he can do so without aggression.

cathartic emotional release, and allowed for discussion of feelings associated with it. I used reflective comments and modeled feelings associated with his actions, which helped to reduce his anger.

In the final three minutes, I taught Jake and practiced the hills and valley finger breathing calming technique. For this activity, Jake used his nondominant hand and with pointer finger on his dominant hand he traces to the top of his thumb while breathing in and then traces down the thumb while breathing out. He repeats this breathing in and out while tracing each finger with a pause between fingers. Jake's homework was to keep practicing finger tracing, teach it to his parents and siblings, and use it as often as possible.

Earlier that day, I saw Jake's parents at the beginning of the school day for a 30-minute session to teach them reflective statements and how to implement natural consequences at home. (See Parent section for more details and additional meetings.)

Session 2

At the beginning of the session, I reviewed the previous week, checked on rehearsal use of the finger breathing, and did a quick practice of finger breathing. I focused on identifying feelings and explained the "What's under the Anger" poster, which shows multiple feelings underneath anger. I encouraged Jake to throw a bean bag at the different feelings and mention a time he felt that way. I provided a handheld mirror for him to see how his face looked while showing the feeling and to check if it was congruent with the chart. We played this for five minutes and the Talking, Feeling & Doing board game for 10 minutes. Jake was then able to have child-led play, which resulted in another abreaction of the uprising using puppets. I used puppets to express empathy and role-modeled appropriate responses and feelings identification. The last few minutes were spent blowing on a pinwheel and taking deep breaths as a coping and calming technique before returning to class. I encouraged Jake to try using his finger breathing at home as homework.

Session 3

After reviewing the previous week, I shared the positive teacher comments that Jake is showing some progress. Jake smiled. We discussed Jake's report about his breathing practice at home, when he used it, and the results. We practiced "I feel" statements. I used a three-headed dragon puppet to show Jake how his thoughts, feelings, and behaviors are related. I explained that the goal was to get the angry, scared thoughts and feelings to lessen, and thereby not get the negative behaviors to come out. We made a feelings thermometer with increasingly larger smiley faces, which Jake colored accordingly. He agreed to use this at home and counseling to show how he was feeling.

Then Jake had 10–15 minutes for self-directed play. Jake decided he wanted to put on a puppet show about being on the playground and a problem he was having with another classmate. I provided empathic responses and role-played problem solving when disagreements and frustration were getting in his way. Jake alternated with me in taking the role of classmate versus himself. The last three minutes were spent on deep breathing using the pinwheel before returning to class. His homework was to practice using "I" statements when needing something or in expressing feelings and using his feelings thermometer at home to show his feelings.

Session 4

Week in review; checked in on trying "I" statements at home and practiced again in session using "I" statements to express his anger. Read *How to Take the Grr out of Anger* and played one round of the Angry Monster Machine board game. Jake had the last 10 minutes for self-directed play. During this play, Jake's play was starting to change. He would build buildings, put miniatures on them, and knock it down, but his aggression was noticeably less. He started to verbalize more empathic feelings toward the figures inside the building, stating, "I feel scared. There are angry people outside. I hope they don't hurt us" as he played out the reenactment. The last few minutes before returning to class were spent with the hills and valley finger breathing, which Jake was also to use at home as homework.

Session 5

Week in review with Jake stating that he liked using his feelings thermometer to show his parents how angry he was feeling. I had Jake trace his left shoe on a large piece of paper, and then his right shoe on it. He was encouraged to stomp on the paper and say the things that make him angry. He was encouraged to let out his angry feelings about school, classmates, parents, and siblings. After about five minutes, Jake was encouraged to say positive things about himself. I led with statements about how great a smile he had and how magical it was in being able to make others smile back. Jake was able to come up with three positives: being a fast runner, able to build things with blocks, and having a loud voice. Jake then spent the next 15 minutes playing with the puppets and putting on a puppet show. He had his puppets talk about being friends, and he and I role-played on making friends and being able to share and not always win. The last five minutes were spent having a cotton ball race. Using two cotton balls, one for Jake and one for me and a straw for each, we took turns in slowly blowing the cotton ball across the table; and then seeing how fast they could roll after taking deep breaths and blowing hard. We repeated this a few times to help teach Jake control and patience. Jake was encouraged to continue working on "I" statements at home and use of his feelings thermometer.

Session 6

Week in review; taught the turtle technique (Feindler, 2009). Jake was told the story using a turtle puppet, of a boy turtle who had problems in school with his classmates with name calling, tattling, and not listening to his teacher. A wise old tortoise shared with the little turtle the secret of being able to calm down. The turtle could pull his head in and count to 10, pretending a red light is shining. Then as he counted down, the turtle would slowly breathe in and out, and the light would change to yellow, and when the turtle felt calm, it would turn to green. Then he could avoid getting himself in trouble. Jake was then encouraged to wrap his arms around himself, put his head down and slowly breathe until he felt calm (green light). This was practiced several times.

During child-led playtime, Jake shifted his play, deciding to use army figures to set up a battle in the sand tray with figures having magical powers to build force fields around themselves to protect themselves from the oncoming army. His battle ended with all parties deciding not to fight.

TABLE 4.2. **JAKE: SESSION 6**

Transcript	Analysis
T: "Today I will teach you the turtle technique to help with calming down and thinking before acting. Watch how I do it, as though I am pulling my head into my shell and slowly breathing."	The goal is to add to the repertoire of techniques Jake can use for affect regulation. By modeling and role-play, Jake will be able to imitate the therapist and try out the technique.
J: "I am a turtle! I can wrap my arms around me and pull my head in. Now I will breathe in and out until I can relax!"	Role-play allows Jake to experience relaxation while trying the technique. Repetition allows for practice in session and mastery to then generalize its use and apply it in other settings.
T: "Now you can use this time to use the toys in the way you would like to play."	Child-led therapy time allows Jake to access unconscious feelings, feel mastery and control while using catharsis to release affect.
J: "I am going to set up my army, and they are going to fight the other guys. But this time my army has a force field to protect them. They have magic."	Power and mastery through use of magic and force field. A shift in the play allowing his army to show strength and have protection.
T: "Your army has magic. They can protect themselves and be safe with their force field."	Empowering Jake and joining in the metaphor of magic and increased sense of protection and safety.
J: "YES! They are safe. No one can hurt them."	Realization that there is safety and that outside forces cannot hurt them. A shift in his cognitive distortions that the world is a dangerous place to feeling that there is safety, and he doesn't have to fear getting hurt.
T: "No one can hurt them. They feel safe."	Reaffirming his realization that there is safety and protection.
J: "The other army cannot win, and they know it. They are deciding not to fight. My army doesn't need to attack them."	Shift in outcome with the armies deciding not to fight, and his side not needing to be aggressive. Jake realizes that aggression and fighting does not have to be the first response and that there are choices and options.

Homework was to practice the turtle technique at home and teach it to his parents. Session ended with Jake using the turtle technique.

Session 7

Week in review. I reviewed progress to date and discussed Jake's upcoming treatment termination with just one session left. We read the book *The Very Angry Day Amy Didn't Have*. I helped Jake with problem-solving skills and taught him the sequence and mantra **STAR—**

1. STOP: What is the problem?
2. THINK: What can I do? Brainstorm solutions; look at all the possibilities.
3. ACT: Try it out and check your answer.
4. REACT: Did it work? Tell yourself, "I did a good job!"

During child-led play, Jake set up the dollhouse and showed what things make him angry at home and how he manages his anger at home. Before ending, Jake picked the turtle technique to practice. Parents were called to check on the progress and remind that next week was the last session.

Session 8

Review of the week; read about termination in *A Child's First Book about Play Therapy*. Coping cards were made, writing the name of each coping and calming technique on separate index cards with Jake drawing pictures on the cards to help remind him what to do. The instructions were written on the back of the card, a hole punched, and a ring attached to them. Jake and I went through each card and practiced each technique twice, reinforcing them, and reviewing his overall progress. I reviewed the problem-solving steps, STAR, with a situation Jake picked about not liking to lose. Jake was given the cards to take home and use whenever he started to feel upset or angry to help him calm down.

Ethical and Cultural Considerations

Ethically, part of informed consent is explaining the limits to confidentiality, which includes serious and foreseeable harm to self or others. To be clear, what a child plays out in a play session does not necessarily indicate that the child will act that out in the community. Clearly, Jake's reenactment of the Capitol violence did *not* indicate that he would do that or enact that at his school. A play therapy guideline is to "allow in fantasy what they cannot do in reality" (Landreth, 2012). His parents and teachers were told that the risks of Jake harming himself or others were minimal at this time but would continue to be monitored throughout treatment. And his parents were made aware of the need to keep any weapons, should they be in the household, safely locked in a gun safe and inaccessible to Jake.

Cultural considerations included ongoing sensitivity and exploration of the parents' conservative religious beliefs and culture of violence that they espoused. Throughout consultation sessions I worked toward being open and accepting of their differing points of view and offered the parents literature on different parenting styles and the impact of viewing violence on television by Jake so that they could better understand how to help Jake regulate his emotions and behaviors.

Parent Consultations

As described above, I met with Jake's parents on a regular basis. The goal was to teach positive parenting skills, help the parents use alternative and more positive means of modifying Jake's behaviors and lessen the negative and aggressive atmosphere in the home that was contributing to Jake's behavioral dysregulation. The parents were receptive and open in working with me and made significant progress over the span of treatment in modifying their interactions with Jake and using suggested techniques.

At the beginning of treatment, the parents were encouraged to "catch Jake being good" by putting a sticker on their watch, and every time they looked at their watch, give positive verbal praise for even the slightest positive behavior at that moment (e.g., "I like how you are sitting so quietly"; "I see how hard you are working on playing nicely with your sister"). I encouraged them to keep a behavioral log and be specific in verbal reprimands, such as "Stop banging the toy in the living room. You can bang it in your bedroom," rather than just saying "stop it" over and over with escalating anger resulting in swatting Jake's bottom. I also taught them natural consequences and encouraged appropriately set limits by stating, "If you continue to bang the toy in the living room, and not play in your room, then you choose to no longer play with that toy for the rest of today." The parents were very receptive to this guidance and willing to implement the suggestions at home.

I also asked Jake's teacher to keep a behavioral log and "catch Jake being good" using the same intermittent reinforcement of randomly focusing on Jake's positive behaviors, which would subsequently increase over responding to negative attention-seeking behaviors.

After the third session, I contacted Jake's parents to share the various self-calming techniques, explain the feelings thermometer, and inquire about the status of behaviors at home. Jake's parents noted that there was progress with Jake listening to them and responding without aggression when they set limits. His interactions with his siblings showed improvement with fewer conflicts, and Jake's nightmares were diminishing. I reviewed with the parents their reflective comments, frequency in "catching Jake being good," and natural consequences used.

In the fifth session Jake's parents came in and reviewed their behavioral log, how they were doing with limit setting and "catching Jake being good." Parents reported positive results in Jake's lessening of behavioral problems, staying more focused, and absence of any nightmares. They stated that he still had occasional temper outbursts when he got frustrated or did not get his way with his siblings, but Jake was responding to using the self-calming techniques. Parents were encouraged to continue their work with Jake, especially giving spontaneous positive reinforcement. Each parent was encouraged to pick a separate night that was designated as Jake's to spend a few minutes before bedtime to read a book, rub his back, and help him settle into sleep. Parents were to keep those designated evenings with Jake regardless of how Jake behaved during the day. The parents wondered how jealous the other children might become in reaction to Jake's exclusive time with a parent. I encouraged the parents to have designated evening times for each of the children, as they, too, could benefit from the positive attention.

In the seventh session, the parents reported Jake's negative behaviors at home were manageable, and interactions were much more positive than negative; all sleep difficulties had ceased, and his interactions with siblings were significantly better. We also discussed termination and my availability in the future should any issues reemerge.

Jake's teacher was contacted periodically regarding progress, and the teacher reported steady positive change. By the seventh session, the teacher reported that Jake's disruptive behaviors had ceased in the classroom and his peer interactions were significantly better. I let the teacher know that the next session would be Jake's last one but that she could contact me in the future should the need arise regarding Jake.

Conclusion

Jake made significant progress in being able to be supportive and cooperative with peers in the classroom, decreased tattling on peers, stayed focused on tasks and completed assignments, and decreased to zero oppositional behaviors in school and at home. He learned coping and calming skills, which he used regularly, and was able to use empathy as well as alter his negative cognitive distortions. Consequently, Jake's relationships with his parents significantly improved, aided by their use of positive feedback and decrease of negative punishment and by altering their lifestyle by lessening TV viewing of violence.

Sample Case Notes

Session 4

Subjective: The previous week was reviewed regarding anger levels and the use of "I" statements at home by Jake. Jake stated that he was using "I" statements when he could remember to use them and that it seemed to help him to slow down and be able to express his feelings with his parents and not become so explosive. Jake's free playtime showed noticeable shifts in not being as aggressive and showing more empathy.

Objective: Read bibliotherapy book *How to Take the Grr out of Anger* and played the Angry Monster Machine board game to help increase understanding about feelings, problem solve, and allow for catharsis.

Assessment: Jake's play is starting to change with noticeably less aggression, with increased verbalization of empathic feelings toward the figures. He was able to express his own scared feelings about potential anger and danger in his world. He is showing more coping strategies and less reactivity.

Plan: Goal is to increase self-soothing and calming resources for Jake to use when upset or angry. Hills and valley deep breathing was taught and homework given to practice this at home.

Resources

For Professionals

The Angry Monster Machine board game—Childswork/Childsplay.

The Talking, Feeling & Doing game—Childswork/Childsplay.

CBT Workbook for Kids: 40+ Fun Exercises and Activities to Help Children Overcome Anxiety & Face Their Fears at Home, at School, and Out in the World by Heather Davidson, PsyD, BCN (2019).

The Mindfulness Workbook for ADHD: Effective Strategies to Increase Focus, Build Patience, and Find Balance by Beata Lewis and Nicole Foubister (2022).

Thriving with ADHD Workbook for Kids: 60 Fun Activities to Help Children Self-Regulate, Focus, and Succeed by Kelli Miller, LCSW, MSW (2018).

Understanding ADHD: A Neurodiversity Affirming Guidebook for Children and Teens by Robert Jason Grant (2022).

For Children

A Child's First Book about Play Therapy by Marc Nemiroff and Jane Annunziata (1990).

How to Take the Grr out of Anger by Elizabeth Verdick and Marjorie Lisovskis (2015).

I Am Stronger Than Anger: Picture Book about Anger Management and Dealing with Kids Emotions and Feelings by Elizabeth Cole (2020).

My Whirling Twirling Motor by Merriam Sarcia Saunders and Tammie Lyon (2019).

The Very Angry Day Amy Didn't Have by Lawrence Shapiro and Charles Brenna (1994).

For Parents

The ADHD Parenting Guide for Boys: From Toddlers to Teens Discover How to Respond Appropriately to Different Behavioral Situations by Richard Bass (2023).

Explosive Children with ADHD: A New Approach to Managing Attention Deficit Disorder in Children to Discipline and Empower Your Super Hero to Achieve Success and Accomplishment by Pansy Bradley (2023).

What Your ADHD Child Wishes You Knew: Working Together to Empower Kids for Success in School and Life by Sharon Saline (2018).

Discussion Questions

1. What contributing factors exacerbated Jake's aggressive behaviors?
2. How would you work in an integrative manner on a short-term basis to address Jake's behavioral issues and ADHD? Would you consider referral for medication?
3. What additional techniques or approaches would you use with Jake going forward if you had more sessions to continue building self-regulation and coping skills?
4. As a mental health professional, how would you talk with the parents about potential possession of guns in the home and personal views about use of violence?

References

Achenbach, T. M., & Rescorla, L. A. (2001). *Manual for the ASEBA school-age forms & profiles.* University of Vermont, Research Center for Children, Youth, & Families.

Afdal, A., Zikra, Z., Sakmawati, I., Syapitri, D., & Fikeri, M. (2022). Psychoeducational intervention in early childhood education: Analysis for children with disruptive behavior. *Advances in Social Science, Education and Humanities Research, 668,* 2–8.

Agus, A. H., Mushfi El Iq Bali, M., & Maula, I. (2022). Role-playing therapy in handling hyperactive children. *Al-Hayati Journal of Islamic Education, 6*(1), 34–42.

Anderson, C. A., Berkowitz, L., Donnerstein, E., Huesmann, L. R., Johnson, J. D., Linz, D., Malamuth, N. M., & Wartella, E. (2003). The influence of media violence on youth. *Psychological Science in the Public Interest, 4*(3), 81–110.

Bandura, A. (1977). *Social learning theory.* Prentice Hall.

Beck, A. T. (1976). *Cognitive therapy and the emotional disorders.* International Universities Press.

Berk, L. E. (2003). *Child development* (6th ed.). Allyn & Bacon.

Browne, K. D., & Hamilton-Giachritsis, C. (2005). The influence of violent media on children and adolescents: A public health approach. *Lancet, 365,* 702–710.

Calvert, S. L. (2006). Media & early development. In K. McCartney & D. Phillips (Eds.), *The Blackwell handbook of early childhood development* (pp. 508–529). Blackwell.

Chen, M., & Chang, K. (2014). A study of the effects of cognitive-behavioral play therapy for ADHD child with disruptive behaviors. https://www.airitilibrary.com/Publication/DetailPrint?DocID=1992

Drewes, A. A. (2009). *Blending play therapy with cognitive behavioral therapy: Evidence-based and other effective treatments and techniques.* Wiley & Sons.

Ellis, A. E. (1971). *Growth through reason: Verbatim cases in rational-emotive therapy.* Science and Behavior Books.

Feindler, E. (2009). Playful strategies to manage frustration: The turtle technique and beyond. In A. A. Drewes (Ed.), *Blending play therapy with cognitive behavioral therapy: Evidence-based and other effective treatments and techniques* (pp. 401–422). Wiley & Sons.

Hirshfeld-Becker, D. R., & Bierderman, J. (2002). Rationale and principles for early intervention with young children at risk for anxiety disorders. *Clinical Child and Family Psychology Review, 5*, 161–172.

Huesmann, L. R., Moise-Titus, J., Podolski, C., & Eron, L. D. (2003). Longitudinal relations between children's exposure to TV violence and their aggressive and violent behavior in young adulthood: 1977–1992. *Developmental Psychology, 39*(2), 210–221.

Jafari, N., Mohammadi, M. R., Khanbani, M., Farid, S., & Chiti, P. (2011). Effect of play therapy on behavioral problems of maladjusted preschool children. *Iranian Journal of Psychiatry, 6*(1), 37–42.

Kasiati, S., Naruvita, S. R., Harti, U., Yulia, I., & Yunitsari, S. E. (2022). Play cognitive behavioral therapy improves the concentration of children with ADHD. *Journal Scientia, 11*(2), 439–443.

Knell, S. M. (2009). CBT: Cognitive behavioral play therapy: Theory and applications. In A. A. Drewes (Ed.), *Blending play therapy with cognitive behavioral therapy: Evidence-based and other effective treatments and techniques.* Wiley & Sons.

Landreth, G. L. (2012). *Play therapy and the art of the relationship* (3rd ed.). Routledge/Taylor & Francis Group.

Lochman, J. E., Powell, N. P., Boxmeyer, C. L., & Jimenez-Camargo, L. (2011). Cognitive behavioral therapy for externalizing disorders in children and adolescents. *Child and Adolescent Psychiatric Clinics of North America, 20*, 305–318.

Murray, A. E. (2015). Evaluating CBPT intervention for kindergarten students with externalizing behaviors [Unpublished doctoral dissertation, Pennsylvania State University].

National Survey of Children's Health (NSCH) Report. (2021). Cfah.org/adhd statistics/2020.

Patterson, G. R. (2002). The early development of coercive family process. In J. B. Reid, G. R. Patterson, & J. Snyder (Eds.), *Antisocial behavior in children and adolescents: A developmental analysis and model for intervention* (pp. 25–44). American Psychological Association.

Perryman, K. (2016). Play therapy in schools. In K. J. O'Connor, C. E. Schaefer, & L. D. Braverman (Eds.), *Handbook of play therapy* (2nd ed., pp. 485–503). Wiley.

Reddy, L. A. (2010). Group play interventions for children with attention deficit/ hyperactivity disorder. In A. A. Drewes & C. E. Schaefer (Eds.) *School-based play therapy* (2nd ed., pp. 307–329). Wiley & Sons.

Rones, M., & Hoagwood, K. (2009). School-based mental health services: A research review. *Clinical Child and Family Psychology, 3,* 223–241.

Siegel, D., & Bryson, T. P. (2012). *The whole-brain child: 12 revolutionary strategies to nurture your child's developing mind.* Bantam Books.

Sukhodolsky, D. G., Kassimnove, H., & Gorman, B. S. (2004). Cognitive-behavioral therapy for anger in children and adolescents: A meta-analysis. *Aggression and Violent Behavior, 9,* 247–269.

Thijssen, S., Ringoot, A., Wildeboer, A., Bakermans-Kranenburg, M., El Marroun, H., Hofman, A., Jaddoe, V., Verhulst, F. C., Tiemeier, H., van IJzendoorn, M. H., & White, T. (2015). Brain morphology of childhood aggressive behavior: A multi-informant study in school-age children. *Cognitive, Affective, & Behavioral Neuroscience, 15*(3), 564–577.

Viranda, C., & Istiningtyas, L. (2019). Bermain Peran (role play) dan Peningkatan Keterampilan Sosial Anak Usia Dini. *Psikostudia: Jurnal Psikologi, 8*(1), 1.

CHAPTER 5

ADHD and COVID-19
Cognitive Behavioral Play Therapy with an African American Child

Lisa Remey

Benjamin is a 6-year-old African American boy living with his mother and father and is a first grader attending public school. Both parents have full-time jobs outside the home. Benjamin has a 4-year-old brother. His parents sought counseling services due to daily teacher reports of incomplete tasks, class disruptions, non-compliance to teacher requests, and classroom outbursts resulting in referrals to the principal's office. An intake session was held with both parents, who shared a history of concerns beginning in kindergarten with some disruptions at home. When asked about day care and/or preschool attendance, parents shared that Benjamin attended day care at 1 year of age; however, when COVID-19 occurred at age 3 and day care closed, he remained at home. During that time, both parents worked from home, navigating parenting and work responsibilities.

For this case study, consider the following:

1. How did the COVID-19 quarantine impact young children with symptoms of Attention-Deficit/Hyperactivity Disorder (ADHD)?
2. What is the rationale for using Cognitive Behavior Play Therapy (CBPT) with Benjamin?
3. Which directive and nondirective strategies seemed to support Benjamin within sessions?

Attention-Deficit/Hyperactivity Disorder

Current research shows that ADHD is the most common childhood neurodevelopmental disorder, which affects 3–9% of school-age children and often persists into adulthood (Ogundele & Ayyash, 2023). The core symptoms of ADHD include pervasive inattention and/or overactivity/impulsiveness and impaired functioning across multiple settings (American Psychiatric Association, 2022).

Additional indicators of ADHD are a short attention span with difficulty sustaining attention due to distraction from extraneous stimuli and internal thoughts. Consequently, it then appears as if children with ADHD are not listening. When children have difficulty focusing their attention, they also have difficulty with follow-through on instructions and completing tasks in a timely manner. Some children with ADHD may have components of hyperactivity as evidenced by high energy levels, difficulty sitting still, impulsivity resulting in disruptive behaviors, difficulty waiting for a turn, and/or interrupting others with questions/comments. Due to these behavioral challenges, children with ADHD tend to have poor social skills and low self-esteem (Ogundele & Ayyash, 2023). They also have decreased working memory, which affects their ability to temporarily store, manipulate, and retrieve information while completing tasks (Wiest, Rosales, Looney, Wong, & Wiest, 2022).

Since the onset of COVID-19, children with ADHD had increases in emotional symptoms (i.e., sadness/depressed mood, loneliness, conduct problems, and sleep problems) compared to before COVID (Segenreich, 2022). Other researchers found that during the COVID-19 quarantine, children with ADHD had increases in anxiety and home learning difficulties (Jackson et al., 2022); deterioration of functional impairment in home life, friendships, learning, and leisure activities compared to children without ADHD (Hall, Partlett, Valentine, Pearcey, & Sayal, 2023); and hyperfocus on the internet with 28% of children with ADHD meeting diagnostic criteria for internet addiction (Kuygun Karci & Arici Gurbuz, 2021).

ADHD symptoms can result in education problems that are predictive of student underachievement and an increased risk of delinquency (Strelow, Dort, Schwinger, & Christiansen, 2021). Because student success requires the ability to attend to tasks, recall teacher instructions, and regulate behavior throughout the school day, children with ADHD need effective treatment.

Cognitive Behavioral Therapy

Cognitive behavior therapy (CBT) has been identified as an approach to support clinical goals associated with treatment for ADHD (Khatoon, Iqbal, & Masroor, 2020). CBT is set in the foundational work of Aaron Beck (2021) and examines how underlying maladaptive beliefs affect emotions and behaviors. Within the CBT framework, change occurs when clients learn to evaluate and shift thinking into more realistic and adaptive patterns, which then increases both positive emotions and behaviors (Beck, 2021). CBT is an empirically researched approach and has been found to be effective in treating children with ADHD (Drewes & Cavett, 2019; Doyle & Terjesen, 2020). Research by von Brachel et al. (2019, as cited in Beck, 2021) showed lasting effects from CBT sessions ranging from 5 to 20 years beyond receiving counseling services.

CBT interventions and approaches are effective for clients from diverse socioeconomic backgrounds, cultures, and ages (Halder & Mahato, 2019). Despite well-defined research, Halder and Mahato (2019) identify clinicians who some-times hesitate to use CBT with children due to minimal levels of young children's language, communication, self-awareness of cognitions, and emotional compe-tencies. However, Halder and Mahato (2019) explain that when working with young children, the focus of CBT is on neutralizing behaviors rather than identi-fying core cognitive errors.

Cognitive Behavioral Play Therapy

Cognitive Behavioral Play Therapy (CBPT) (Knell, 1993) merges CBT's theoret-ical foundation with the foundational aspects of play therapy to meet children's developmental level in communication and awareness. When CBT is blended with the therapeutic powers of play, children can communicate without verbaliz-ing thoughts explicitly (Kaduson, Cangelosi, & Schaefer, 2019). Through thera-peutic play and concrete examples, CBPT builds social-emotional understanding and positive self-talk before negative patterns take root (Drewes, 2009; Knell & Dasari, 2010). It also supports CBT essentials of building client awareness of emotions and the ability to discriminate thoughts, behaviors, and feelings. CBPT uses the CBT framework of reinforcement techniques to achieve the desired change in the client's behavior (Halder & Mahato, 2019).

Knell (1993) outlines six aspects of CBPT:

1. treatment that involves play;
2. a focus on the client environment, fantasy, thinking, and feeling;
3. strategies to develop adjusted behaviors and thinking;
4. structured and goal-oriented sessions;
5. using a combination of empirically demonstrated techniques; and
6. allowing collaborative control of treatment.

Razak, Johari, Mahmud, Zubir, and Johan (2018) explained that CBPT addresses problematic behaviors arising from maladaptive thinking by using play activities and engaging children in verbal and nonverbal communication. This play-based approach positively affects children's feelings and behaviors. CBPT uses both directive and nondirective approaches to address treatment goals. It involves structured and unstructured activities to support the child in generalizing and learning adaptive behaviors (Friedberg & McClure, 2018; Knell, 2015).

In both traditional nondirective play therapy (e.g., Child-Centered Play Therapy) and CBPT, therapists establish a positive therapeutic relationship with children by having a play therapy room that is a safe place so children can communicate through play (Knell, 2015). Both types of play therapists provide therapeutic responses to increase children's understanding during their play and fantasy (Razak et al., 2018). In contrast to traditional nondirective play therapy, CBPT therapists focus on goals and provide selected activities as well as instruc-tion to shape behaviors (Razak et al., 2018).

Collaborative Session Structure

CBPT provides session structure, but the play therapist does not solely lead this structure. The therapist puts the session structure in place and then collaborates with the client to meet current needs and treatment goals (Knell & Dasari, 2010). With this said, in CBPT, the therapist maintains a similar structure each session. This can begin with a client check-in, consisting of a mood check, reconnection, review of the previous session to bridge sessions, review of concerns, updates from the client about their week, and establishing a session plan (Okamoto, Dattilio, Dobson, & Kazantzis, 2019). In a CBPT session, check-in includes a self-report of the week's positive and negative parts. This time helps facilitate discussion regarding choices the client made and build rapport by accepting and normalizing both positive and negative experiences. The check-in allows time for problem solving and learning new strategies. Session planning is collaboratively created during check-in with input from both counselor and client to determine activities and interventions aligned with treatment goals (Knell, 2011). At first glance, session structure may appear rigid. However, the process ebbs and flows based on the client's need and can be as short or as long as appropriate based on client age, abilities, and developmental stage. Okamoto et al. (2019) state that adhering to a collaborative, predictable, yet flexible session structure is related to positive response toward treatment goals.

Strategies

CBPT therapists use a variety of treatment strategies. Common CBPT strategies are self-expression and abreaction as part of nondirected play; direct/indirect teaching; stress inoculation; behavioral rehearsal/role-play; creative problem solving within therapist-directed interventions; and psychoeducation to increase children's awareness of their strengths and weaknesses (Knell, 2011). Other activities and experiential learning using varied techniques to enhance client self-regulation, attention, and flexibility have been identified by Doulou and Drigas (2022). CBPT strategies help children develop positive core adaptive cognitions that prevent maladaptive automatic thoughts and self-talk from taking root in the child's development. The strategies also assist children in creating adaptive self-statements as a coping strategy and boosting adaptive thoughts and behaviors (Drewes, 2009). Coinciding play therapy with psychoeducation and parent sessions reinforces adaptive core beliefs and coping self-talk beyond the play therapy sessions (Knell & Dasari, 2010).

During nondirective play, the CBPT therapist provides facilitative responses to reflect observed actions, raises hypotheses around client thoughts, brings awareness to problem solving, and states observed processing demonstrated by the client. These play therapy facilitative response skills relate directly to CBPT theory in that reflective and tracking statements focus on thoughts, feelings, and actions, which can shift children's awareness and lead to alternative outcomes. Common reflective responses may include "I wonder what happens next," or "I noticed you stopped and thought." The specific facilitative responses made by the therapist align with the client's treatment goals while also considering the individual development and progress of the client. Example response statements for a treatment goal of increasing body awareness may include "Your body really was able to stop right then," "I noticed how you were really focused on where your body was stepping," or "Your pause tells me you are thinking about what to do next." During nondirected play, the therapist gains a sense of how children's thoughts and perceptions are merging with their skills and strategies. Balancing unstructured client-led activities and structured counselor-led interventions is an important aspect of the CBPT process (Knell & Dasari, 2010).

Case Study Application

I will apply CBPT concepts and strategies in Benjamin's play therapy sessions to support him in reducing negative teacher reports, behavioral outbursts, noncompliance, and incompletion of tasks. During the intake session with both parents, they reported that Benjamin's ADHD symptoms increased at school and home as well as with peers during and after the COVID-19 quarantine. I collaborated with his parents to develop treatment goals and objectives as follows.

Treatment Goals: Reduce impulsive actions, increase focus and completion of low-interest activities, and develop effective emotional and behavioral regulation.
Objectives:

1. Identify feelings and connect thoughts, feelings, and actions to choices.
2. Learn thinking and problem-solving skills before acting on the first impulse.
3. Apply skills and increase compliance with rules in the classroom and at home.

I will use CBPT treatment strategies of psychoeducation as well as social-emotional and communication skill development to address Benjamin's impulsivity, self-esteem, compliance, executive functioning, and working memory. I will conduct parent sessions to build parent skills and strategies to support Benjamin. The treatment process begins in Benjamin's initial session. I will work to build rapport and assess Benjamin's recognition of concerns, areas of desired changes, ability to recognize and identify feelings, and his awareness of the effects of his choices on relationships with others. Session structure in an initial session will mirror the structure of future sessions to have session consistency of expectations.

Session 1

I began the initial session with Benjamin using a check-in to briefly explain counseling as a place to explore feelings and problems and develop problem-solving skills. Benjamin shared that he is currently getting in trouble at school and desires to no longer be in trouble with his teacher. After checking in, I introduced the playroom and session structure.

My directive intervention for the first session consisted of a prompt for a kinetic family drawing with the goal of learning about Benjamin and his family, building rapport, and assessing coping with directives and transitions. A timer is used at the end of each session. I set the timer when there are 5 minutes left in the session and let Benjamin know that when it rang, it was time to clean up the playroom and end the session. Using the timer supports building skills and treatment goals of coping with transitions, building compliance, completing tasks, and using self-control.

TABLE 5.1. BENJAMIN: SESSION 1A

Transcript	Analysis
T: "In the playroom, there are many things you can do; if there is something you cannot do, I will let you know. Sometimes you will choose what to do; other times, I will choose. Today you can start by choosing what to play, and later, I have a few things for us to do."	Introduction of the play therapy room and structuring the session provide expectations for this and future sessions.
B: "Okay."	Benjamin explored the room, distracted by toys, with some difficulty deciding what to choose. This response is not uncommon during the first session. Allowing time to explore while providing facilitative responses helps Benjamin build familiarity with the playroom while building rapport.
T: "Your pause tells me you are thinking about what to do next."	Tracking, reflecting, and attunement to Benjamin to meet initial session goals.
T: "In five minutes, I have something for us to do. I will set this timer so we will know when to change activities."	The use of a timer provides structure as well as a cue for transitioning activities. Children with ADHD often have difficulty transitioning tasks, and building transitions into sessions provides opportunities to cope with transition and compliance.

TABLE 5.2. BENJAMIN: SESSION 1B

Transcript	Analysis
T: "The timer rang. Do you remember what that means?"	Prompt to assess working memory as well as bringing awareness to expectations and structure
B: "It means it is time to clean up. But I want to keep playing."	
T: "You wish you had more time to play. However, our time is done for today. I wonder what you will choose next week?"	Limit setting stating client desire, limit, and opportunity to plan.

Session 2

The second session began with a client check-in with Benjamin. As Benjamin shared about his week, I reflected his feelings, understanding of experiences, and choices made while exploring together whether his choices helped make problems bigger or smaller. In doing so, I helped process his feelings, choices, consequences, and thoughts as well as built his self-efficacy.

After check-in, I introduced the concept of a "pause button," explaining how pausing to think through and/or take two breaths can shift choices made, often resulting in reducing negative outcomes.

After the "pause button," I introduced and engaged him in a new game. The Bubble Pause game consisted of using a bubble blower to produce bubbles all over the room with a prompt to pop all the bubbles he could until I said "pause." Once "pause" is said, Benjamin would freeze until I said "un-pause," and then he returned to popping bubbles. While playing the game, my facilitative responses focused on Benjamin's actions, self-control, and abilities.

Once the game was completed, Benjamin was invited to choose what to play. During his play, my facilitative responses focused on reflecting choices, feelings, and observations of pausing to think by Benjamin and/or play characters (such as deciding what to do next or problem solving). These facilitative responses brought awareness to times when Benjamin naturally used his pause skill in decision making and within his play, helping to bring awareness to bridge and expand skills within and outside of sessions. I used a timer to indicate 5 minutes left in the session and when the timer rang, Benjamin and I cleaned up the playroom.

TABLE 5.3. BENJAMIN: SESSION 2A

Transcript	Analysis
T: "Before we play today, let us begin with a check-in. Tell me some good and not-so-good parts of your week."	Building session structure and demonstrating will be exploring both positive and negative choices in which clients experience positive regard from the therapist as well as problem solving and applying to treatment goals.
B: "I don't know."	Clients can often be uncertain how to respond in the beginning phase of treatment.
T: "Okay, let us start with something not-so-good that happened this week either at school or home."	Provide guidance and prompt.
B: "I got in trouble for talking during work time."	Builds trust and rapport when negative aspects are shared and accepted.
T: "One not-so-good thing this week was when you were talking instead of working. Okay, what is something good that happened this week?"	Reflecting and accepting both positive and negative parts of the week equally creates safety within the session and acceptance.

TABLE 5.4.　BENJAMIN: SESSION 2B

Transcript	Analysis
T: "I want to share with you about using a "pause button" to stop and think before making choices. This often can help in pausing before acting. What color would you like yours to be?"	A pause button is a tool I use to practice self-control and the ability to stop and think with the goal of reducing impulsivity and increasing self-awareness and intentional choices.
D: "I pick blue; it's my favorite color."	A pause button is drawn on Benjamin's and my hand.
T: "Let us practice. When I say 'pause,' we push the pause button and freeze until I say 'un-pause,' then we continue with what we are doing."	This makes it a fun game to incorporate into sessions.

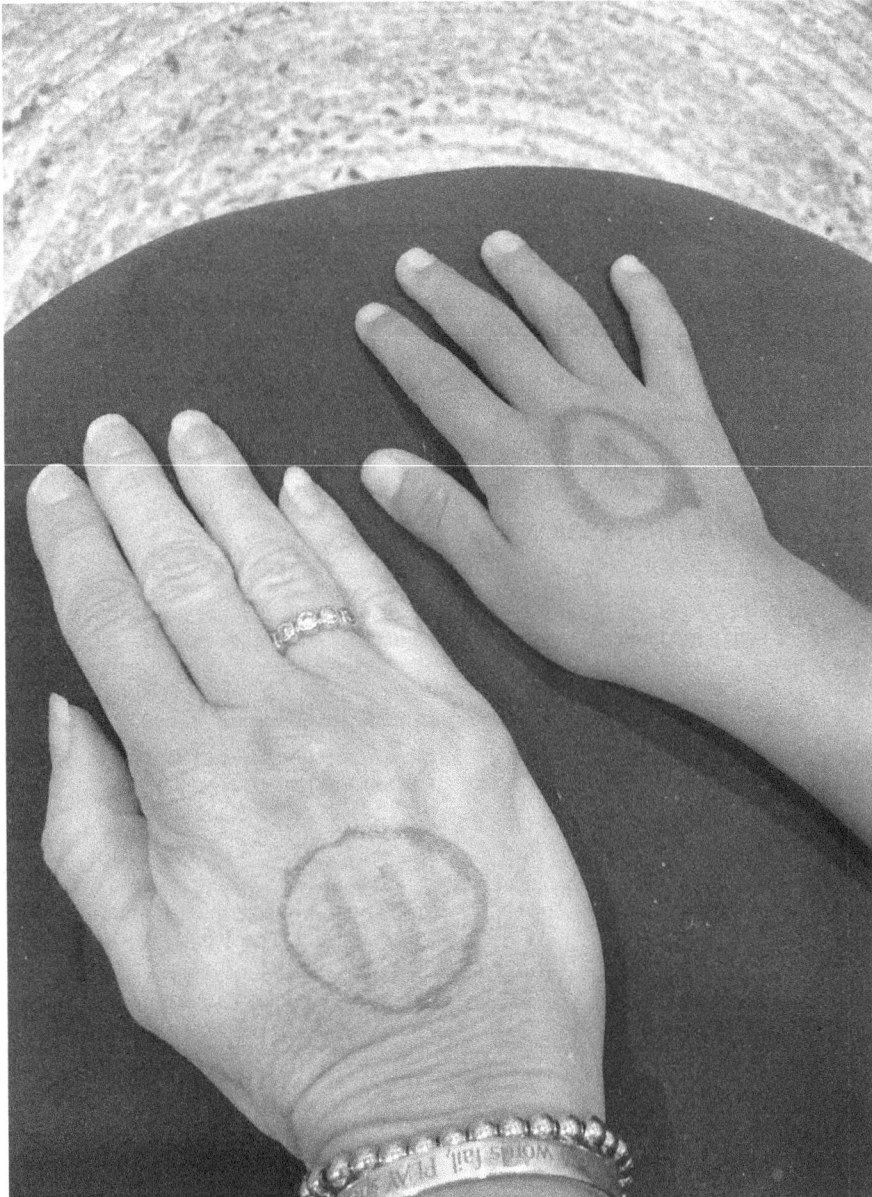

Figure 5.1.　Pause Button Photo courtesy of Lisa Remey.

TABLE 5.5. **BENJAMIN: SESSION 2C**

Transcript	Analysis
T: "You are really getting all the bubbles"; "Nice pause, you got your whole body to stop quickly"; "That can be hard to stop in the middle of something, but you did it!"	These facilitative responses build positive reinforcement as Benjamin builds self-control and body awareness.

Session 3

Benjamin's third session began with a check-in. He shared using the pause button during the week.

After the check-in, we drew pause buttons on our hands, and I introduced the Self Control song (Kisor, 2009). The song is an action song in which children follow along, practicing body awareness and control, moving their body fast, slow, and stopping. During the intervention, I reflected on Benjamin's ability to control his body and follow the song's directions. The remainder of the session was nondirective play chosen by Benjamin. I intermittently prompted him to "pause" and "un-pause," practicing pausing our actions and word.

TABLE 5.6. **BENJAMIN: SESSION 3**

Transcript	Analysis
B: "This week, I had some trouble listening during group time."	Reflective listening and acceptance of the client demonstrated.
T: "I wonder if there is a way the pause button could help you during group time?"	Prompt to apply strategy and build coping skills.
B: "I could push the pause button and remember to listen to the teacher, so I don't get in trouble."	He demonstrated the benefits of the strategy and the ability to apply it to other settings.
T: "Good idea; I wonder if using the pause button and reminding yourself to listen will help?"	Returning responsibility and decision making.
B: "Yes, because then I will get to have recess."	Demonstrating awareness of the effects of choices and benefits of using skills.

Session 4

On the fourth session during check-in, Benjamin shared drawing a pause button on his hand each day before school. He then shared using the pause button often without prompting, such as on the playground at recess. Another example was when he became distracted while the teacher talked and used the pause button to focus on teacher-directed tasks. After check-in, I introduced the My Pleasure game. I created this game using a Thumball™, a softball with panels consisting of printed phrases, words, or images for throwing or rolling, with prompts such as "take 5 giant steps." The ball was gently tossed between Benjamin and me. I read the prompt my thumb landed on when catching and requested that Benjamin complete the task. Prior to completing the task, a crucial rule of the game that I had is for the player to first respond with "no problem," "yes, ma'am/sir," or "my pleasure." The game addresses both working memory and self-control through the steps of gameplay reinforcing pausing and thinking prior to taking the action identified on the Thumball. Benjamin enjoyed playing the game and needed reminders of the rules as he learned the steps. After game completion, Benjamin was provided an opportunity for nondirective play with a timer used to indicate the end of the session and clean-up time.

Ethical and Cultural Considerations

Benjamin's family sought counseling services due to experiencing school difficulties and not meeting the expectations of his classroom environment. I obtained written informed consent from his parents and written permission to contact his teacher. To honor his family's culture, during the intake session, I explored his parents' family rules, expectations, and parenting style to support and blend strategies to meet treatment goals at home and school.

When using the My Pleasure game intervention, it is important to consider family and cultural expectations for understanding tasks and compliance. For example, Benjamin lives in a southern state where it is common for children (and adults) to respond with "yes, ma'am" or "yes, sir," and this may be expected within the culture and community. However, this approach may not fit cultural norms in other communities and may appear authoritative. As the therapist, I take these aspects into consideration and adjust game response options accordingly. At times, I engage the child in collaboratively deciding appropriate response options that indicate understanding and compliance.

Parent Consultations

Parent session goals consist of reviewing play therapy sessions and how they relate to addressing treatment goals and Benjamin's progress observed in sessions. Parents are provided with details of how interventions support Benjamin's gaining skills to process and cope with experiences and feelings, bring awareness to choices, increase self-control, and build sense of mastery. I shared how Benjamin can pause his activity and then pick up where he left off, demonstrating increased self-control. His parents shared about his progress at school with reduced acting-out behaviors in class. I discussed parent strategies to implement a behavior management system to identify choices made at school, create a plan to encourage and reinforce positive choices, and reward Benjamin's use of coping skills and strategies. Using a system to chart progress supports increasing parental observation of behavioral shifts and changes made and will also build Benjamin's self-esteem and mastery. To support parents in enhancing reflective listening and limit setting at home, I recommended the book *How to Talk So Children Will Listen and Listen So Children Will Talk* (Faber & Mazlish, 2013) and discussed it in future parent sessions.

Conclusion

After four sessions, Benjamin increased his ability to comply with tasks at school, demonstrated his ability to pause before acting on impulses, and increased his awareness of his feelings and experiences. Working with Benjamin taught me how younger children can increase awareness of internal cognitions as a part of learning new skills. Benjamin's ability to express using his pause button on his own without prompting, as well as then sharing no longer needing the pause button, further taught me how children can quickly work through the process to build awareness, make positive changes, and formulate positive cognitions. Benjamin's excitement at the process and observing his own increase in self-esteem shows me the effectiveness of the CBPT process.

Sample Case Notes

Parent Consultation Session

The initial parent consultation session was an intake session with both parents reviewing their history of concerns and currently seeking counseling due to Benjamin's difficulty at school. Parents reported some noncompliance at home. However, goals consist of supporting Benjamin to increase school compliance with his teacher and decrease outbursts when given directives for undesired tasks. Benjamin has a diagnosis of ADHD from his pediatrician. The treatment goals identified are to increase self-control and compliance, build social-emotional skills and ability to cope with feelings, and increase positive choices to undesired tasks. Parents are open to learning parent strategies and skills to support their son. Parent sessions are to be scheduled after four therapy sessions.

Session 1

Initial session with Benjamin, who eagerly entered the playroom and was engaged with me. I did a check-in with Benjamin describing the play therapy process and counseling goals, with Benjamin identifying a goal of not getting into trouble with the teacher. I had Benjamin complete a kinetic family drawing, which he did, and shared enjoying swimming with his family. His play choice was to explore the animal bins. I used facilitative responses focused on building rapport, feeling identification, decision making, and mastery. Timer used at the end of the session to prompt end of the session and picking up the playroom with initial hesitation from Benjamin followed with compliance.

Session 2

Benjamin smiled and entered the session, engaging with me. Check-in completed, with Benjamin sharing positive and negative aspects of his week. Psychoeducation of introducing and exploring how choices make problems bigger or smaller. Interventions included teaching Benjamin how to use a "pause button" to stop and think about choices. I then drew a pause button on his hand, practicing the skill. Gameplay of Bubble Pause game to continue practicing the skill and building self-control. Benjamin's play choice was floor play, creating a scene with vehicles. My facilitative responses focused on choice, feelings, and decision making, and when Benjamin naturally paused and thought about choices. The timer signaled the end of the session, with Benjamin responding to the prompt, acknowledging it as the time to clean up the playroom.

Session 3

Benjamin eagerly entered the session and engaged with me. During check-in, he shared using the pause button during the week and having difficulty listening during group time. I reflect on experiences with inquiry to ideas of how Benjamin could improve listening to the teacher. He identified using the pause button during group as a coping strategy. Interventions of drawing pause buttons on our hands, practicing pausing and unpausing during the session, and actively listening to the Self-Control song. The remainder of the session consisted of Benjamin's nondirective play selecting blocks, vehicles, and people to create a scene. Session focus and my facilitative responses addressed choices, feelings, self-control, body awareness, and building self-efficacy. A timer was used at the session's end with no prompts needed. Benjamin demonstrated his ability to understand and comply with the session structure.

Session 4

Benjamin was involved in the session and with me. During check-in, he shared drawing a pause button on his hand during the week and using it without prompting at school as well as to increase focus during group time. Intervention was of teaching Benjamin the My Pleasure game. I provided prompts as he learned the rules of the game, with Benjamin showing interest and desire to comply with the game rules. I observed and reflected on Benjamin having difficulty remembering the steps of gameplay. Plan to play My Pleasure game in future sessions with the goal of building working memory, increasing focus, and ability to complete multiple-step tasks. Benjamin's play choice of floor play, with a battle scene created with the theme of good versus bad. The timer used at the end of the session.

Resources

For Professionals

Kisor, D. (2009). Self-control. *I Can Settle Down: Songs of Self Control.* Kisor Music Studios, Fort Thomas, KY.

Mother May I Thumball™ [toy]. (2014). Maple Shade, NJ: Answers in Motion LLC.

For Parents

Faber, A., & Mazlish, E. (2013). *How to Talk So Kids Will Listen and Listen So Kids Will Talk.* Lagom.

Discussion Questions

1. How would you consider working with Benjamin moving forward to continue building and internalizing skills?
2. What other parenting skills and strategies would you work on with Benjamin's parents?
3. How can facilitative responses build client skills during nondirective play?
4. How could different cultures, socioeconomic statuses, and/or beliefs influence working with a client such as Benjamin?

References

American Psychiatric Association. (2022). *Diagnostic and statistical manual of mental disorders* (5th ed., text rev.). https://doi.org/10.1176/appi.books.9780890425787

Beck, J. S. (2021). *Cognitive behavior therapy: Basics and beyond.* Guilford Press.

Doulou, K., & Drigas, A. (2022). ADHD: Causes and alternative types of intervention. *Scientific Electronic Archives, 15*(2). https://doi.org/10.36560/15220221514

Doyle, K. A., & Terjesen, M. D. (2020). Rational-emotive and cognitive-behavioral treatment for attention-deficit/hyperactivity disorder among youth. In M. Bernard & M. D. Terjesen (Eds.), *Rational-emotive and cognitive-behavioral approaches to child and adolescent mental health: Theory, practice, research, applications* (pp. 285–310). Springer Nature Switzerland AG. https://doi.org/10.1007/978-3-030-53901-6_14

Drewes, A. A. (2009). *Blending play therapy with cognitive behavioral therapy: Evidence-based and other effective treatments and techniques.* John Wiley & Sons.

Drewes, A., & Cavett, A. (2019, September). Cognitive behavioral play therapy. *Play Therapy, 14*(3), 24–26.

Friedberg, R. D., & McClure, J. M. (2018). *Clinical practice of cognitive therapy with children and adolescents: The nuts and bolts.* Guilford Press.

Halder, S., & Mahato, A. K. (2019). Cognitive behavior therapy for children and adolescents: Challenges and gaps in practice. *Indian Journal of Psychological Medicine, 41*(3), 279–283. https://doi.org/10.4103/ijpsym.ijpsym_470_18

Hall, C. L., Partlett, C., Valentine, A. Z., Pearcey, S., & Sayal, K. (2023). Understanding the impact of home confinement on children and young people with ADHD and ASD during the COVID-19 pandemic. *Child Psychiatry and Human Development.* https://doi.org/10.1007/s10578-022-01490-w

Jackson, A., Melvin, G. A., Mulraney, M., Becker, S. P., Bellgrove, M. A., Quach, J., Hutchinson, D., Westrupp, E. M., Montgomery, A., & Sciberras, E. (2022). Associations between anxiety and home learning difficulties in children and adolescents with ADHD during the COVID-19 pandemic. *Child Psychiatry and Human Development.* https://doi.org/10.1007/s10578-022-01338-3

Kaduson, H. G., Cangelosi, D., & Schaefer, C. E. (Eds.). (2019). *Prescriptive play therapy: Tailoring interventions for specific childhood problems.* Guilford Publications.

Khatoon, A., Iqbal, N., & Masroor, U. (2020). Efficacy of cognitive behavioral play therapy (CBPT) for children with attention deficit hyperactivity disorder (ADHD). *Clinical & Counselling Psychology Review, 2*(2), 16–27.

Knell, S. M. (1993). *Cognitive-behavioral play therapy.* Rowman & Littlefield.

Knell, S. M. (2011). Cognitive-behavioral play therapy. In C. E. Schaefer (Ed.), *Foundations of play therapy* (pp. 313–328). J. Wiley.

Knell, S. M. (2015). Cognitive-behavioral play therapy. In K. J. O'Connor, C. E. Schaefer, & L. A. Braverman (Eds.), *Handbook of Play Therapy* (pp. 119–133). https://doi.org/10.1002/9781119140467.ch6

Knell, S. M., & Dasari, M. (2010). Cognitive-behavioral play therapy for preschoolers: Integrating play and cognitive-behavioral interventions. In C. E. Schaefer (Ed.), *Play Therapy for Preschool Children* (pp. 157–178). https://doi.org/10.1037/12060-008

Kuygun Karci, C., & Arici Gurbuz, A. (2021). Challenges of children and adolescents with attention-deficit/hyperactivity disorder during the COVID-19 pandemic. *Nordic Journal of Psychiatry.* https://doi.org/10.1080/08039488.2021.1980610

Ogundele, M. O., & Ayyash, H. F. (2023). ADHD in children and adolescents: Review of current practice of non-pharmacological and behavioural management. *AIMS Public Health, 10*(1), 35–51. https://doi.org/10.3934/publichealth.2023004

Okamoto, A., Dattilio, F. M., Dobson, K. S., & Kazantzis, N. (2019). The therapeutic relationship in cognitive–behavioral therapy: Essential features and common challenges. *Practice Innovations, 4*(2), 112–123. https://doi.org/10.1037/pri0000088

Razak, N. H., Johari, K. S., Mahmud, M. I., Zubir, N. M., & Johan, S. (2018). General review on cognitive behavior play therapy on children's psychology development. *International Journal of Academic Research in Progressive Education and Development, 7*(4). https://doi.org/10.6007/ijarped/v7-i4/4842

Segenreich, D. (2022). The impact of the COVID-19 pandemic on diagnosing and treating attention deficit hyperactivity disorder: New challenges on initializing and optimizing pharmacological treatment. *Frontiers in Psychiatry, 13.* https://doi.org/10.3389/fpsyt.2022.852664

Strelow, A. E., Dort, M., Schwinger, M., & Christiansen, H. (2021). Influences on teachers' intention to apply classroom management strategies for students with ADHD: A model analysis. *Sustainability, 13*(5), 2558. https://doi.org/10.3390/su13052558

Wiest, G. M., Rosales, K. P., Looney, L., Wong, E. H., & Wiest, D. J. (2022). Utilizing cognitive training to improve working memory, attention, and impulsivity in school-aged children with ADHD and SLD. *Brain Sciences, 12*(2), 141. https://doi.org/10.3390/brainsci12020141

CHAPTER 6

Anxiety and Asian Hate
Adlerian Play Therapy with a Chinese American Child
Kristin K. Meany-Walen

Huan is an 8-year-old, second-generation, Chinese American, second-grade girl who lives with her parents, maternal grandmother, and 6-year-old brother in a small town in the Midwest United States. Huan and her classmates were in kindergarten when COVID-19 pandemic protocols began in the United States. When discussing COVID-19 with her grandmother, Huan said children at school told her that she and her "people" are murderers and responsible for the pandemic. Huan is now experiencing anxiety, manifested by crying and not following directions to get ready when going to school and public outings. At school, she keeps to herself and has stomachaches when she must do group projects. Huan's parents are seeking counseling to "help her do the right thing."

For this case study, consider:

1. What is the intersectionality of Huan's age, culture, family, school, peers, local community, global pandemic, and political context? How do these contribute to Huan's anxiety?
2. What is the rationale for using Adlerian play therapy with Huan? Which strategies in each of the Adlerian play therapy phases seemed to help Huan?
3. What are culturally responsive strategies for working with Huan and her family? How do Huan's parents and teachers help her?

Chinese Culture and Virtues

Core Chinese virtues include Ren, Yi, Li, Zhi, and Xin (Yu & Xie, 2021). Ren is the foundation of humanness and includes kindness, love, and benevolence. Yi is righteousness or doing the right thing even at the sacrifice of self. Li is the virtue of being civil, humble, and respectful. It is considered the primary method of achieving social harmony and peace. Zhi and Xin support the other three and involve lifelong learning and integrity. These virtues create a foundation for living within Chinese culture and influence the daily lives of Chinese people as they interact with family, friends, school peers, coworkers, and members of their faith community.

Children's academic achievement is emphasized in Chinese families because Chinese values link education with financial and social success. Children are responsible to their parents, which creates pressure for children to perform well so they can bring pride to their parents and family (Quach, Epstein, Riley, Falconier, & Fang, 2015). These pressures can create distress for children, resulting in mental health concerns such as anxiety. Parental warmth and support were shown to moderate negative effects for the pressure and serve as a protective factor for ongoing negative mental health symptoms (Quach et al., 2015).

Anxiety

Anxiety is on the rise in Chinese children between the ages of 8 and 13 and is rapidly becoming a top health concern (Gao, Liu, Xu, Mesman, & van Geel, 2022). As Chinese children acculturate to US values and become more independent, anxiety becomes maladaptive, preventing them from achieving social and academic competencies. Unfortunately, the traditional Chinese parenting style, which is authoritarian in nature, contributes to Chinese American children's anxiety (Gao et al., 2022). As generations become more acculturated in the United States, an autonomy-supportive parenting style rather than a controlling parenting style helps decrease anxiety in Chinese American children. Parents who maintain high expectations, consistent with Chinese culture, and can also allow for children's autonomy to create ideal environments for children to thrive in their current culture.

COVID-19 had a profound impact on children's functioning and mental health (Litam & Oh, 2021). In the United States, people of color experienced challenges of COVID-19 beyond that of their White counterparts. Many Chinese people experienced COVID-related racial discrimination, which increased the likelihood for this population to have diagnosable mental health concerns and lower levels of life satisfaction (Litam & Oh, 2021). Asian children were particularly susceptible to loneliness, low self-esteem, and social anxiety due to COVID-related discrimination (Chen & Qin, 2020).

Adlerian Play Therapy

Adlerian play therapy (AdPT) is based on the theoretical tenets of Alfred Adler's Individual Psychology or Adlerian theory (Kottman & Meany-Walen, 2016). Adler contended that people's childhood influences their perceptions of how they fit with others and their beliefs about themselves, others, and the world. He also described the role of play in the lives of children, stating that it was their way of communicating and learning (Adler, with Ansbacher & Ansbacher, 1928/1956). However, he did not specifically describe how to work therapeutically with children. Terry Kottman developed AdPT to meet the developmental communication and learning style of children while using Adlerin theory as the foundation for understanding and intervening with children (Kottman & Meany-Walen, 2016).

View of Children

Adlerian play therapists believe that children—and all people—are socially embedded, creative, and goal oriented (Kottman & Meany-Walen, 2016). From the time of birth, people strive to belong and find significance, or how they matter in the world. Their original social group is their family, followed by extended family, neighborhoods, schools, spiritual or religious influences, and other communities or organizations. The family constellation and family atmosphere are significant contributors to lifestyle. Family constellation is how it *looks*, similar to the representation of a genogram. This includes parental relationships (married, divorced, widowed, same sex parents, adopted, etc.), birth order, sex or gender roles and order, attachment breaks or deaths, blended families, and so forth. Family atmosphere is how it *feels* to be in this family, which could include, for example, anxious, athletic, achieving, outdoing, relaxed, chaotic, disengaged, enmeshed. Because people are socially embedded, they must be understood in relation to their social context and roles.

Children are creative. They create unique and individualized "lifestyles," or patterns of thinking, behaving, and feeling, based on their perceptions of how they belong and gain significance within their family and then within other social spheres (Kottman & Meany-Walen, 2016, 2018). They create beliefs about themselves, others, and the world and then interact in the world as if their beliefs are true. Lifestyles are the amalgamation of multiple components that include such concepts as *personality priorities*, *goals of misbehaviors*, *life tasks*, and *Crucial Cs*, which will be described later in this section.

Adler believed that children are goal directed, and their behaviors are purposeful; the goals and behaviors are often out of people's awareness (Adler, 1927/1998). Their behaviors have the goal of meeting their perceived needs, and others' reactions to their behaviors reprove what they already believe to be true about themselves, others, and the world. They continuously seek—and find—feedback that supports their lifestyles, which reinforces their thoughts, emotions, and behaviors. Most often, without intervention this loop continues over time and across situations.

According to AdPT, children and all people react to life from an encouraged (well) or discouraged (unwell) lifestyle (Kottman & Meany-Walen, 2016). People who are discouraged have lifestyles that are not socially advantageous and are potentially destructive. Because the lifestyles are consistent, they will continue until they receive feedback or have experiences that disprove what they already believe. Counseling and play therapy can be an experience that disproves someone's lifestyle and creates new and encouraged beliefs, emotions, and behaviors toward self, others, and the world (Kottman & Meany-Walen, 2018).

One of the hallmarks of Adlerian theory is *social interest*, or community feeling. Social interest is people's emotions, beliefs, and behaviors that provide evidence that they care about their community and environment, make choices that are in the best interest of the greater population, and act with compassion and empathy toward others and the world (Kottman & Meany-Walen, 2016). The degree to which a person shows social interest is the indicator of a person living an encouraged or discouraged life. Adler believed that people who acted selfishly were unwell and had a greater degree of mental illness. A primary goal of therapy is to increase a client's social interest.

Four Phases of AdPT

AdPT moves through four phases of Adlerian theory:

1. building an egalitarian relationship with the child (and family, teachers, or other important people in the child's life);
2. investigating the child's lifestyle;
3. helping the child gain insight; and
4. reorienting/reeducating the child to new ways of feeling, thinking, and behaving.

Alderian play therapists do this using foundational play therapy skills as well as directed interventions such as creating art, making metaphors, telling stories, playing games, using puppets, and cleaning the room together (Kottman & Meany-Walen, 2016). Because people are unique and creative, the therapeutic process is individualized and responds to the individuality of each client's lifestyle.

In the first phase, building an egalitarian relationship, the Adlerian play therapist works with the child to develop a collaborative and shared partnership in which the client feels respected and a part of the process, rather than feeling as a recipient of interventions (Kottman & Meany-Walen, 2016). In the second phase, investigating the child's lifestyle, the play therapist's goal is to learn how the child makes sense of their world and finds significance. Specifically, the Adlerian play therapist uses nondirected play and directed intervention aimed to discover the child's personality priorities (Kfir, 2011), goals of misbehavior (Dreikurs & Soltz, 1964), life tasks (Mosak & Maniacci, 2008), Crucial Cs (Lew & Bettner, 1998, 2000), and assets (Kottman & Meany-Walen, 2016).

Personality priorities are a pattern of beliefs and behaviors that help a person to navigate through and predict life. The four personality priorities are pleasing, control, superiority, and comfort (Kfir, 2011). Personality priorities each have assets and liabilities; none is better or worse than another. Although people have characteristics of each priority, people primarily operate from two priorities. The first priority is used most consistently and is how people structure their daily life. The second priority is how people respond to stress. Play therapists use this information to help inform their interventions and treatment planning.

The four goals of misbehavior are attention, power, revenge, and proving inadequacy (Dreikurs & Soltz, 1964). The goal of misbehavior answers the questions "What is this child trying to gain from this behavior?" "What does this behavior communicate to others and reveal about the child?" Children use misbehavior because they feel discouraged and believe socially constructive behavior is unable to meet their needs, or they have not had experience and support to develop socially constructive behaviors.

The five life tasks are family, love/friendships, work/school, self, and spirituality (Mosak & Maniacci, 2008). All people are challenged with these tasks throughout life. People meet these tasks with different degrees of success, and some tasks can prove more challenging than others at different points of life. Children in therapy often experience greater challenges in the life tasks of family, friendships, and/or school.

Unlike the other elements of lifestyle described in this chapter, Crucial Cs are the assets or the qualities people must possess to handle the challenges of life (Lew & Bettner, 1998, 2000). The four Crucial Cs are count, connect, courage, and capable. A child must believe that he or she *counts* or matters in the world, is able to *connect* with others in meaningful ways, has *courage* to make mistakes and be imperfect, and is *capable* of handling hardships and uncertainty. The play therapist seeks to discover the child's current Crucial C functioning, encourage positive change, and strengthen areas that are lacking.

Nondirected play and directed interventions such as sand tray, storytelling, doll play, puppets, dance or movement, and art among other strategies can be used to help Adlerian play therapists learn about the child (Kottman & Meany-Walen, 2016, 2018). Counselors use what they have learned about the child's personality priorities, goals of misbehavior, functioning at life tasks, Crucial Cs, and assets as well as family constellation and atmosphere, support and resources, and other information to develop their conceptualization of the child. The client conceptualization provides a framework from which Adlerian play therapists develop treatment plans (Kottman & Meany-Walen, 2016).

Next, the Alderian play therapists move into the third phase, helping the child gain insight. Here, therapists create interventions that are intentionally geared toward helping children become aware of their lifestyle characteristics (Mosak & Maniacci, 2008). As children become more aware of their typical patterns of emotions, thoughts, and behaviors, they are more able to make informed decisions about the changes they want to make and how they want to make those changes (Kottman & Meany-Walen, 2016).

During the last phase of AdPT, helping the child gain insight, therapists teach and/or provide opportunities and experiences for the child to replace destructive patterns with constructive patterns (Kottman & Meany-Walen, 2016). Therapists capitalize on the resources, assets, and interests of the child to help teach and practice new skills. Some children need specific instruction and repeated opportunities to try new ways of being. Other children naturally begin to implement new patterns of emotions, thoughts, and behaviors in and out of play therapy sessions.

Case Study Application

Client Conceptualization

From an AdPT perspective, Huan is an 8-year-old girl who is developing her lifestyle through her interactions with family, peers, schools, and others in her community. The dyadic and collective relationships between Huan and her family as well as the intersectionality of her familial culture, her acculturation, her geographical location, and the current significant social and political events contribute to her lifestyle. Her familial culture holds to most traditional Asian virtues of Ren, Yi, Li, Zhi, and Xi. They place particular importance on academic achievement, interdependence, and "saving face" or representing the family positively. Huan has acculturated to some Midwest values of individuality, independent achievement, and "Midwest nice" or being agreeable, friendly, and avoiding conflict.

Huan's family constellation includes living with biological parents and maternal grandmother; she is the oldest sibling and identifies as female. As the oldest child, she is responsible, caring, and helpful. She feels obligated to make her parents proud. Her family atmosphere is one of safety and connection between family members, with an expectation of seriousness and achievement. In addition, they distrust and are cautious with people who are outside their culture. The grandma and parents also emphasize the importance of the traditional Asian concept of "saving face" and representing the family well in social settings.

Huan's primary personality priority is pleasing, and secondary is control. The pleasing personality priority is characterized with a desire to be accepted and liked and with a fear of rejection. Huan often worries about what others think of her and her family. She strives toward being perceived as a "good girl" with her peers and teachers. At times she sacrifices her own needs and boundaries to avoid rejection. For example, she lets children go in front of her in line, avoids asking too many questions of teachers, and frets about upsetting someone to the point of anxiety and self-isolation.

Huan is well-behaved and has no history of problematic behaviors at school, other than her anxiety. Proving inadequacy is Huan's goal of misbehavior and presents as avoidance of interactions and attempting new things. Her teachers and grandmother have noticed a change in Huan's behaviors in the past few months. She had been willing to ask questions, made attempts at answering questions, tried new activities or games with friends at school, and approached other children with relative ease. As of late, Huan avoids new activities and people. She completes her schoolwork but no longer asks the teacher for help or makes attempts at answering questions or trying new activities. The teacher reported that Huan moves sluggishly and slowly in the classroom, chooses to sit alone at recess and lunch, and tries to be unnoticed during class.

As an 8-year-old, Huan is naturally engaged in the life tasks of family, friendship, and school. She holds and values her family's spirituality practices and teachings, and she is steadily growing in her understanding of self. The spiritual and self life tasks are not of significant concern at this point. Her family relationships are strong and supportive. The family can be a source of support as she struggles in other areas. She experiences more challenges with friendships and school at the present time. She isolates from peers and friends, and reports feeling shame and guilt because of their accusations. School has become a challenge as Huan has increasingly become uninvested and disengaged in academics.

Huan showed the greatest strengths in the Crucial Cs count, connect, and capable and a low level of courage. Huan had a history of collaborative and supportive dynamics within her family and school relationships. She integrated feedback and experiences that supported her knowing that she was able to succeed. Her perceptions of those experiences helped strengthen her Crucial Cs of count, connect, and capable. Huan showed a reduced sense of courage over the past year. Due to COVID-19 and its tertiary societal impact, which included negative comments and behaviors from her peers, Huan has a fear of making mistakes and causing problems. She becomes nearly stagnant in her ability to take risks and try new things because of her belief that she will fail or cause harm to herself, family, or others.

Huan has developed beliefs about herself, others, and the world that are discouraged and unproductive to developing and employing social interest. She has the mistaken beliefs that she is bad, is dangerous, and does not belong; others are better than she is, are the deciders of good and bad, and belong in her community; and the world is unkind, doomed, and a scary place.

Treatment Goals and Objectives

The primary concerns of Huan's parents, grandmother, and teachers are (a) a lack of motivation and effort put into schoolwork, (b) withdrawn and anxious behaviors in peer social interactions, and (c) reduced classroom participation and engagement. Huan's primary concern is her fear of hurting people and being disliked. The primary pattern of thoughts, emotions, and behaviors suggested that Huan experienced symptoms of anxiety that was initially related to the impact of COVID-19 and has become more generalized in nature. In addition to these concerns and symptoms, Huan has started to fidget, complain of stomachaches and headaches, and request for herself and her family to wear protective masks.

The treatment goals were collaboratively created between Huan, her parents, and the therapist. The therapist took into consideration family and cultural values and expectations, Huan's current state of functioning and reasonable expectations, Huan's lifestyle and development.

Two treatment goals with accompanying objectives were identified:

1. Huan will demonstrate motivation and academic engagement at home and in school.

To meet this goal, Huan will

a. Develop a collaborative relationship with the therapist in which she can initiate play activities.
b. Cocreate a story that includes a character with courage who overcomes challenging and unpredictable circumstances.
c. Engage in activities that create opportunities for Huan to take risks, receive encouragement, and feel proud of herself (e.g., balancing a peacock feather, juggling scarves, helping the therapist solve "problems").

Huan will demonstrate success by:

a. Doing homework and/or studying for a minimum of 20 minutes, 5 days a week.
b. Reporting a minimum of two things she learned/discussed at school to parents or grandma.
c. Answering one question or prompt to the teacher in the morning and one in the afternoon. This can be done in front of the class or one-on-one.

2. Huan will improve her self-confidence and internal locus of evaluation.

To meet this goal, Huan will:

a. Do directed play activities focused on what is within her control and what is outside of her control.
b. Create a "insecurity/security" blanket.
c. Engage in activities that create opportunities for Huan to take risks, receive encouragement, and feel proud of herself (e.g., balancing a peacock feather, juggling scarves, helping the therapist solve "problems").

This is demonstrated by:

a. Being able to identify negative self-talk and replace it with positive self-talk statements.
b. Showing appropriate risk-taking behaviors such as approaching peers, asking questions, and speaking in front of others.
c. Initiating play activities during sessions.

Strategies used during play sessions to accomplish these goals and objectives included child-led play, storytelling and metaphor, art, movement, and directed play activities.

Treatment Process

Huan's mother called me at the recommendation of Huan's school counselor and teacher. I held an initial meeting with Huan's parents and grandmother to gather background information about Huan, including Huan's development, parents' perceptions of the problem, identified concerns from the school, and their observations of Huan over the past couple of months.

Phase 1

In addition to gathering information, my goal was to initiate a relationship (phase 1) with the significant adults in Huan's life as described in the parent and teacher consultation section below. I built an egalitarian and collaborative therapeutic relationship (phase 1) with Huan by using nondirective play, asking and answering questions, leading directed play activities, and using foundational play therapy skills. I understood that setting clear and direct expectations is traditional in Huan's family and may facilitate comfort. I also knew that experiences in school or other settings in predominantly the White, midwestern United States often allow for children to be rather autonomous and to make choices, which could contribute to Huan's anxiety in school. I started the session using a nondirective strategy and allowing Huan to explore the playroom independently. I was prepared to make modifications to this plan as necessary.

This exchange was paced slowly to match Huan's affect. Based on what I knew about Huan's presenting concerns and culture, I made the intentional and therapeutic decision to be clearer and more direct about the expectations of the play sessions while also allowing for and encouraging Huan to make choices.

TABLE 6.1. **HUAN: PHASE 1A**

Transcript	Analysis
T: "Huan, this is our playroom. Here you can play with all the toys. Sometimes I'll decide what we play and other times you'll decide what we play."	Introduction to the playroom and the play therapy process.
H: [Wringing her hands, fidgeting with her clothes, avoiding verbal interactions, and avoiding taking initiative. She either stared at toys without touching them or tentatively held a toy without playing.]	Demonstrated her anxiety. It can be common for children to feel uncertain or anxious in their first session(s). This is a new and likely unusual experience for children.
T: "You're looking at all the toys."	Tracking her behaviors and communicating to her that I notice, and I am paying attention.
H: [Stood in the middle of the room and blankly looked at the toys]	This gives me clues to her lifestyle. I take mental note that this might indicate anxiety, a desire to do the "right" thing, fear of making mistakes, or wanting to please.
T: "You notice that there are a lot of toys in this room."	Tracking to communicating understanding and to normalize this experience.
H: [Nodded slowly while standing in the middle of the room and looking at the toys]	I take mental note of her cautious, hesitant, slow movements as these can be helpful in creating her lifestyle conceptualization and treatment plan.
T: "Sometimes kids aren't sure where to start."	Normalizing her experience.
H: [Nodded slowly]	
T: "There's a lot of new things going on and it can feel a bit scary." [Pause] "You're feeling unsure."	Reflecting feelings and doing so with an accepting tone. I want to create a space where it is okay to not know what to do.

TABLE 6.2. **HUAN: PHASE 1B**

Transcript	Analysis
T: "When people are nervous it can be hard to make decisions. You could start by playing with the toys or you could play with the art materials."	I took advantage of the learning opportunity by providing information (phase 4) about making decisions. Because our main focus was building a therapeutic relationship (phase 1), I moved on to giving choices with the intent of increasing comfort and reducing her anxiety.
H: [Moved slowly to the art table and reached for paper and colors. She looked at me and slid another paper to the side of the table.]	Huan was easing into the process. Adlerians believe that all behavior is purposeful and goal directed. The goal of this behavior was to invite me to draw with her.
T: [Followed Huan's lead and sat down] "You decided to draw, and you want me to draw with you."	I tracked her behavior and meta-communicated about the goal of her behavior.

Huan and I drew pictures. Huan drew pictures of a rainbow, trees, flowers, and sun. I wanted to eliminate the suggestion of competition or any expectation that they need to do the same thing, so I drew pictures of overlapping shapes. I focused my verbal attention on Huan and her work. I reflected feelings, tracked, and used encouraging statements. By the end of the session, Huan voluntarily, and with some enthusiasm, showed me her picture and explained what she drew.

The primary emphasis during the next two sessions was to continue building a collaborative relationship in which Huan felt safe, valued, and respected. Throughout the treatment process, the therapeutic relationship was fostered and maintained. Therapy generally moves through the subsequent phases in order; however, it is not a strictly linear process. Phases may overlap throughout sessions as new information is revealed and opportunities to gain insight and practice new strategies emerge in the session. For example, in the first session I provided information, which is a focus of phase 4.

Phase 2

In phase 2 (investigating the client's lifestyle), I continued to give Huan choices and would sometimes have a directed activity planned. Huan still presented with anxiety, but those behaviors reduced as she became more comfortable. My goal was to gather enough information about Huan that I could create a lifestyle conceptualization and treatment plan.

I started the third session by exploring Huan's perception of her family.

Adlerian play therapists take notice of the product (what the child creates) and the process (how the child goes about creating) of play and activity. At times Huan would appear to be unsatisfied with her drawing. She turned over the page or asked for another sheet of paper. I reflected feelings, encouraged, tracked, and allowed for silence. I meta-communicated about Huan's goals of behaviors.

I was attentive to *how* Huan went about an activity, *how* she handled challenges, and *how* she perceived herself. Huan showed a desire for things to be just

TABLE 6.3. **HUAN: PHASE 2A**

Transcript	Analysis
T: "Today I have an activity planned. I want to learn more about your family. You can choose to draw a picture, or you can choose to do a sand tray. Which do you choose?"	I specifically wanted information about her family. Therefore, I gave choices about *how* an activity was done as opposed to *if* an activity was done.
H: She hesitated for one minute before pointing at the colors and paper and said quietly, "Draw a picture."	Huan has colored in session before. She feels comfortable with this task, which is why I offered it as a choice. I also consider this as I develop her treatment plan. Coloring may be a self-soothing activity for her. It may also be something I avoid in future sessions so she can practice courage.
T: [Used a bit of animation and still nearly matched Huan's tone] "You decided you'd draw a picture. With these materials, please draw a picture of everyone in your family doing something."	I used encouragement to emphasize that she made a choice and had agency. I lifted my voice slightly in an attempt to connect with her while also respecting her soft demeanor.

TABLE 6.4. **HUAN: PHASE 2B**

Transcript	Analysis
T: "I noticed you turned the paper over and appeared disappointed. I'm guessing you're dissatisfied with what you've drawn."	Meta-communicated about her behaviors and reflected her feelings.
H: "Yes. This isn't good enough, and I forgot to include my grandfather who died."	Huan is demonstrating the cultural values of Ren and Li.
T: "Your grandfather is really important to you, and you want to make sure you include him. You feel bad that you forgot him."	Reflecting her feelings about her grandfather and her feelings toward herself for forgetting.
H: [Nodded]	
T: "You can decide if you start over or if you keep going with your picture."	I could have sat quietly and waited for her to proceed in whatever direction she chose. I made the therapeutic judgment to offer two choices. I believed it was more therapeutic to see what she decided and how she moved forward as compared to sitting in ambiguity and anxiety.

as she expected, a limited flexibility in handling challenges, and a critical view of herself when she makes mistakes.

Phase 3

Huan and I gradually moved from phase 2 to phase 3 (helping the child gain insight). Here, my goal was to help Huan understand patterns of her thoughts about herself, others, and the world; how she belongs; and how she believes she gains significance. I helped Huan develop insight into the goals of her behaviors and how they have or have not been working for her. I used what I learned about Huan to develop a conceptualization and treatment plan. In addition to the skills I used in previous phases, I used more meta-communication and directed activities to help Huan develop awareness.

Through previous sessions, I learned that Huan had internalized messages from peers and believed she and her family were responsible for COVID-19 and its impact such as the shutdown of schools and business, requirement of masks and quarantine, loss of jobs, and death rates. She became overwhelmingly worried of doing anything without a predictable and guaranteed outcome for fear of wreaking havoc and embarrassing her family and culture. She had mistaken beliefs that she made bad things happen because of who she was, and believed that if she were good enough, she could keep people safe. She believed it was her responsibility to be good and keep people safe.

I intentionally designed various interventions to help Huan become aware of her mistaken beliefs and discouraged lifestyle patterns. Huan admired Disney princesses, particularly Elsa with her fair skin and blonde hair. Knowing this, I created an intervention that drew upon the comparisons between Elsa and Huan such as feeling guilty and alone, believing they are responsible for damage to people and communities, and forsaking themselves to protect their family and others. In later sessions, I came back to this intervention to recognize their differences and assets particularly related to appearance, culture, self-acceptance, and their beliefs about others' perception.

TABLE 6.5. HUAN: PHASE 3A

Transcript	Analysis
T: [In response to the hula hoop game] "It's really important to you that you are careful in making decisions."	Meta-communicated about how she makes decisions.
H: "Yes. Kids told me it's my fault that bad things happened to their family."	An example of COVID-related discrimination.
T: "You're worried that if you're not careful, more bad things will happen."	Reflecting feelings and meta-communicated about her fears.
H: "Uh-huh."	
T: "You decided to believe what other kids said."	I wanted to gently make notice that she had the choice to believe or not believe other kids without belaboring the point.

TABLE 6.6. HUAN: PHASE 3B

Transcript	Analysis
T: "It's hard to trust yourself."	Reflecting feelings and meta-communicating.
H: "Yes. Kids told me it's my fault that bad things happened to their family."	
T: "I can understand why you might think this way. You decided that if you stay away from people and you work really hard at being perfect and always doing the right thing, you'll be able to make sure nothing bad ever happens again."	Meta-communicating about her thinking patterns and goals of behavior.

I implemented a movement game with hula hoops (see "Hoops of Control" on page 91) in which Huan could gain awareness of what was within and outside of her control.

I chose to use these specific words because I wanted to gently create awareness that Huan had a choice. It was subtle and may have been missed by Huan. I would not know for sure. Thinking ahead to phase 4, I started to make these soft statements consistently and periodically with the goal of creating "aha" opportunities and potentially planting small changes in her perspective.

Phase 4

The goal of reorienting/reeducating the client (phase 4) is for the client to learn new perspectives, ideas, or skills and/or practices new ways of thinking, feeling, and behaving. Some of the changes are made and practiced in session. Others are developed outside of session such as at home or school. I attempted to use what I knew about Huan to make the best use of time and resources. For example, one intervention (taking risks) could be useful in both goals, or connecting things that happen in session with things that happen at home or school (refuting mistaken beliefs about her role in COVID-19).

In the sessions, I created challenges Huan could complete and feel successful and challenges that would require her to handle adversity. This responded to Huan's treatment goals in which she would take appropriate risks and develop courage to be imperfect, and she would try new things without a guarantee of success. Examples of these interventions are juggling scarves; drawing pictures with her nondominant hand; balancing a peacock feather; and creating a sculpture with recycling, odds and ends and leftover materials such as egg cartons, straws, cereal boxes, tape, and so forth.

I provided materials for Huan to create an "insecurity/security" blanket (described below). This intervention was started in the play sessions and later was taken back and forth between home and therapy. This allowed Huan to practice positive self-talk between sessions.

I believed Huan's parents and grandmother would be best suited to give their experiences and perspectives of the pandemic as well as how they had been impacted because of their shared cultural experience and family values. Huan's family and I found statistics and evidence to counter Huan's belief that their family was responsible for COVID-19 and its effects.

Huan's teacher was also made aware of Huan's beliefs and the peer interactions at school. The teacher created lessons that allowed all students in her class to research facts about the pandemic and other current events. The goal was to educate all students on this matter, create opportunities for students to express their concerns, and to dispel inaccuracies and misunderstandings between students. Huan was also able to use this as study time at home and as a point of discussion with her family, both of which are in her treatment plan.

Ethical and Cultural Considerations

Ethically, it was my duty to be culturally responsive to Huan and her family. Although I had limited experience working with clients from Asian cultures, I did know that making the initial call was likely very stressful for Huan's mother as seeking outside help is not typical for Asian families. I wanted to create an atmosphere of comfort and trust, so I prepared myself by researching information, seeking professional consultation, and broaching the topic of culture and values with the family.

Parent and Teacher Consultations

Approximately every two weeks, I conducted parent consultations in order to maintain the therapeutic relationship with the parents (phase 1) as well as to gather more information (phase 2); provide information about Huan's lifestyle and potential dynamics within the family (phase 3); and assess progress, provide suggestions or information, and help the family to adjust to any changes that may occur when any family member makes changes. In phase 4, I enlisted Huan's parents and teachers in reeducating Huan on accurate facts about the COVID-19 pandemic so that she could change her belief from "my people and I caused deaths" to "Each person is capable and can have courage to work together with others to be as healthy as possible."

I conducted consultations with Huan's teachers and school counselor. Consequently, they provided opportunities for Huan to practice and reestablish friendships with peers. They implemented general lessons on tolerance, diversity, empathy, and kindness, which helped all students develop their social interest and friendship life tasks.

Conclusion

Huan developed a more logical awareness of the global pandemic, its origins, and its impact. Huan practiced courage in the playroom, developed friendships in the classroom, and reduced her sense of responsibility for the effects of the pandemic. Then, she naturally started to take appropriate risks in the classroom and engage more in academic work.

Our treatment plan targeted only a few specific areas of concern (academic motivation and courage). At the end of fourteen sessions, Huan was regularly showing courage to be imperfect. She took initiative and appropriate risks in the play sessions, she laughed more and was silly at times as well. Huan's parents and teachers reported that she took appropriate academic and social risks, and she was tending to schoolwork at home as parents desired. Huan's fidgety and avoiding behaviors faded without any direct attention to them. Likewise, she was able to set boundaries by communicating her needs and limits in social situations, which suggested that her pleasing personality priority was being managed in a more encouraged manner than before. With the collaborative approach to

Huan's treatment that included her family, teachers, and school, Huan was able to develop skills that helped her thrive.

Session Notes

Huan, 1/26/2023, 4 p.m.

Huan was present and engaged in the play therapy session. As is consistent for Huan, she asked permission before initiating any play activity. For most of her session, she chose to play with the dress-up clothes and medical kit. Huan took turns being the patient and the doctor. She showed themes of empathy and relationship, control, mastery, and being capable.

Huan appears to be practicing Crucial Cs courage and capable. She showed *courage* by being vulnerable as the patient and by being willing to engage with and help others by being the doctor. She also showed *capable* by believing that she was able to help patients, which mitigates her goal of misbehavior, proving inadequacy.

Huan strives for belonging by pleasing others. She has the mistaken beliefs that she is responsible for the pandemic and for bad things happening. Huan overcompensates for her mistaken beliefs by striving to be perfect and having a lack of courage. She believes that if she is perfect and does not make any mistakes, she will not cause any more harm.

I will continue to allow Huan to make choices in the playroom, with the goal of her practicing courage and experiencing positive feedback and natural consequences. We will also play Hoops of Control next session to help her gain insight into what is within her control and what is out of her control.

Hoops of Control

Age/Participants: 5 or older; 1–100 participants
Purpose: Participants will be able to identify situations that are within their control and situations that are out of their control.
Materials: One hula hoop for every 1–3 participants. Rope, tape, or other markers to section off different areas on the floor could be used in place of hula hoops.
Considerations: participant mobility, space, number of participants
Directions:

1. Place hula hoops on the floor.
2. One person will read a list (below) of scenarios. After each scenario, participants jump inside the hula hoop if it is *within* their control, and they will jump on the outside of the hoop if it is *out* of their control.
3. Repeat through all the scenarios.

Processing Questions:
Take a mental note of participants' hesitancy, mistakes, or other reactions during the game and refer to these during the processing questions.

1. How do you know if something was in your control or out of your control?
2. Which ones were difficult? Easy?
3. What about (scenario) made it difficult or easy to know if it was within your control?
4. In cases where the participant said, "It depends" (or something similar), what were your thoughts about this scenario? What would your answer depend on?
5. How do you feel when you do/don't have control?
6. What are things in your life that are in your control? Out of your control?
7. What things do you wish you had control of?

Sample Scenarios: Due to space limitations, only a brief list for young kids was included.

Make additions and adjustments as needed to fit your clients' experiences. Interweave serious and silly scenarios, pointed and general scenarios.

1. You have a substitute teacher.
2. It's raining, and you can't go outside for recess.
3. You didn't brush your teeth.
4. You did your homework.
5. You are sad because you lost a toy.
6. You yelled at your parents because you were sad.
7. Who your friends choose to be friends with. Or how your friends act toward others.
8. Your bedtime, chores, or routines at home (or other home expectations).
9. Your principal colored their hair pink.
10. How you treat/react to other people.

Security/Insecurity Blanket

(T. Kottman, personal communication, January 4, 2007)
Age/participants: 5 and older; individual, family, or group sessions
Purpose: To help participants gain insight into mistaken beliefs or negative self-talk. To identify assets and positive qualities.
Materials: blanket or comparable size cloth such as fleece material, fabric markers
Directions:

1. Explain that a security blanket is something that people use as comfort. They wrap up in their security blanket when they feel sad or scared, or when they want to feel cozy and loved. Define "security" and "insecurity" if necessary. The counselor can explain that sometimes people focus on their insecurities even if they aren't true or don't feel good. We're going to focus on both (or see modifications).
2. On one side of cloth, the participant writes or draws her insecurities. For participants who have difficulty thinking of them or putting them into words, be prepared to give examples that you think are true for the participant.

3. On the other side, the participant does the same as in step 2 with securities. Have a list of these prepared as well.
4. This can be a multi-session activity.

Processing Questions:

1. Which list was easier?
2. Which do you think of more often?
3. Which of the securities or insecurities do you think is most true?
4. What are your top three insecurities that would you like to erase or change?
5. What securities would you like to have on there that aren't there yet?
6. What securities or insecurities do you think others would say about you?
7. Do you think it's possible for anyone to have only securities and no insecurities?
8. How can insecurities be helpful or motivating?
9. Where/how do you think you came up with your insecurities? Securities?
10. Which of the insecurities is/are not true, even though it/they feel true?
11. Which of the securities are you most proud of or thankful for?
12. How can you erase or change insecurities?
13. How do you add more securities?

Modifications:

1. Counselor makes a blanket for the participant.
2. Focus on one area (security or insecurity).
3. Write the insecurities with washable markers so when washed only securities remain.
4. Make a smaller version for the participant to be able to keep in her pocket as a transitional or comfort object.
5. Participants (or counselors) solicit securities from their family and/or friends to reinforce assets.

Discussion Questions

1. Only two areas of concern were directly addressed through the treatment process, despite other areas being identified as potentially problematic such as Huan's over-functioning *pleasing* personality priority and *proving inadequacy* goal of misbehavior. Yet, these areas improved over the course of treatment. What may account for these changes? What are your thoughts about not specifically addressing these areas? What areas would you have addressed or not addressed?
2. How has COVID-19 impacted your beliefs about self, others, and the world? Why is this awareness important?

3. Huan lived in a rural community, Midwest United States. How does this impact your understanding of the client and the treatment plan? How did culture influence Huan's lifestyle?

4. How has your family of origin, atmosphere, and constellation influenced who you are and how you believe you belong and find significance in the world?

References

Adler, A. (1998). *Understanding human nature.* Oneworld Oxford. (Original work published in 1927.)

Adler, A. (with Ansbacher, H. L., & Ansbacher, R. R.). (1956). *The individual psychology of Alfred Adler: A systemic presentation in selections from his writings.* Harper & Row. (Original work published in 1928.)

Chen, C., & Qin, J. (2020). Emotional abuse and adolescents' social anxiety: The roles of self-esteem and loneliness. *Journal of Family Violence, 35,* 497–507. doi: 10.1007/s10896-019-00099-3

Dreikurs, R., & Soltz, V. (1964). *Children: The challenge.* Hawthorn/Dutton.

Gao, D., Liu, J., Xu, L., Mesman, J., & van Geel, M. (2022). Early adolescent social anxiety: Differential associations for fathers and mothers' psychological controlling and autonomy-supportive parenting. *Journal of Youth and Adolescence, 51,* 1858–1871. doi: 10.1007/s10964-022-01636-y

Kfir, N. (2011). *Personality and priorities: A typology.* Author House.

Kottman, T., & Meany-Walen, K. K. (2016). *Partners in play: An Adlerian approach to play therapy* (3rd ed.). American Counseling Association.

Kottman, T., & Meany-Walen, K. K. (2018). *Doing play therapy: From building the relationship to fostering change.* Routledge.

Lew, A., & Bettner, B. L. (1998). *Responsibility in the classroom: A teacher's guide to understanding and motivating students.* Connexions Press.

Lew, A., & Bettner, B. L. (2000). *A parent's guide to understanding and motivating children.* Connexions Press.

Litam, S. D. A., & Oh, S. (2021). Effects of COVID-19 racial discrimination on depression and life satisfaction among young, middle, and older Chinese Americans. *Adult Lifespan Journal, 20*(2), 70–84. doi: org.proxy.lib.uni.edu/10.1002/adsp

Mosak, H. H., & Maniacci, M. (2008). Adlerian psychotherapy. In R. J. Corsini & D. Wedding (Eds.), *Current psychotherapies* (8th ed., pp. 63–106). Thomson Brooks/Cole.

Quach, A. S., Epstein, N. B., Riley, P. J., Falconier, M. K., & Fang, X. (2015). Effects of parental warmth and academic pressure on anxiety and depression symptoms in Chinese adolescents. *Journal of Child Family Studies, 24,* 106–116. doi: 10.1007/s10826-013-9818-y

Yu, L., & Xie, D. (2021). Measuring virtues in Chinese culture: Development of Chinese moral character questionnaire. *Applied Research in Quality of Life, 16,* 51–69. doi: 10.1007/s11482-019-09745-w

CHAPTER 7

Autism and Neurodivergence
Group Play Therapy with Children
Robert Jason Grant

Six boys, ages 11 to 13, were referred for counseling services. Four of the boys had been diagnosed with Autism Spectrum Disorder (low support needs), and two had been diagnosed with Attention-Deficit/Hyperactivity Disorder with some suspicion of other neurodivergence-related diagnoses. According to their parents, all the boys had difficulty with peer connection and social navigation. I will refer to these boys as Andres, Brian, Cody, DeShaun, Ezekiel, and Farrell. Each boy presented with a variety of strengths and needs. I sought to properly understand each child individually to learn about their social connection strengths and the needs that may require support.

In my experience and through networking with other therapists, social connection groups are often sought after in communities. These types of groups can help children and adolescents recognize they are not the only person who identifies a certain way or struggles with a particular component. These groups offer the prospect of connecting with peers and building friendships with other children and adolescents. As a result, children can gain a level of self-identified social success. In the group, children practice and address social connection in a more natural, affirming, less dysregulating environment. I am highlighting a case study that showcases the many benefits of implementing group-play therapy, rather than individual social-focused approaches, for preteens with autism and other neurodiversity.

For this case study, consider:

1. What are important tenets and paradigms when working with autistic children? What is the rationale for using an integrative process?
2. What are the procedures for implementing play-group work with autistic children? What was the outcome of social connection for the autistic children in this play group?
3. What are the unique ethical and cultural issues that need to be considered?

Autistic and Other Neurodivergent Children

The Centers for Disease Control and Prevention (2020) estimates that 1 in 44 children in the United States has an autism spectrum disorder diagnosis. Autistic children fall within the identity of neurodivergent, which includes those with a diagnosis of attention-deficit/hyperactivity disorder (ADHD), sensory differences, learning differences, developmental disabilities, and so forth. It has been roughly estimated that 1.2 billion of the world population is neurodivergent (Grant, 2023).

Often, the misinterpretation is that autistic children prefer to be alone. Autistic individuals typically want to have meaningful social relationships, but social situations can be difficult and anxiety provoking, so they may choose to withdraw instead (Grant, 2021). Studies have shown that compared to neurotypical children, autistic children are less involved in group play and social activities, engage in fewer play behaviors, and experience social rejection (sometimes bullying) from peers (Chester, Richdale, & McGillivray, 2019). Jamison and Schuttler (2017) proposed that social navigation and engagement can involve a complex set of skills that evolves over the course of human development. Autistic children may find the social functioning world confusing, frustrating, and even scary.

Group Approach

Before children or adolescents begin participating in a social group, it is essential to assess their current social strengths and needs (Radley, Dart, Moore, Battaglia, & LaBrot, 2016; Grant, 2017). For the group experience to be as smooth and successful as possible, it is important that the children and adolescents participating be similar in their social strengths and needs. If the gap in social presentation between the group members is too great, it will become challenging to improve social navigation and may create further issues with children and adolescents being uncomfortable in the group. This could affect group members' willingness to participate (Grant & Turner-Bumberry, 2020).

Hull (2014) noted that the role of the therapist in neurodivergent focused groups is to provide relationship. Further, the therapist can help model in an affirming manner for group members a safe and natural way of learning what they need or want to see in their life. Sweeney, Baggerly, and Ray (2014) espoused that the group-play therapist has a crucial role in the functioning and success of the group process. It is important for the therapist to model what is expected and exhibit a belief in the process as well as communicate this belief to group members.

Integrative Play Therapy

In the group I facilitated, I decided that an integrative play therapy approach seemed best to support the social and connection preferences as well as needs of each group member. Given the spectrum of presentation that exists among autistic and other neurodivergent children, providing an integrative philosophy would produce the best outcomes. An integrative therapy approach can be traced back to the 1930s (Seymour, 2011). Integrative therapy is defined as an approach to therapy that involves selecting the techniques from different therapeutic orientations best suited to a client's particular problem. By tailoring the therapy to the individual, integrative therapists hope to produce the most significant effects (Cherry, 2021). Integrative play therapy offers promise in its flexible use of integrating play therapy theory and techniques so clients can experience the best therapy for their presenting problems (Grant, 2023; Drewes, Bratton, & Schaefer, 2011).

AutPlay Therapy

AutPlay Therapy as an integrative family play therapy approach designed to address the mental health needs of neurodivergent children (Grant, 2023). The foundation of AutPlay Therapy consists of seminal play therapy theories and approaches integrated within a neurodiversity affirming framework. This seemed like a good basis for my group design as the process of integrating play therapy theories and approaches while staying committed to neurodiversity affirming practices is already established in the AutPlay framework.

AutPlay Therapy has an outlined play-group process. Grant and Turner-Bumberry (2020) stated that AutPlay Therapy groups provide a sense of belonging for children. Many autistic and other neurodivergent children are left out of groups and activities that involve neurotypical peers. In AutPlay Therapy groups, children can develop relationships, practice navigation, and have positive recreational experiences. Children and adolescents can gain a feeling of acceptance and optimism about social situations, especially social situations with peers. They may also discover they are not alone and that other peers have the same needs they do. For guidance with my group, it felt important to follow the AutPlay Therapy play and social groups affirming tenets:

- The group should be a safe and supportive environment for children and adolescents to interact in a way they feel comfortable.
- Group processes should promote a natural and playful opportunity to learn and practice connection and social navigation.
- The group experience should provide opportunities to build self-esteem and confidence, especially in social situations.
- The group should provide an opportunity to establish friendships.
- The group should also provide a supportive environment for parents.

As the therapist, I am the most important component of the AutPlay Therapy group process. My affirming beliefs, attitudes, interactions, and selection of protocols would provide the foundation for a successful group experience. I understood that the children participating in the AutPlay group would need me to be flexible and adaptable, switching smoothly from child-led relationship building to psychoeducational teaching while maintaining a neurodiversity affirming stance. This would require me to be a participant, a role model, and a guide—staying present with the happenings of each group member.

The Neurodiversity Paradigm

In my design of the group protocol, it was essential that I stay committed to the neurodiversity paradigm and neurodiversity affirming processes. Walker (2021) defined the neurodiversity paradigm as a specific perspective on neurodiversity. It is a perspective or approach that embodies three fundamental principles:

1. Neurodiversity is a natural and valuable form of human diversity.
2. The idea that there is one "normal" or "healthy" type of brain or mind, or one "right" style of neurocognitive functioning, is a culturally constructed fiction, no more valid (and no more conducive to a healthy society or to the overall well-being of humanity) than the idea that there is one "normal" or "right" ethnicity, gender, or culture.
3. The social dynamics that manifest regarding neurodiversity are similar to the social dynamics that manifest in regard to other forms of human diversity (e.g., diversity of ethnicity, gender, or culture). These dynamics include the dynamics of social power inequalities, and the dynamics by which diversity, when embraced, acts as a source of creative potential (Walker, 2021, pp. 34–46).

Throughout the group process it was critical that I not only maintained a consistent neurodiversity understanding but also avoided ableist processes—which stand in direct opposition to the neurodiversity paradigm. Scuro (2018) described ableism as a harmful bias, which is often trivialized but can be very damaging. The embeddedness in cultural conditioning and societal system is widespread and somewhat menacing. Often ableist constructs are put forth (without awareness) by well-intended and even established, respected, individuals and institutions. Ableism would deny neurodiversity, instead insisting that there is one right type of brain and one correct way to process, respond, communicate, and navigate.

Although neurodiversity applies to the totality of the human race, most attention is focused on those who are neurodivergent. Grant (2023) proposed that neurodivergent refers to an individual who has a less typical (societally considered "normal") cognitive variation. "Neurodivergence" is the term for people whose brains function differently in one or more ways than what society considers standard or typical. Neurodivergence is neither good nor bad. It is just different. In this group case study, the members of the group were children who had received a diagnosis of autism, ADHD, and/or sensory differences and were all considered neurodivergent.

My challenge in working with the neurodivergent population in a group setting was to provide an atmosphere that helped the children improve their well-being and success while respecting their neurodivergence. This required me to be mindful in implementing neurodiversity-affirming processes—carefully assessing needs versus trying to make the neurodivergent children look neurotypical. This proved to be an especially critical awareness for me because neurodivergent children who may have needs with social navigation can easily find themselves in programs or therapies that promote ableist concepts (Turner-Bumberry & Grant, 2022).

Case Study Application

I met with the six boys in 10 one-hour group sessions. Previously, I prescreened each boy by reviewing paperwork and consulting with his parents to ensure that each boy was a good fit for the group. In the first group meeting, my goal was to create a safe and familiar atmosphere. I was expecting that there would be anxiety and possibly some dysregulation due to being in a new setting with new people. Through pre-group screening processes, it was clear that all the boys shared common interests in Minecraft, LEGO bricks, and constructive play. I planned to use their special interest to help create relationships, nurture connection, and facilitate social navigation. I copied images of Minecraft characters on pieces of paper for coloring. This was to be used as an introduction activity and to help the boys begin to feel comfortable in the group atmosphere.

Session 1

The group began with me introducing myself and sharing a bit about the group goals (i.e., connecting, building relationships, and having fun). I also communicated that the group was a safe place to be yourself and covered a few basic group rules (i.e., different is okay, no bullying, participate at your own comfort, and keep group happenings confidential). After explaining the group rules, I introduced the Minecraft coloring activity.

TABLE 7.1. **AUTPLAY GROUP: SESSION 1**

Transcript	Analysis
T: "Welcome to the group, everyone! I am so glad you all are here! We are going to start with a Minecraft activity to help us get to know each other a little better. We have several Minecraft coloring sheets here; pick the one you want and color it any way you like. Feel free to color and/or draw on it to represent yourself."	It was important to establish an atmosphere of safety and welcome. Many neurodivergent children will experience heightened anxiety in new places and around new people. I wanted to provide the boys with an activity that they would all be familiar with (align with their special interests) and thus help them relax.
C: "What if I don't want to color and just draw on it?"	Some neurodivergent children have specific and strong preferences for how they do something; the way they learn or process the best. I knew it would be important to be flexible and let each child produce in the way he felt most comfortable
T: "You can draw on it, write on it, color it, anything you like that feels like the way you want to do it."	I reaffirmed that each child had choice in what to do with his own paper. This permissiveness was intended to decrease anxiety.
E: "I am doing a Zombie Pigman; they are my favorite."	The freedom provided facilitated spontaneous communication.
T: "For this activity, you can do anything you want. All choices are okay."	I reflected often so the boys could feel empowered to make choices and know that differences were okay. This became an important ongoing message in the group for social navigation and feeling empowered in their own identity.

(continued)

TABLE 7.1. *(CONTINUED)*

Transcript	Analysis
T: "It looks like everyone is finished. Let's try going in a circle and sharing yours with the group. You can show and say anything you want about it. You can also decide not to share anything. I will go first. I colored Steve, but I gave his clothes colors that I like to wear myself. I also gave him a hat because I like to wear hats. I like Steve because he seems very resourceful and can figure out what to do. Andres, do you want to share?"	Due to the different ways neurodivergent children may communicate and the varying anxiety issues, it was important that I communicate clearly that sharing in any way and not sharing at all are okay. Forcing a neurodivergent child to do something different from the way he navigates or ignoring his anxiety can increase his resistance and anxiety. Further, it was important that I complete the activity as well and that I go first in sharing my creation. This helped the boys feel more relaxed and provided a model for what I was asking them to do.
A: "I choose Steve because he is the main character, and he builds things and fights the Zombies."	
B: "Mine is Enderman because it is the best one. I made it all black."	
E: "I like your Enderman."	
T: Ezekiel, you like Brian's Enderman. I like it also, and I like Andres's Steve."	I linked the boys' interests and provided affirmation for A so he would not feel dismissed but, rather, included.
C: "I did a Wither because it is the most powerful character in Minecraft."	
E. "No it's not!"	
B: "Disagree! Sorry, not sorry!"	Some neurodivergent children (as was the case with this group), may have needs with perspective taking. They find it challenging to understand that it is okay when others' feelings and thoughts are different from themselves.
T: "Cody, you feel that Wither is the most powerful, but Ezekiel and Brian, you do not think so. We can all have different thoughts and opinions; we do not have to feel the same way. It is okay to let someone feel differently from us. Some things we will agree on and some we will not; we can still enjoy each other."	This was a natural opportunity to address perspective-taking issues in social navigation. I reflected the different options and validated that each child could have his own opinion, and this was okay. There does not have to be a right or wrong, and we can still have fun together with different opinions. This was an ongoing reflection throughout the 10 group meetings.
T: [after each child had shared] "Thank you all for sharing. I really enjoyed seeing what everyone did and hearing what you said about it. I think it is fun that we all like Minecraft. I think you all have a lot of things in common. I am looking forward to us all having a fun group experience together."	I closed the group with an appreciation for each boy and what he had done and shared. I also wanted to acknowledge what they had in common with each other and that our group experience was going to be fun. I did this to further the group connection and help the boys feel comfortable participating in the group.

Later Sessions

In the next few sessions, we continued to complete various Minecraft-themed interventions that promoted connecting with each other. In session 4, we engaged in a role-play activity of having each boy choose a character and then we acted out scenes from Minecraft. Each boy got to create a short scene for all of us to play out together. My goal for session 5 was to transition to some LEGO activities. I introduced creating a Minecraft environment using Minecraft LEGO bricks. The boys all worked together on a large table to create a LEGO Minecraft world. They communicated to establish what they wanted and how it would be designed.

TABLE 7.2. AUTPLAY GROUP: SESSION 5

Transcript	Analysis
T: "Today we are going to use all these Minecraft LEGO bricks and work together to create a Minecraft world. It can be anything you all want, but you must work together with everyone having a chance to contribute. I will just be watching and provide help if needed."	I wanted to transition from Minecraft-themed interventions to LEGO-based interventions. This stayed consistent with the identified special interest of the boys. I provided less detailed instructions as we were moving along in the group because I wanted the boys to take more ownership of their social navigation with each other.
B: "I'm ready!"	
C: "What are we going to build?"	
B, D, and E: [already starting to build without saying anything]	This activity highlighted the different spaces (variance) of social navigation and communication that each of the boys possessed.
T: "Some people are already starting to build, and others are asking what to do?"	I reflected what I was seeing regarding the different approaches and comfort levels of interaction and communication.
B: "Just build what you want; you can choose."	
T: "Brian, you think everyone can start building what they like."	I reflected what "B" said to help communicate the concept of perspective—each person can build as he likes, and this is okay.
A, C, D: "Yes."	
T: [Observed that for the majority of the time, the boys worked more in parallel play while building. Occasionally someone would ask for a LEGO or how to build a particular thing, and someone would answer him.]	Parallel play can be common in autistic and other neurodivergent children. It is a way of playing that can feel very connecting for autistic children. This was certainly observed in this activity with the group. I would periodically make a reflective comment such as "It looks like everyone is working on it together" or "Everyone is doing what he wants to do, and we are all here together."

Last Session

My goal for session 10 (the final group session) was to have the boys reflect on their group experience and think about what they wanted to remember and take with them from the group. I also wanted to celebrate each of them and their time in the group and end the group on a positive feeling. I introduced an intervention called All of Us Chain. In this intervention we each have seven strips of paper. There is a strip of paper for each group member and for me. We signed the strips of paper and wrote or drew something on each strip of paper that we wanted to give to the other members. Once everyone received their strips of paper from each member, each member used glue to link the strips received from others to form their own individual chain. The end product was each of us having a chain of seven links with things written or drawn on each one from our other group members.

TABLE 7.3. AUTPLAY GROUP: SESSION 10

Transcript	Analysis
T: "For our final group, we are going to complete an activity to share something with each other about our group time." [I provided the boys with the instructions and materials for completing the All of Us Chain intervention.]	I knew it would be necessary to have a closure activity at the end of the group that would help the boys say good-bye and remember what they had gained. I also wanted them to have a tangible, visual item to take with them as a reminder.
T: [I observed the boys being mostly quiet and each one completing his paper strips for each other. Some wrote words, and some drew pictures.]	
T: [After all the boys had finished the intervention] "It looks like we are all finished and have our own chain links created. Does anyone what to comment on his links?"	I wanted to give the boys a chance to share any thoughts or feelings they were having. This helped the boys continue in their connection with each other.
B: "I do not want the group to end" [a comment that was then echoed by other group members].	I had expected this to be the reaction of the boys, as the group had become a positive social interaction space for each of them. I also knew it would be important for me to hold space for these feelings and allow the boys to express these feelings.
T: "It is OK to feel sad about the group ending. It is good that you had a positive time."	It was important that I reflect and acknowledge the boys' sad feelings about the group ending. They could see that these feelings were okay.
T: "We now know that we can have positive social connections and look for other opportunities in our lives. What are some things you can do moving forward to continue to have positive social connection times?"	I wanted to help the boys move forward and take the group experience as empowerment to find more spaces in their lives for positive social connection.
T: [I wrote down a list of ideas that the boys shared and some I added of ways they could continue to have positive social connection. As the group ended, I gave each boy a copy of the list and a card thanking him for his participation and encouraging him to move forward in his social navigation.]	I did this to provide something concrete that the boys could take with them to encourage them to continue their social connection journey.

Ethical and Cultural Considerations

For ethical considerations I stayed informed about group ethical guidelines established by my state licensing board. Further, I familiarized myself with the best practices and ethical guides highlighted by the Association for Play Therapy (APT) *Best Practices* (2023) considerations for play therapists conducting group work:

> The play therapist selects clients for group play therapy whose needs are compatible and conducive to the therapeutic process and well-being of each client. Play therapists using group play therapy take reasonable precautions in protecting clients from physical and psychological trauma. Play therapists explain to group members, and/or their legal guardians (when the group includes those who are legally under guardianship) the importance of maintaining confidentiality outside of the group, instruct them in methods for doing so and make special efforts to ensure confidentiality in settings where it may be more readily compromised, such as schools or inpatient/residential treatment settings. Rules for the group and consequences of breaking the rules should be clear to all group members. If a member of the group cannot abide by the rules of the group, consequences need to be enforced for the protection of others. (p. 6)

My focus in this group was on neurodivergent children and valuing neurodivergence as an identity. As such, I conceptualized neurodiversity and more specifically, the cultural and diversity needs of neurodivergent individuals, within the greater diversity awareness paradigm. An understanding of racism, discrimination, prejudice, bigotry, and so forth provided for a greater understanding of what neurodiversity means and how neurodivergent people and their allies are leading efforts in the neurodiversity movement to help improve acceptance and inclusion in societies that have historically lacked neurodivergent affirming constructs (Grant, 2023).

Parent Consultations

AutPlay Therapy functions ideally as a family play therapy approach involving both the child and the parent in the therapeutic process. In AutPlay groups, parents participate in initial meetings with the therapist to assess the child's best fit in a group. I gave instructions to the parents on how the group would progress through 10 meetings. I encouraged parents to take an active role in promoting connection and social navigation with their child. At the end of each group meeting, I provided the parents with an information sheet that described what had been implemented and processed in the group. I further encouraged the parents to connect with each other outside of group meetings to facilitate social opportunities.

Conclusion

Autism cannot be labeled as one thing, one "look," or one manifestation of symptoms. It is a vast and varied spectrum. The differences between two individuals with the same autism diagnosis can be many. As a professional working with autistic and other neurodivergent children, it is important for me to remember the individuality of the diagnosis and strive to understand each child with whom I am working. This was especially true as I facilitated this group of six boys with social connection goals. In this group, the children varied in their social navigation needs and strengths, how socially capable they felt, and what particular social situations were difficult. Despite these differences, the group of boys were able to find social connections and navigate with each other through various interventions with a positive outcome.

Sample Case Notes

Group Meeting 1

Subjective: The group members shared their Minecraft drawings and some brief information about themselves. Each member shared something, and a couple of members expressed excitement about being in the group. E: "I love this group!" B: "This is going to be a fun group!"

Objective: Initially, each group member appeared to be reserved, likely anxious about the new experience. The group members were slow to begin talking and interacting.

Assessment: From an AutPlay and Neurodiversity Paradigm perspective, this first group meeting looked typical. Neurodivergent children often have needs with social navigation and connection. These processes can create high levels of anxiety, fear, and confusion. It was expected that the members would be anxious and reserved, needing time and opportunity to feel comfortable and sure about the process. The Minecraft intervention was chosen because it represented each member's special interest and would likely help them feel more comfortable sharing about themselves. The whole group did relax some and were able to begin interacting through the Minecraft intervention.

Plan: Structured play interventions that align with the group members' special interests will be implemented to encourage connection and positive social interaction. This will be meshed with therapist reflections that support social navigation and neurodiversity affirming principles.

Group Meeting 5

Subjective: The group members worked together to create a Minecraft world from LEGO bricks. The group members worked mostly independently in parallel play. Occasionally, a member would ask if something could be moved or added or ask for help finding a LEGO piece. Communication such as "Can I use that piece?," Does anyone have this piece?," and "Can I add to this or move this?" were made throughout the creation time with responses given.

Objective: The group members seemed to value each other's space and ideas in creating the world. When members needed to work together or needed help, they communicated in appropriate ways. Once the creation was completed, all the group members seemed pleased with the process and the final outcome.

Assessment: From an AutPlay perspective, the group showed progress from the first session. They were now able to navigate some social situations on their own without the therapist's instruction. The LEGO creation provided an opportunity for the members to work together, requiring them to interact and communicate. Overall, the process went well and showed group members' growth.

Plan: Structured play interventions focused on the group members' special interest in LEGO. Interventions will progress requiring more social group interaction and less facilitation from the therapist.

Resources

For Professionals

Grant, R. J. (2023). *The AutPlay therapy handbook: Integrative family play therapy with neurodivergent children*. Routledge.

Silberman, S. (2015). *Neurotribes: The legacy of autism and how to think smarter about people who think differently*. Allen & Unwin. AutPlay Therapy. https://autplaytherapy.com/

For Children

Congratulations, you're autistic! by Katie Bassiri (2022).
Some brains: A book celebrating neurodiversity by Nelly Thomas (2020).
Understanding autism: A neurodiversity affirming guidebook for children and teens by Robert Grant (2021).

For Parents

Autistic Self Advocacy Network, https://autisticadvocacy.org/
Autistic Women & Nonbinary Network, https://awnnetwork.org/
Sincerely, your autistic child: What people on the autism spectrum wish their parents knew about growing up, acceptance, and identity edited by Morénike Giwa Onaiwu, Emily Paige Ballou, & Sharon daVanport (2021).

Discussion Questions

1. What were some of the reasons for focusing on connection and social navigation with a group of neurodivergent children?

2. Why was it important to understand the boys' special interests and use the special interests in focusing on group goals?
3. As a therapist, what neurodiversity affirming constructs and cultural issues would you need to be aware of to effectively facilitate a group of neurodivergent children? Give specific examples.
4. What would be some of the benefits of an integrated group approach with this population?

References

Association for Play Therapy. (2023). *Play therapy best practices.* https://www.a4pt.org/page/Research

Centers for Disease Control and Prevention. (2020). *Autism spectrum disorder.* https://www.cdc.gov/ncbddd/autism/data.html

Cherry, K. (2021). *What is integrative therapy.* Very Well Mind. https://www.verywellmind.com/integrative-therapy-definition-types-techniques-and-efficacy-5201904

Chester, M., Richdale, A. L., & McGillivray, J. (2019). Group-based social skills training with play for children on the autism spectrum. *Journal of Autism and Developmental Disorders, 49,* 2231–2242.

Drewes, A. A., Bratton, S. C., & Schaefer, C. E. (2011). *Integrative play therapy.* John Wiley and Sons.

Grant, R. J. (2017). *AutPlay therapy for children and adolescents on the autism spectrum: A behavioral play-based approach* (3rd ed.). Routledge.

Grant, R. J. (2021). *Understanding autism: A neurodiversity affirming guidebook for children and teens.* AutPlay Publishing.

Grant, R. J. (2023). *The AutPlay therapy handbook: Integrative family play therapy with neurodivergent children.* Routledge.

Grant, R. J., & Turner-Bumberry, T. (2020). *AutPlay® therapy play and social skills groups: A 10-session model.* Routledge.

Hull, K. B. (2014). *Group therapy techniques with children, adolescents, and adults on the autism spectrum: Growth and connection for all ages.* Jason Aronson.

Jamison, T. R., & Schuttler, J. O. (2017). Overview and preliminary evidence for a social skills and self-care curriculum for adolescent females with autism: The girls night out model. *Journal of Autism Developmental Disorders, 47,* 110–125.

Radley, K. C., Dart, E. H., Moore, J. W., Battaglia, A. A., & LaBrot, Z. C. (2017). Promoting accurate variability of social skills in children with autism spectrum disorder. *Behavior Modification, 41*(1), 84–112. https://doi.org/10.1177/0145445516655428

Scuro, J. (2018). *Addressing ableism: Philosophical questions via disability studies.* Lexington.

Seymour, J. W. (2011). History of psychotherapy integration and related research. In A. A. Drewes, S. C. Bratton, & C. E. Schaefer (Eds.), *Integrative play therapy* (pp. 3–18). John Wiley & Sons.

Sweeney, D. S., Baggerly, J. N., & Ray, D. C. (2014). *Group play therapy: A dynamic approach*. Routledge.

Turner-Bumberry, T., & Grant, R. J. (2022). AutPlay therapy play groups for high needs autistic groups. In C. Mellenthin, J. Stone, & R. J. Grant (Eds.), *Implementing play therapy with groups: Contemporary issues in practice*. Routledge.

Walker, N. (2021). *Neuroqueer heresies: Notes on the neurodiversity paradigm, autistic empowerment, and postnormal possibilities*. Autonomous Press.

CHAPTER 8

Grief after COVID-19 and Gun Violence
Sand Tray Therapy with a Mexican American Child
Clarissa L. Salinas and Jennifer N. Baggerly

Salvador is a 9-year-old Mexican American boy with a learning disability who lives with his mother, father, and 3-year-old sister in a town on the Texas–Mexico border. In 2021, Salvador's grandmother died due to complications with COVID-19. Due to limited income, she could not afford to stop her work in a factory and contracted COVID-19 from an infected coworker. However, because Salvador's grandmother was undocumented, she did not have insurance and was afraid to go to the hospital. She died in their family home. Afterward, Salvador experienced fear of dying and grief but did not receive counseling due to quarantine restrictions. In 2022, Salvador's favorite older cousin, Rubin, was shot and killed by a semiautomatic gun during community violence at a school-sponsored soccer game. Afterward, Salvador expressed his anger by being extremely disrespectful to teachers and other adults in the community; avoided playing soccer, which he loved; perseverated on "what-if" scenarios regarding Rubin and his grandmother; and stopped trying at school because "what's the use since I may die soon, too?" Salvador's school counselor recommended that his parents seek counseling to address his compound grief.

For this case study, consider:

1. How do children's symptoms of grief differ from traumatic grief?
2. What is the rationale for using sand tray therapy with Salvador?
3. What unique ethical and cultural guidelines need to be considered?

Grief and Traumatic Grief

COVID-19

According to the United States Centers for Disease Control (CDC, 2023), the number of people who died in the United States from COVID-19 as of June 3, 2023, is 1,131,439. The race/ethnicity percentages of these deaths were first, White, non-Hispanic at 64%; the second largest race/ethnic group was Hispanic/Latino at 16.8%, followed by Black at 12.6%, Asian at 3.3%, and American

Indian/Alaska Native at 1.1%. People over the age of 65 represented 75.9% of the deaths from COVID-19 (CDC, 2023).

With more than a million deaths by COVID-19, conceivably a million US children experienced grief due to the loss of a loved one. Early in the pandemic, December 2021, estimates of children who lost a parent or in-home caregiver to COVID-19 were already at 167,082 (Treglia et al., 2021), and that was before another surge of deaths in January 2022. Non-White children lost care-giving adults at higher rates than their White peers. Treglia et al. (2021) reported:

> Some of the cruelest pain has come to a group with the least capacity to understand and cope with it. . . . For these children, COVID-19 has done more than hurt their lives; it has ended their world. . . . The sudden, seemingly unexplainable departure of a caregiver leaves a void of affection and direction that each child will struggle to fill. And the outcome of that struggle will determine much about their future. The traumatic loss of a caregiver has been associated with depression, addiction, lower academic achievement, and higher dropout rates. It represents lost potential for individuals and our society. (p. 4)

Grief

Grief is a normal process following the loss of a loved one (Treglia et al., 2021). Grief in children after a family member's death can result in an array of typical responses such as sadness, loneliness, anxiety, guilt, anger, and helplessness. Grief can cause changes in thoughts (e.g., disbelief or protest, imagining alternative scenarios); behaviors (e.g., avoiding grief triggers, inability to connect with others); emotions (e.g., guilt, anger); and physiology (e.g., stomachaches, headaches) (Center for Prolonged Grief, n.d.). Children's ability to recover from grief is based on several factors such as their age, support systems, and circumstances surrounding the family member's death. Although many children's sense of security, relationships, and meaning are challenged after the death of a loved one, positive personal growth is possible if emotional support is provided (DeAngelis, 2022).

Unfortunately, during the COVID-19 pandemic, many children had caregivers who were also stricken with grief, hindering their ability to provide emotional support. In addition, quarantine impeded interaction with other support systems such as school staff, community members, and counselors. These circumstances increased the likelihood of children's atypical grief response of Prolonged Grief Disorder (PGD), defined as "intense yearning or longing for the deceased (often with intense sorrow and emotional pain), and preoccupation with thoughts or memories of the deceased (in children and adolescents, this preoccupation may focus on the circumstances of the death)" (APA, 2022). PGD is persistent and pervasive and interferes with functioning (Center for Prolonged Grief, n.d.). About 10% of children experience traumatic, complicated, or prolonged grief for which clinical therapy may be required (Treglia et al., 2021).

Community Violence

According to the CDC National Violent Death Reporting System, 20,663 people were victims of homicide in 2020, with the most common method being firearms (Liu et al., 2023). "Violence erodes entire communities—reducing productivity, decreasing property values, disrupting social services, and making people feel unsafe in the places where they live, work, and learn" (CDC, n.d., p. 1). The National Child Traumatic Stress Network (NCTSN, n.d.a) stated that chronic community violence can destroy children's sense of safety, put them in survival mode, make them ready to gear up for fight or flight, and dampen their outlook on the future as well as their sense of control.

Traumatic Grief

Community violence that results in a sudden and unexpected death of a loved one can cause childhood traumatic grief that is severe or prolonged and interferes with children's functioning (NCTSN, n.d.a). In addition to grief symptoms discussed above, traumatic grief is characterized by intrusive memories about the death (e.g., nightmares, guilt, horrifying thoughts about the death); avoidance and numbing (e.g., withdrawal, avoiding reminders of the person or events related to the death); and physical or emotional symptoms of increased arousal (e.g., irritability, anger, trouble sleeping, increased vigilance, and fears about safety for oneself) (NCTSN, n.d.a). Unfortunately, any thoughts, even happy ones, about the person who died can trigger fears and upset the child. Reminders that may trigger distress are trauma reminders (e.g., places, situations, people); loss reminders (e.g., photos, special occasions previously enjoyed with the person who died); and change reminders (e.g., situations, people, or things that change such as no longer attending a sporting event). Intervention is needed to prevent ongoing mental health problems in children with Prolonged Grief Disorder and Traumatic Grief.

Sand Tray Therapy

Prolonged grief and traumatic grief are often treated with Cognitive Behavior Therapy and Trauma-Focused Cognitive Behavior Therapy (Center for Prolonged Grief, n.d.; Cohen, Mannarino, & Deblinger, 2006), which are both well described in other chapters in this book. However, the American Psychological Association recommends tailoring treatment to meet the developmental and cultural needs of a particular client (DeAngelis, 2022). Given Salvador's developmental level and Hispanic heritage, I (first author) believe he will also benefit from sand tray therapy for several reasons. First, due to Salvador's developmental level and learning disability, he has difficulty with abstract concepts and prefers hands-on activities but "not baby toys" (his perception of the standard playroom). Second, Salvador does not like to talk about things as his traumatic grief tends to limit his verbal ability, so he needs nonverbal engagement to activate his experiences in a non-threatening manner. Third, sand tray has been shown to be a desired modality with children who are Latinx and/or struggling with grief (Deligiannis & Pinilla, 2022; Salinas, 2021; Thanasiu & Pizza, 2019).

Sand tray therapy is a child-centered technique created by Lowenfeld (1979). Also known as "The World Technique," this child-centered approach consists of a tray of sand, water to be added into the sand tray, if the client chooses, and miniatures of various items for the client to create an imaginative and symbolic world in the sand tray to reflect their inner experiences (Lowenfeld, 1979). The World Technique is based on the principles of psychoanalysis, particularly the concept of the unconscious mind and the symbolic nature of play (Lowenfeld & Brittain, 1982). During a sand tray session, the child is invited to create a "world" in the sand tray, using the miniature figures to represent various elements of their inner and outer worlds. The therapist encourages the child to freely express himself through the placement and manipulation of the figures within the sand tray.

Sand tray is particularly helpful for children with traumatic grief as it allows for posttraumatic play to help them process death and unconsciously reenact trauma in an effort to self-soothe (Webb, 2010). When children use miniatures in the sand tray, they project feelings, thoughts, and experiences onto miniatures, creating a safe distance to process death emotionally and cognitively (Homeyer & Sweeney, 2022; Salinas, 2021). Children can relive memories of their loved one who died and re-create what they would like to have said or done. Children's symbolic play in the sand tray allows counselors to view what a child understands and thinks about the death, and it gives counselors an opportunity to intervene appropriately (Webb, 2010). The burying theme is often seen in sand tray of children who are grieving (Green & Connolly, 2009). It metaphorically allows children to play out the burial of their loved one. It also allows avoidance of the painful emotion when recalling and making sense of a death (Green & Connolly, 2009).

As described by Lowenfeld and Brittain (1982), sand tray materials include the following:

1. Sand: The central component of a sand tray, typically a fine-grain, clean sand is used. It should be easily moldable and provide a suitable texture for creating landscapes and designs.

2. Sand Tray: A container or tray specifically designed for the sand play. It is usually shallow, rectangular, and made of durable materials such as wood, plastic, or metal. The sand tray is standardized at approximately 75 cm x 50 cm x 7 cm and painted blue to create an image of sky or water that contains the sand (Hutton, 2004). A tray that is too small can quickly be filled and overwhelm a child who has been traumatized, and thus should be avoided (Mattson & Veldorale-Brogan, 2010).

3. Miniature Figures: These are small, three-dimensional objects that represent people, animals, objects, and symbols. They are placed in the sand tray to create scenes and narratives. Miniature figures can include humans of different ages, genders, and occupations; animals of various species; vehicles; natural

elements (trees, rocks); and symbolic objects (bridges, fences). They offer a wide range of options for the child to express her thoughts and experiences.

4. Natural Elements: Additional natural materials such as twigs, leaves, shells, and stones can be provided to enhance the sand tray experience. These materials can be used to create landscapes, add details, or provide a sensory aspect to the therapy.

5. Other Props: Depending on the therapeutic goals or specific interventions, additional props may be included that target the client's individual experience, such as tombstones, religious items, beer bottles, cars, or hospital bed. These props can provide opportunities for role-playing, storytelling, or exploring specific themes.

It is important to note that the selection of sand tray materials may vary based on the therapeutic approach, the child's age and preferences, and the therapist's assessment and goals for the session. In addition, ensuring the safety and cleanliness of the materials is crucial to maintain a hygienic and secure therapeutic environment.

When conducting sand tray, my role with the client is to

1. develop a warm relationship where he feels accepted and valued,
2. give him the freedom to lead in his sand tray creation,
3. accept his feelings and behavior unconditionally, and
4. encourage his self-expression (Homeyer & Sweeney, 2022; Lowenfeld & Brittain, 1982).

My goal with the client is to help him readjust to life without his grandmother and cousin. Additional goals include helping him to process the fear he has related to his own death and build coping skills for times that he feels sad or is reexperiencing trauma symptoms.

Sand tray treatment procedures and strategies that will be helpful to Salvador are (1) introduction and explanation, (2) free play, (3) intentional prompts, (4) symbolic play and storytelling, (5) processing and reflection, and (6) closure and integration (Homeyer & Sweeney, 2022; Lowenfeld & Brittain, 1982). First, it is important to explain the purpose of sand tray to Salvador in a mature manner so that he does not confuse it with the idea of just playing in the sand. This is important because he thinks he is "too old for kid toys." Next, it is important that Salvador has unstructured time to freely explore the sand tray and select miniature figures to which he feels connected. Prior to the start of the session, the counselor should equip the room with miniatures that Salvador can relate to, given his loss—for example, a miniature mask to represent life during COVID-19, a miniature soccer ball to represent his passion for the game, and a miniature gun to represent the community violence leading to his cousin's death. Having a well-thought-out array of miniatures can allow the client to engage in symbolic play in the sand, act out scenes, and create narratives. Further, the counselor may use specific prompts or themes to guide the client's play in the sand tray. These prompts can be related to the client's current concerns or therapeutic goals. For example, I suggested that Salvador create a scene in the sand of himself and his family.

Finally, after the sand tray is created, the counselor should facilitate a reflection and discussion with the clients, allowing them to share their thoughts and feelings about their creation. The counselor encourages the client to explore the connections between the sand tray and real-life experiences, promoting integration and understanding. The counselor also assists clients in summarizing their sand tray experience. This can involve identifying insights gained, discussing coping strategies, and setting goals for future sessions or outside the therapy context.

Case Study Application

With this deeper understanding of grief, traumatic grief, and treatment approaches, we can now apply them to Salvador. From a sand tray therapy perspective, I conceptualize Salvador as a 9-year-old Mexican American male struggling with traumatic grief because he has not been able to safely express his thoughts and emotions to the point of integration and understanding. His parents also identify as Mexican American and are grieving the loss of their mother and nephew. Further, the family has a strong belief in the Catholic religion. It is important to note that many Mexican Americans value family as a source of strength, which supports their preference for interpersonal relationships, known as *personalismo* (Garza & Bratton, 2005). Parents usually have very close relationships with their children, especially mothers with their children. When death occurs in Mexican American families, counselors can build rapport with their clients by identifying support systems for the family to rely on (Doran, 2002). Along with having a sense of family, most Mexican Americans value religion as a source of strength. Counselors can benefit from understanding their client's cultural connection to religion and spirituality. For example, in the event of a death, a new relationship with the deceased may be created, and families may gather to pay respects and remember the deceased during Día de los Muertos (Day of the Dead).

Session 1

My goals for the first session were to develop rapport, assess Salvador's working diagnosis, identify his treatment goals, facilitate his expression, and provide some beginning coping skills. I prepared by providing a room with a sand tray and hundreds of miniatures categorized as described above. After introducing myself, obtaining informed assent including limits of confidentiality, I invited Salvador to engage with the sand tray.

After the sand tray, I asked what he would like to accomplish in our counseling together. We agreed on the following:
Treatment Goal: Decrease grief, anger, and disrespect and increase effective emotional and behavioral regulation.

TABLE 8.1. **SALVADOR: SESSION 1**

Transcript	Analysis
T: "Hi, Salvador. Today we are going to use the sand tray. I have lots of miniatures here for you to explore and choose from to include in your sand tray. Take your time to look at all the miniatures available, and when you are ready, I want you to create a scene in the sand of you and your family. I will sit here quietly until you finish your sand tray."	Introduction of the sand tray and invitation to choose miniatures. This informed the client that he gets to take the lead in his sand tray.
S: "Okay. How many miniatures can I choose?"	Children often look for rules in new situations.
T: "You can choose as many or as few miniatures as you would like."	Therapist returned responsibility to the client. Here, the therapist encouraged Salvador to make up his own mind about how many miniatures to use.
S: [Quietly Salvador selects an adult male and female miniatures and a young girl. He lines them up in the sand tray and then goes back to select a young male miniature and older male. He looks at his sand tray and pauses before announcing that he is done.]	Salvador felt safe to create a scene in the sand. He was unsure whether he was finished with his scene as evidenced by his pause.
T: "It sounds like you are done with your sand tray. Still, I'll give you another second or two to decide if you would like to make any changes or if it is good as is."	Reflection of content. This helped Salvador feel heard. Therapist gives client permission to take additional time to finish his scene if needed.
S: "It is good as is."	Salvador used his voice and was assertive when he assured the therapist that he was finished.
T: "Okay. Please tell me a story about your sand tray."	Invitation for client to share his sand tray with therapist.
S: [Salvador points to each miniature as he narrates] "This is my dad, my mom, my baby sister, and my grandpa."	Depending on the developmental age of children, they may either tell you a story about their scene using metaphor or be literal in describing who each miniature represents. Salvador, given his developmental age of 9, appropriately shares who each miniature represents.
T: "Ahh, I see. In your family is your mom, dad, sister, and grandpa. I notice a couple people missing that you mentioned earlier in our appointment were in your family—your grandma and cousin Rubin."	Reflection of content helps Salvador feel heard. Therapist reflects discrepancy between the information given at intake about client's family and how it is portrayed in the sand tray. It is an invitation for client to elaborate on his grief.
S: "Yes they were in my family, but they died."	Salvador felt comfortable sharing his confusion about whether to include his grandmother and cousin in the sand tray.
T: "It sounds like you are unsure if they can still be part of your family because they died."	Reflection of feeling and meaning. Here, the therapist acknowledged Salvador's grief.

Objectives:

1. Express grief related to his grandmother and cousin and develop a restorative understanding of their deaths.
2. Identify and connect experiences, emotions, and perceptions underlying grief and anger.

3. Replace thinking errors with balanced thoughts.
4. Develop effective coping and communication skills.

I also want to give Salvador at least two practical coping strategies for some symptom relief. I explain and demonstrate box breathing and suggest that he direct his upset feelings toward a soccer ball and kick it as hard as he can. See Session 1 Note for a summary.

Session 2

My goal for the second session was to continue to develop rapport with Salvador, understand the relationship he had with his grandmother and cousin, and help him work through the pain of grief. By session 4, Salvador began to identify his feelings related to grief, and his anger intensified as he talked about his loved ones who died.

In the next few sessions, Salvador began to speak more openly about missing his grandmother and cousin. He was able to identify feelings that made up his grief, which included anger, sadness, shock, confusion, and joy. He also began

TABLE 8.2. SALVADOR: SESSION 2

Transcript	Analysis
T: "Today, I want to invite you to create a scene in the sand of the moment you found out Rubin died."	This directive prompt is geared at helping the client begin to work through the pain of his grief.
S: [Salvador quietly brings to the sand tray a car, cellphone, people, and road signs. He creates a scene in the sand of him and his family driving home from dinner. Before he can announce that he is done, Salvador destroys his scene and buries the miniatures in the sand.] "I don't want to do this anymore!"	Working in the sand can elicit unconscious feelings for the client. As Salvador reflected on his memory of learning about Rubin's death, he was flooded with anger. He then refused to continue working in an effort to avoid his anger.
T: "I can see that you are angry. Thinking about Rubin is difficult."	Reflection of feeling and meaning. Here, the therapist acknowledged Salvador's anger.
S: [Salvador remains silent]	Children are often unsure how to respond to reflections of feelings.
T: [Matches Salvador's silence]	I gave Salvador space to sit with his thoughts.
S: "I wish he was still here."	After giving Salvador time to process his thoughts, he expressed his yearning for Rubin.
T: "You wish Rubin was still alive. It's okay to be angry. I noticed you working hard in the sand tray until something upset you."	Reflection of content. Therapist normalized Salvador's feelings of anger and then reflected his nonverbal behavior to elicit a response.
S: "Yeah, I remember my mom getting a phone call from my tía on our drive home, and she was screaming. I heard everything. She said Rubin had been shot and was rushed to the hospital, but he did not make it."	Salvador felt comfortable and safe with the therapist to describe his memory.
T: "So, you remember being in the car when you got the news and hearing your tía's pain. Wow, that must have been a lot for you to take in."	Reflection of content helps Salvador feel heard. Therapist empathized with the client.
S: "Yeah, I do not like thinking about it. I should have been there with him."	Salvador makes deeper meaning of feeling guilt for not being present when his cousin died.

to adjust to life without his grandmother and cousin. The counselor provided Salvador a prompt, "On one side of the sand tray, create a scene of 'family time' before your loved one died, and on the other side, create a scene of 'family time' now after your loved one died." Salvador was able to understand that he could be happy even after his loved ones died and that playing soccer was a great way to honor his cousin rather than it be reminder of his death. Once Salvador practiced his coping skills and better understood his grief, his disrespect toward teachers also decreased.

Ethical and Cultural Considerations

One major ethical consideration in Salvador's case is the health inequities that occurred during COVID-19. The CDC (2022) stated, "The population health impact of COVID-19 has exposed longstanding inequities that have systematically undermined the physical, social, economic, and emotional health of racial and ethnic minority populations and other population groups that are bearing a disproportionate burden of COVID-19." Many low-income Hispanic families, especially with undocumented family members, did not receive needed health services during the COVID-19 pandemic. According to the American Counseling Association advocacy competencies (Toporek, Lewis, & Ratts, 2010), counselors are to engage in social justice advocacy on behalf of or preferably with clients. I did this by helping Salvador write a letter to his state and US Congress representatives asking them to (a) fund public health clinics and agencies for Latinx families, regardless of immigration status, and (b) enhance gun control by banning semiautomatic guns.

An important cultural consideration was to honor Salvador's Mexican American cultural values of familism (i.e., family is a source of support and guidance, and family needs come before one's needs) and respect (e.g., youth must respect their elders) while recognizing the stigma associated with counseling (Choi et al., 2023; Knight et al., 2010). As a counselor, I worked to engage in "*la plática*" (i.e., small talk) to build rapport; demonstrated respect to Salvador's parents by addressing them as *Señor* and *Señora* and asking *con permiso* (for permission) to work with Salvador; and explained that counseling helps typical children with difficulties to decrease the stigma. In addition, I recognized that the Mexican American emphasis on machismo for males seems to have contributed to Salvador's misperception that because he is a "man," he should have demanded care for his grandmother and stopped his cousin's shooting. I reminded him that the events leading up to his grandmother's and cousin's death were not in his control, but he does have control in helping to make his community better.

Parent Consultations

I collaborated closely with Salvador's parents by meeting with them at the beginning of each session while Salvador drew or colored a mandala in the waiting room. Recognizing that his parents were also grieving, I gave them resources described below, encouraged them to practice positive coping strategies with Salvador, use a thermometer scale to illicit the intensity of his feelings on a regular basis, talk with him about grandmother and his cousin, and engage in religious rituals (e.g., lighting candles at church).

Conclusion

Salvador made remarkable progress in understanding his grief and expressing it to others. Sand tray provided him an expressive outlet to process his experiences and create hopeful scenes of the future. Salvador accepted that the deaths were out of his control, but he could control how he coped with the loss. Salvador and his parents decided together to honor his grandmother and cousin on their birthday anniversary by doing a balloon release. This encouraged Salvador to stay connected to his family even after death and send them messages of love.

As a therapist, I learned to trust the process of grief work. During some sessions, Salvador was too angry to participate in sand tray, at which point I allowed him to engage in free play. There were also sessions in which we did not discuss grief at all. It was important for Salvador to be in control of his grief journey and open up when he was ready.

Sample Case Notes

Session 1

Subjective: Client expressed his perception of his family unit in the sand tray. He included adult male and female miniatures to represent his mom and dad, young girl and boy miniatures to represent his sister and himself, and an older adult miniature to represent his grandfather. Client did not include his grandmother or cousin in his sand tray. Client reported that his grandmother died from COVID-19, and his cousin was shot and killed. Client also reported to have a close relationship with his grandmother and cousin. Client's parents report him to be disrespectful toward his teachers and is displaying anger. Identified treatment goals include expressing grief and coping with anger.

Objective: Client was cooperative and displayed appropriate affect. He was cautious when working in the sand tray but displayed developmentally appropriate behavior. He was oriented to time, place, and situation.

Assessment: Client presents with traumatic grief and is having outbursts at school. He currently reports low motivation to attend school and play soccer; however, he is motivated for treatment.

Plan: Provided weekly individual therapy. Work through Worden's 4 Tasks of Mourning in the sand tray. Next session, focus on helping client work through the pain of his grief by having client share memories of his loved ones in the sand.

Session 4

Subjective: Counselor provided client prompt for sand tray, "create a scene in the sand of the moment you found out Rubin died." The goal of the prompt was to help client work through his pain of grief. Client included a car, cellphone, people, and road signs in the sand. Client became angry while working in the sand and buried miniatures. He reported learning about his cousin's death while driving home with his family. Client realized that he had guilty feelings for not being with his cousin when he died. Counselor demonstrated box breathing to client in which he draws the outline of a box with his finger and takes a deep breath in and out each time he draws out a line. Also, counselor and client agreed that it might help client to focus his anger on a soccer ball and kick it as a way to cope.

Objective: Client became angry during session as evidenced by him burying his miniatures. Then, he displayed sad affect when talking about his cousin. His behavior was developmentally appropriate. Client was oriented to time, place, and situation.

Assessment: Client is working through the pain of his grief and remains motivated for treatment.

Plan: Next session, help client adjust to life without the deceased according to Worden's task 3 by providing directive prompt for sand tray. For example, on one side create a scene of life before grandmother and cousin died, and on the other side create a scene of life now. Process with client.

Resources

For Professionals

Creative Interventions for Bereaved Children by Liana Lowenstein (2006).

NCTSN. *Cultural and Contextual Considerations in the Treatment of Childhood Traumatic Grief.* https://www.nctsn.org/resources/cultural-and-contextual -considerations-treatment-childhood-traumatic-grief

Sandtray Therapy: A Practical Manual, Fourth Edition by Linda E. Homeyer & Daniel S. Sweeney (2022).

For Children

NCTSN. *Ready to Remember: Jeremy's Journey of Hope and Healing.* https:// www.nctsn.org/resources/ready-remember-jeremys-journey-hope-and-healing

NCTSN. *Taking Care of You.* https://www.nctsn.org/resources/taking-care-of-you

When Someone Dies: A Children's Mindful How-To Guide on Grief and Loss by Andrea Dorn (2022).

For Parents

NCTSN Video and Resources. *I Don't Know How to Support My Child through Loss: Multigenerational Cultural Perspectives.* https://www.nctsn.org/

resources/i-dont-know-how-to-support-my-child-through-loss-multigeneratio
nal-cultural-perspectives

NCTSN. *Rosie Remembers Mommy: In Her Heart Forever.* https://www.nctsn
.org/resources/rosie-remembers-mommy-forever-her-heart

NCTSN. *Información en Español.* https://www.nctsn.org/resources/informacion-
en-espanol?search=&resource_type=All&trauma_type=All&language
=86&audience=29&other=All

Discussion Questions

1. What were some of Salvador's unique experiences and needs as a result of his compound grief?
2. How did sand tray facilitate the achievement of Salvador's treatment goals? Give specific examples.
3. As a therapist, what beliefs, biases, and/or emotions would you need to bracket to effectively work with Salvador and his family?
4. What actions could you take to promote social justice advocacy related to medical services for undocumented families and gun violence?

References

American Psychiatric Association. (2022). *Diagnostic and statistical manual of mental disorders* (5th ed., text rev.). https://doi.org/10.1176/appi.books .9780890425787

Centers for Disease Control and Prevention. (2022). *CDC COVID-19 Response Health Equity Strategy: Accelerating Progress Towards Reducing COVID-19 Disparities and Achieving Health Equity.* https://www.cdc.gov/coronavi-rus/2019-ncov/community/health-equity/cdc-strategy.html

Centers for Disease Control and Prevention. (2023). *COVID data tracker.* https:// covid.cdc.gov/covid-data-tracker/#datatracker-home

Centers for Disease Control and Prevention. (n.d.). *National violent death reporting system.* https://www.cdc.gov/violenceprevention/datasources/nvdrs/resources .html

Center for Prolonged Grief. (n.d.). *Complicated grief.* https://prolongedgrief .columbia.edu/professionals/complicated-grief-professionals/overview/

Choi, N.-Y., Li, X., Crossley, R., Gibbs, J., & López-Harder, J. (2023). Mental health and attitudes toward seeking counseling in Mexican Americans: Exploring values and social class. *Counseling Psychologist, 51*(4), 560–589. https://doi.org/10.1177/00110000231160766

Cohen, J. A., Mannarino, A. P., & Deblinger, E. (2006). *Treating trauma and traumatic grief in children and adolescents.* Guilford Press.

DeAngelis, T. (2022). *Thousands of kids lost loved ones to the pandemic. Psychologists are teaching them to grieve, and then thrive.* American Psychological Association. https://www.apa.org/monitor/2022/10/kids-covid-grief

Deligiannis, A., & Pinilla, M. (2022). Migratory phenomenon and expressive sandwork in vulnerable populations. *Journal of Analytical Psychology, 67*(1), 88–104. https://doi.org/10.1111/1468-5922.12751

Doran, G. (2002). *Family grief experience at the death of a child in the Mexican American community* [ProQuest Information & Learning]. In *Dissertation Abstracts International: Section B: The Sciences and Engineering* (Vol. 63, Issue 5–B, p. 2578).

Garza, Y., & Bratton, S. C. (2005). School-based child-centered play therapy with Hispanic children: Outcomes and cultural considerations. *International Journal of Play Therapy, 14*(1), 51–80. https://doi.org/10.1037/h0088896

Green, E. J., & Connolly, M. E. (2009). Jungian family sandplay with bereaved children: Implications for play therapists. *International Journal of Play Therapy, 18*(2), 84.

Homeyer, L., & Sweeney, D. (2022). *Sandtray therapy: A practical manual* (4th ed.). Routledge.

Hutton, D. (2004). Margaret Lowenfeld's "world technique." *Clinical Child Psychology and Psychiatry, 9*(4), 605–612.

Knight, G. P., Gonzales, N. A., Saenz, D. S., German, M., Deardorff, J., Rossa, M. W., & Updegraff, K. A. (2010). The Mexican American cultural values scale for adolescents and adults. *Journal of Early Adolescence, 30*, 444–481. https://doi.org/10.1177/027243161609338178.

Liu, G. S., Nguyen, B. L., Lyons. B. H., Sheats, K. J., Wilson, R. F., Betz, C. J., & Fowler, K. A. (2023). Surveillance for violent deaths—National violent death reporting system, 48 states, the District of Columbia, and Puerto Rico, 2020. *Morbidity and Mortality Weekly Report*, (SS-5), 1–38. http://dx.doi.org/10.15585/mmwr.ss7205a1

Lowenfeld, M. (1979). *Play in childhood*. Free Association Books.

Lowenfeld, M., & Brittain, W. L. (1982). The world technique. In L. McMahon (Ed.), *The handbook of play therapy* (pp. 313–338). Routledge.

Mattson, D. C., & Veldorale-Brogan, A. (2010). Objectifying the sand tray: An initial example of three-dimensional art image analysis for assessment. *Arts in Psychotherapy, 37*(2), 90–96.

National Child Traumatic Stress Network (n.d.a). *Community violence*. https://www.nctsn.org/what-is-child-trauma/trauma-types/community-violence/effects

National Child Traumatic Stress Network (n.d.b). *Traumatic grief*. https://www.nctsn.org/what-is-child-trauma/trauma-types/traumatic-grief

Salinas, C. L. (2021). Playing to heal: The impact of bereavement camp for children with grief. *International Journal of Play Therapy, 30*(1), 40–49. https://doi.org/10.1037/pla0000147

Thanasiu, P. L., & Pizza, N. (2019). Constructing culturally sensitive creative interventions for use with grieving children and adolescents. *Journal of Creativity in Mental Health, 14*(3), 270–279. https://doi.org/10.1080/15401383.2019.1589402

Toporek, R. L., Lewis, J. A., & Ratts, M. J. (2010). The ACA advocacy competencies: An overview. In M. J. Ratts, R. L. Toporek, & J. A. Lewis (Eds.), *ACA advocacy competencies: A social justice framework for counselors* (pp. 11–20). American Counseling Association.

Treglia, D., Cutuli, J., Arasteh, K., Bridgeland, J., Edson, G., Philips, S., & Balakrishna, A. (2021). *Hidden pain: Children who lost a parent or caregiver to COVID-19 and what the nation can do to help them.* COVID Collaborative. https://www.hiddenpain.us/

Webb, N. (2010). *Helping bereaved children: A handbook for practitioners.* Guilford Press.

CHAPTER 9

Family Stress
Filial Therapy with an Indigenous American Family
Risë VanFleet

Kallik was an 8-year-old boy who originated from arctic Alaska. He bore a traditional Inuit name, although the one here is substituted to preserve his privacy. His tribal affiliation is not included here, either, for privacy reasons. His father had been killed in a fishing accident two years prior, and when his 16-year-old sister attempted suicide, his mother, Kanani, moved both her children to the "lower 48" to live near her sister and her family. This represented a considerable change from their close-knit arctic village to an East Coast town of 50,000 people. Kallik had difficulty adjusting to his new physical and cultural environment. He was sometimes heard crying during the night, and he resisted going to school. In school he often refused to do his work and said very little when asked what the problem was. The school counselor asked Kanani if she would seek help for him. His sister was already in treatment for her own issues. Kallik had not made many friends and often stayed in his room at home. Kanani said she was unable to get him to talk about what was on his mind. Kanani then contacted some key people in her former Native Alaskan district who directed her to me.

For this case study, consider:

1. How did Kallik's new environment contribute to his behavior problems at school?
2. Why is Filial Therapy an appropriate intervention for Kallik and his family? How is it culturally appropriate?
3. What did Kallik's play reveal about his experience? How did his mother facilitate his change through Filial Therapy?

Indigenous Cultural and Environmental Context

There were no therapists from Kallik's culture, or even from Alaska, who practiced within 100 miles of the family's new location in the northeastern United States. The family had learned of another professional who was from a different indigenous culture, but she was prohibitively far away. I (author) had been recommended to them by an Alaska Native program for whom I had provided several training workshops in Filial Therapy (FT) in the past and who thought the method would be very useful for this family.

Because Kallick's withdrawn behavior at home and the various problems reported at school were new behaviors, it seemed that the grief over his father's death, the attention given to his sister's attempted suicide, followed by the move from his familiar home community to a very foreign environment had a cumulative detrimental effect on Kallik's psychosocial well-being. These factors all needed to be considered in this case and should be borne in mind by readers.

The family stress must be considered as well. Kanani certainly had her own feelings about the loss of her husband and her daughter's suicide attempt, and they seemed to have prompted her to move from her home community to be closer to her sister. She was worried because of the high rate of suicide among young people in arctic villages and believed that a different environment might prevent further attempts by her daughter. She was carrying a lot of family stress on her shoulders, and that, too, is an important consideration in her decisions and the subsequent therapeutic process for her family.

Significant cultural and social factors also need to be considered. As happened with many indigenous peoples in the United States and elsewhere, indigenous Alaskan villages experienced an erosion of their cultural integrity and heritage when confronted by Westerners who assumed power over their traditional lands, engaged in heinous acts, and removed much of their sovereignty and agency (Rosita, 2010). Core beliefs and ways of living with the land and each other were affronted and disregarded in a manner that had devastating impact that continues as intergenerational trauma. The historical and continuing difficulties faced by this family's village and neighboring communities and indigenous people throughout the United States are relevant as they influence many factors important for mental health and a sense of belonging. The loss of land and culture was accompanied by the loss of language, traditions, spiritual beliefs, and how people lived their daily lives with each other (Donovan et al., 2015; Stringer, 2018). The separation of children from their families and other physical and psychological atrocities left their mark as well.

This child and his family had experienced these challenges in their own community in arctic Alaska, and now they had been uprooted in an effort to protect the children and in hopes of providing them more opportunities. Kanani also wanted to connect her children with other family members who had moved from the community about a decade earlier and appeared to be doing well.

Bronfenbrenner (1979) proposed the Ecological Systems Theory of child development. This theory offered a broader and deeper framework from which to understand child development and things that interfere with it, posing challenges to child and family adjustment. It provides a useful frame to consider the difficulties that Kallik and his family faced. In it, Bronfenbrenner looked at the impact of different levels of "systems" in which the child was embedded. These

nested environmental structures included (a) the microsystem of the child's immediate settings and relationships, such as family, school, friends, and neighbors; (b)
the mesosystem of interrelationships between and among these settings directly
involving the child such as the intersection of family and school, family and the
child's friends and neighbors; (c) the exosystem of events and interactions that
have indirect impact on the child and family, such as the parents' employment,
extended family, social media, local governments; (d) the macrosystem of wider
systems that also have indirect influence such as social norms, socioeconomic
status, political systems, culture, laws; and finally, (e) environmental changes
that take place throughout the child's and family's life, including planned and
unplanned events (Bronfenbrenner, 1979; VanFleet, 1985). It is clear in Kallik's
case that factors at each level were operating, and careful consideration of them
would potentially influence the success of any intervention.

Filial Therapy

Filial Therapy (FT) is a systematic and time-limited family intervention created and developed by Drs. Bernard and Louise Guerney over the past 60 years
(Guerney & Ryan, 2013; Topham & VanFleet, 2011; VanFleet, 2014; VanFleet
& Guerney, 2003). Based on a psychoeducational model, FT empowers families in direct ways. The therapist trains and supervises parents as they learn
to conduct one-to-one nondirective play sessions with their own children. As
parents develop competence in the four play sessions' skills of structuring,
empathic listening, child-centered imaginary play, and limit-setting, they begin
to understand more clearly the meaning of their children's play themes, from the
children's points of view. This allows them to deepen their empathy and demonstrate fuller understanding of their children's dilemmas, worries, and problems,
as well as their hopes, desires, and dreams. FT has been shown through contin-
uous research on the Guerneys' family model as well as several derivative programs to be effective in ameliorating children's problems while strengthening
the family (Bratton, Ray, Rhine, & Jones, 2005; Guerney & Ryan, 2013; Van-
Fleet, 2014). It has also been shown in controlled research that the most dysregulated children and most dysregulated parents show the greatest gains with FT
(Topham, Wampler, Titus, & Rolling, 2011).

FT is based on an elegant integration of multiple theories. It includes psychodynamic, humanistic, behavioral, interpersonal, cognitive, developmental/attach-
ment, and family systems perspectives and applications. Its core values include
genuineness, empathy, relationship, empowerment, collaboration, humility, and
playfulness, among others (VanFleet, 2014). Its reliance on nondirective parent-
child play sessions makes it particularly well suited for children ages 3 to 12
years, but it can be adapted for adolescents as well. Ideally, all children in the
family are involved.

The therapist typically trains parents how to conduct the play sessions in three
training sessions, and then observes five or six sessions in person. Each training

activity and each play session is followed by the therapist going through a collaborative feedback process with the parent in which they cover the things that the parent has done well followed by just one or two things to work to improve the next time. As parents gain skills, additional discussion about the play themes and parent reactions are included. Parents typically can become very skilled in these play sessions.

When the parents are competent in conducting the play sessions, they are moved to the home setting. The parent conducts the sessions on their own and then meets with the therapist to discuss what went well, what presented problems, the primary play themes, and parent feelings about the sessions and the play. All of this is processed with parents in an empathic, supportive manner while monitoring the child's progress. FT focuses not only on empowering the child through the play sessions, but on building self-efficacy in the parents through this collaborative process.

Because FT is a process-oriented, relationship-centered approach, it has many complexities that are sometimes overlooked by those unfamiliar with it. These subtleties are critical so that the parents feel understood and supported, just as the FT process helps them become more empathic and supportive of their children. Limits are used sparingly during the play sessions but are important in reestablishing parental authority in some cases. Problems typically begin to show resolution within four to six sessions, and this in turn increases parental motivation to continue. Near the end of the FT process when parents are conducting weekly half-hour play sessions with each of their children, the therapist helps them generalize what they have learned to daily life. By this time, the parents are quite skilled, and this generalization to the more complex realm of daily life is done with relative ease.

FT can be used in conjunction with other forms of play therapy or behavioral intervention, depending on the nature and severity of presenting issues. It is a flexible approach that has been used successfully in many countries and cultures, in large part because family is so important to human existence everywhere, and play is universal in children.

I have trained countless professionals throughout the world to conduct FT. Within North America, this has included more than 90 indigenous American/Inuit professionals representing approximately 20 different tribal affiliations. I have been invited repeatedly by several native organizations to offer FT to indigenous professionals and paraprofessionals through the years. Many have noted the compatibility of the approach with their cultural values. Frequently, during professional training sessions, when I showed a listing of the FT values next to documents detailing tribal and cultural values, participants' suspicions of yet another intervention ill-suited to tribal social values dissipated. During one such workshop, all the participants asked for copies of both documents and later confirmed that their experiences with FT bore out the harmony of the method with their families. Glover (1996, 2003), who applied and researched a variation of FT with Native American parents on the Flathead Reservations in Montana, noted the empowerment of parents as the change agents for their own children and the FT emphasis on parent-child relationship over individual child problems as aligned with indigenous American parenting values.

Case Study

Case Conceptualization

Using Bronfenbrenner's Ecological Systems Theory, Kallik and his family had experienced trauma and pressure from virtually all of the system levels within which they were embedded. Within the microsystem of the immediate family, they had experienced the unexpected and traumatic death of Kallik's father and the suicide attempt by his sister. Kallik had struggled in school, and his mother was at a loss as to how to reach and help him. The teacher meetings suggested that no one knew how to help Kallik, and they seemed to expect Kanani to "fix" the problem. Kallik also had few opportunities to make new friends.

On the mesosystem level, because of their relocation, Kanani had good support from her sister and family, but she felt displaced from the village she had lived in her entire life and disconnected from her culture. The indirect influences on Kallik included Kanani's job, which was low paying while her expenses had mounted, and she was away from home longer due to having to commute to it. On the exosystem level, Kanani was unsure of the impact of social media on both her children, and she worried they could come under bad influences because she was not there to monitor them. The economic pressures only compounded the stress Kanani felt and added to her feelings of helplessness. Within the macrosystem, she said she felt like she was in a totally different country where she did not understand what was expected of her. She also had experienced occasional overt racist remarks when in the vicinity of her work. Although she tried to provide love and care for her children, she felt inadequate to the task when immersed in such a different environment.

Treatment Goals

The treatment goals were set after an individual meeting between Kanani and me followed by a family play observation, one of the assessment methods used in FT. I also conducted a nondirective play session demonstration with Kallik that Kanani observed, and she and I discussed it afterward. I then held another meeting with Kanani individually so we could discuss all questions she had, the play session she had observed, and my recommendation of Filial Therapy as the primary intervention. I recommended FT because of its alignment with the family's cultural values, as Kanani readily recognized, and its potential to build family empowerment, not only for the children, but also for Kanani. Because Kanani's sister was an important support, and their traditional values emphasized extended family and community, I asked if Kanani would like her sister to participate as well, and we could have all the children in the two families participate in the FT play sessions. Kanani quickly accepted this idea, and her sister was immediately accepting of it as well. For the sake of brevity, this chapter focuses only on the FT sessions held with Kanani and Kallik, but both entire families were involved eventually in the one-to-one parent-child play sessions and discussions with me.

Goals were developed through a collaborative process with Kanani, and later with Kallik and his sister. Kanani had clearly stated her goals from the start, so they were discussed in more detail, and plans to meet them were set in place. For Kallik, goals were to help Kallik overcome his discomfort of going to school, and for him to participate in some neighborhood events and play with his cousins, in hopes that this would facilitate his making new friends. Goals for Kanani included learning the FT skills and applying them in her play sessions with Kallik, and her modified FT sessions with her daughter. Family goals were to strengthen all their relationships, help them all feel understood, foster their adjustment to their new life, and find ways to have fun together. Kanani also wanted to find opportunities through which she and her children could engage in traditional cultural rituals, practices, and games.

FT Treatment Process

Beginning Training Sessions

Filial Therapy was implemented in the usual sequence. After the play session demonstration that I held with Kallik, we moved into the parent training phase. This entailed three sessions with Kanani and her sister. I discussed the four skills of structuring, empathic listening, child-centered imaginary play, and limit-setting and gave examples of them drawn from the prior play demonstration. I then asked Kanani and her sister to take turns practicing the empathic listening skill with me playing the part of a child playing by myself. I stopped periodically to give them positive feedback and immediately returned to my child role. At the end, I went through the usual FT feedback process to tell each parent what they had done well and making suggestions for one or two things to work on. This first training session was followed by two more in which I helped them practice all four skills in mock play sessions. Once again, I pretended to be a child and played in ways that allowed each parent to individually practice all the skills.

Once again, I gave quick ongoing feedback in the midst of this play and more dedicated feedback at the end of it. As is usually the case, I injected some humor into the play, which helped ease the performance pressure that parents sometimes feel. Kanani laughed during her practice sessions, but she caught onto the skills quickly, as did her sister. They both commented at the end of the mock play sessions that the nondirective nature of the play fit their cultural parenting beliefs and practices very well. They commented that they could see how it allowed the child (me) to open up more.

TABLE 9.1. KANANI: TRANSCRIPT/ANALYSIS

Transcript	Analysis
FT: "Now I'll pretend to be the child, and Kanani, you can focus on empathic listening and child-centered imaginary play."	Naming the specific skill before role-playing is less overwhelming for Kanani and helps parents develop that specific skill.
K: "Okay. I think I remember what you taught us. I will feel embarrassed, but I'll try."	Kanani's hesitation and embarrassment are common when beginning.
FT: "You're a little anxious about it but willing to give it a try. You have more wisdom than you think. Everyone is nervous at first. My role is to be supportive and kind to you." [Pretending to be child]: "Mom, this stuff is stupid. I don't know what to do."	Genuine empathic listening of Kanani's feelings helps her feel understood, and identification of her strengths and reassurance of support facilitate trust in the FT and process.
K: "Well, just try."	This response shows Kanani's commitment to the FT process, although she missed the feeling and child-centered imaginary play.
FT: "Watch my face and see if you can tell how I am feeling. Then tell me what that is. Let's try that again." [Exaggerating facial expression this time] "I don't want to do this stuff—it's stupid." [Turning to Kanani] "What am I feeling?" [FT pauses while Kanani tries, then adds], "That's terrific—you got that I was unhappy about it."	It is important to set parents up for success. This process of modeling possible child reactions and exaggerating facial expressions and tone of voice as needed help parents develop skills more naturally. Giving Kanani an opportunity to say a more accurate response strengthens parent confidence. Reinforcing her attempts while gently shaping them builds parents' motivation and enjoyment of the process.
FT: [Later in the roleplay, using puppets] "I am a hungry polar bear. You are a little seal."	FT clearly explains the roles at the start of this imaginary play skill practice.
K: [Holding the seal puppet] "Oh, no! A polar bear! I have to find a place to hide from the bear!" FT smiles, quickly says, "That's it!" [and continues with the role-play].	Kanani demonstrates the imaginary play skills and follows the "child's" lead well. Kanani's accurate responses and the FT's positive feedback increase her confidence.

During my initial play session with Kallik, he had played without speaking with me, and Kanani had seen how I had responded by never requiring him to speak. While I fully expected that Kallik would eventually talk more with his mother than he had with me, I prepared Kanani in our next mock session how to respond if he remained quiet, but also how to handle various limits and other challenging situations.

We also discussed what play items might make the playroom more culturally familiar to Kallik. I already had some items from my many trips to Alaska, such as bears, moose, and caribou, as well as two authentic Alaska native-made yo-yos (igruuraak, Inupiaq), sometimes called Eskimo yo-yos, that I had purchased from the Alaska Native Hospital gift shop in Anchorage. Kanani suggested adding a few more drums, some sled dogs and a sled, snow machines, a kayak, a seal, whales, some white material that could represent snow, traditional hunting implements, and traditional clothing items. I acquired those items and included them in the playroom for all future sessions.

Office-Based Parent-Child Play Sessions

After the three training sessions with Kanani and her sister, we were ready to begin their nondirective parent-child play sessions with their children, one at a time. With Kanani's daughter, we decided to wait to involve her in some special times after we got started with Kallik. She was already receiving therapy, so a short delay did not seem to be problematic.

Kanani held her first play session with Kallik the following week. He had played during the play session demo but had not spoken, and often he had turned his back on me. I had reflected that he didn't want me to see what he was doing, and he nodded very slightly. When I could see what he was doing, I made sure my empathic listening responses were short and worded in my own way so he would not feel as if I was intruding. He mostly had explored the various toys in the room, picking them up, looking at them, and in a few cases seeing how they worked. When he had his first parent-child play session with Kanani, he was immediately more animated, showed his mother some of the items in the play-room, and quietly spoke to her. He continued exploratory play and pulled out more toys to look at or use for a short while. Kanani held a skilled first session, remaining in empathic listening mode as he explored and showed her items. He did not engage in any imaginary play, nor did he break any limits. During my feedback session alone with Kanani afterward, she commented that it had felt good to her to see how he wanted to show her items of interest to him and that she had found it easier to show empathy than she had expected. We briefly discussed his play themes, and I explained that exploratory play is very common in the early play sessions. They were off to a good start.

In the next session, Kallik's play shifted from exploratory play to a longer focus on the animal figures in the room. He positioned together a group of animals consisting of deer, caribou, elephants, and moose. A second grouping included a lion, a bear, and a rhinoceros. He played briefly and intensely as the first group moved around the playroom while the second group followed them around, yelled at them, and told them they should fight. This play shifted suddenly to quieter play where he ran his fingers through the sand and made some tracks in it. He told his mother that this was the very long road to danger. Kanani followed his lead most of the time, and my feedback was overwhelmingly positive and specific. I suggested that she watch a bit more for Kallik's feelings, or the feelings of his characters, and to reflect them. I gave her examples of this: "That group is saying some unkind things to the first group. . . . It looks like the first group is moving around a lot and aren't sure how to get away from the other ones." Or "You've put a road in the sand, and it goes to a risky place. . . . A road to danger. It's hard to find a safe place." When talking about possible play themes, I asked Kanani what she thought. She suggested that maybe this all had something to do with their move and the bullying he had experienced. I confirmed that that was a possibility and added that it seemed he was dealing with perceived or real threats and danger. I explained to her that she should not ask him about this part of his play at home as he would likely reveal more to us in subsequent sessions.

Indeed, that is what happened. In the next two sessions that I observed directly, he continued this theme, although it took different forms, sometimes in the sand tray, sometimes with puppets, and sometimes with the animal groups. The animal groups engaged in battles with each other, and usually the "bully animals" prevailed. Kanani's skills grew rapidly as she reflected more of the characters' feelings, narrated the battles, and followed his play beautifully.

His play during his fifth filial play session took another turn. He pulled out one of my conga drums and sat on the floor and tapped it. He found another drum and asked his mother to join him. She followed his lead with the rhythms without being asked, but it appeared that that was precisely what he had intended. He gathered his animal groups once again and then whispered something to the "vulnerable" group. Kanani told me later he had said they needed better ways to protect themselves. He then moved back and forth between the animals and playing some rhythms on the drums. Once again, he asked Kanani to join him. At this point, he asked Kanani to keep playing the drums, and he gathered the animal group that had been bullied and moved around the playroom while he made dancing movements with them in his hands. During the next battle, the bullied animals scared off the bully animals by telling the drummer (Kanani) to drum very loud and fast. The bully animals ran away in fear.

For the first time, Kallik laughed aloud. Kanani commented, "Oooh, that felt good to see how those bullies were so afraid." As the play continued, she had other excellent empathic listening responses that were very accurate, such as, "Those animals don't have to be afraid anymore. They know they are strong! The bullies were full of hot air." Kanani had been very skilled throughout the session, and she immediately noted the themes when I asked her impressions. She saw that the threat theme had morphed into one of power and mastery over the bullies. She also commented on the drumming and how Kallik had once heard some well-known and impressive high school drummers in a program at the Alaska Native Heritage Center in Anchorage.

We decided to hold one more play session in my presence before she would transfer the play sessions to home. Before we headed into the sixth play session, Kanani asked to talk with me privately. She excitedly told me that Kallik seemed to be doing much better at school and had proudly walked away from one of the other students who had called him names in the past. He had begun talking more at home, seemed more relaxed, and smiled much more frequently. He had also asked his mother if they could get some drums so that he and his cousins could play with them together. There had been other reparative play themes besides the ones mentioned here, but after just five filial play sessions, he had made notable improvements at home. During the sixth session, Kallik involved his mother in nearly everything and used the human figures to create a family in front of the dollhouse. At the end of the session, he proudly showed his mother his skills with the Alaska Native–made yo-yo and then turned to me (in the corner of the room "doing my work" as usual) and showed me his skills. Both his mother and I reflected how proud he was of his ability to use them.

Home-Based Parent-Child Play Sessions

From this point on, Kanani held the play sessions at home with Kallik and reported to me or showed me portions of videos she had taken. We continued to discuss his play themes, her pleasure in seeing his confidence and interest in life return, and her enjoyment in holding the sessions. She was surprised that he had made progress so quickly, but I reminded her that it was because of her relationship with him that he could feel safe so quickly and because of her empathy that he could reveal and play through the issues that had been bothering him.

When Kanani and I met to discuss his home sessions, we also began work on her generalizing her skills to the rest of their daily lives. She excelled at the skills by now, so this was an easy process. We also began thinking about activities that they could do together to help Kallik learn about and identify with his cultural heritage. Kanani produced most of the ideas, and then we discussed the best ways of implementing them. She ordered books at his reading level about their indigenous group affiliation; she ordered some traditional clothing items from their home village, and Kallik asked his teacher if he could talk about life in the arctic among his people during a show-and-tell time with his class. His confidence continued to grow. When his classmates heard of his Alaska Native traditions and all he knew about survival as well as his Eskimo yo-yo skills, they were impressed. His mother also took him to the National Museum of the American Indian in Washington, DC (part of the Smithsonian Institution), and he told her he would need to come back many times. Kallik's sister also enjoyed these outings, and Kanani began holding special "fun times" with her individually as well.

No other interventions were necessary, and I discharged Kallik and his mother after their fifth home play session, the fifteenth session total. Kanani and Kallik continued to have play sessions at home, and Kallik made a much better adjustment to his new life, which was sustained when I did a 4-month follow-up call to Kanani.

Ethical and Cultural Considerations

When facilitating FT with indigenous families, the most crucial ethical and cultural consideration is to begin with cultural humility, which is the therapist valuing and being a learner of the client's culture and experience (Hook et al., 2016). Maintaining cultural humility and a working alliance results in fewer microaggressions toward indigenous people, particularly from nonnative and White people (DeBlaere et al., 2023). To increase my cultural humility and cultural responsiveness, prior to meeting Kanani I contacted a colleague and friend in Alaska who had the same tribal affiliation as Kanani and asked questions to refresh and extend my understanding. I also reviewed general information about mental health among Alaska Natives available at https://www.ncbi.nlm.nih.gov/books/NBK539588/ and https://store.samhsa.gov/sites/default/files/sma08-4354.pdf and reread two books I had been given when I attended a meeting in an arctic village with the same native affiliation as Kanani's several years before. Throughout my sessions with the family, I asked them to let me know if I said or did something that was not accurate or honoring of their culture. They were eager to share their culture, history, and stories with me, and the partnership grew as a result of this dialogue.

Conclusion

Filial Therapy was particularly useful with this family, in part because its values and practices were a good match with the traditional values and parenting/family practices of this family. Empowerment of parents as change agents for their own children coupled with empowerment of children through nondirective play worked well in this case as both mother and son found their way in their new home. Because FT honors and engages family members as *individuals* and as *partners*, parent and family input about their own unique backgrounds and cultural identity is incorporated easily into the process. One of the great strengths of FT is that parents already have a relationship with their children; and even though they might struggle, children and parents alike want to have a healthy, secure attachment with each other. The therapist provides some guidance and encouragement in learning the skills to create this, but the content of the sessions belongs to the family members themselves. The flexibility of FT conducted with a true partnership between therapist and family makes it possible to capitalize on indigenous values and traditions in unique ways that empower and serve families well.

Sample Case Notes

Kanani held her third play session with Kallik. She followed his lead beautifully throughout, empathically listening when he chose to play alone and engaging in child-centered imaginary play when he asked her to play a role. She told me she felt more confident with the skills and was excited to see how Kallik was expressing himself. She commented that storytelling was an important part of their culture and that letting Kallik lead the way allowed him to tell his own story. I responded that I thought that was a wonderful parallel that she had noticed.

During the play session, Kallik engaged in a hunting theme. He walked around the playroom looking for game and then shot a pop gun at an imaginary moose. He played rather intensely, and Kanani responded with lovely empathic responses such as, "You're on the hunt, looking for something. . . . Oh! You just spotted a moose! . . . Pow! You got him! That makes you very happy." Kallik nodded as she said this and then told her to be quiet, so she stopped saying anything as he wished. He then enacted tracking the moose, and Kanani reflected again about his stealth and care in finding the moose. After he had dragged the imaginary moose across the floor to the kitchen set, he announced, "*Now* we will have food for the winter." Kanani responded, "That was very hard work, but you are proud you got a moose to feed everyone."

Kanani and I discussed possible play themes from this, and for the first time she asked, "He saw his father and our whole village hunting. Do you think he is filling in for his father?" We discussed this as a possibility and decided it would be good to monitor the development of his play themes in the next session.

The play themes seem to relate to the goals of identity and relating to his culture, working through the loss of his father, and development of competence and confidence through traditional skills. For Kanani, this session showed her skill development to be at a high level as she followed this powerful play. She also expressed how touched she was that he was finally opening up and how his indigenous heritage was so important to him. She reported that they were talking and playing more in general at home, and the presenting problems were lessening as Kallik seemed to be more "himself."

The plan is to observe two to three more play sessions to see how the play and the relationship develop.

Resources

For Professionals

Alaska Native Tribal Health Consortium. https://www.anthc.org/what-we-do/behavioral-health/

Children of the First People: Fresh Voices of Alaska's Native Kids (Children of the Midnight Sun) by Tricia Brown (2019).

Filial Therapy: Strengthening Parent-Child Relationships through Play (3rd ed.) by Risë VanFleet (2014).

For Parents

A Parent's Handbook of Filial Therapy: Building Strong Families with Play (3rd ed.) by Risë VanFleet (2022).

Discussion Questions

1. What did you learn about working with indigenous people and Alaskan natives that you did not know?
2. Which parts of Kallik's play were particularly revealing or moving to you? What impressed you about Kanani's responses to Kallik?
3. How will you show cultural humility when working with indigenous people and Alaskan natives?

References

Bratton, S. C., Ray, D., Rhine, T., & Jones, L. (2005). The efficacy of play therapy with children: A meta-analytic review of treatment outcomes. *Professional Psychology: Research and Practice, 36*(4), 376–390.

Bronfenbrenner, U. (1979). *The ecology of human development.* Harvard University Press.

DeBlaere, C., Zelaya, D. G., Dean, J.-A. B., Chadwick, C. N., Davis, D. E., Hook, J. N., & Owen, J. (2023). Multiple microaggressions and therapy outcomes: The indirect effects of cultural humility and working alliance with Black, Indigenous, women of color clients. *Professional Psychology: Research and Practice, 54*(2), 115–124. https://doi.org/10.1037/pro0000497.supp (Supplemental)

Donovan, D. M., Thomas, L. R., Sigo, R. L. W., Price, L., Lonczak, H., Lawrence, N., Ahvakana, K., Austin, L., Lawrence, A., Price, J., Purser, A., & Bagley, L. (2015). Healing of the canoe: Preliminary results of a culturally tailored intervention to prevent substance abuse and promote tribal identity for native youth in two Pacific Northwest tribes. *American Indian and Alaska Native Mental Health Research, 22*(1), 42–76. https://doi.org/10.5820/aian.2201.2015.42 https://www.ncbi.nlm.nih.gov/pmc/articles/PMC4374439/

Glover, G. J. (1996). *Filial Therapy with Native Americans on the Flathead Reservation.* [Unpublished doctoral dissertation, University of North Texas, Denton, Texas.]

Glover, G. (2003). Filial therapy with Native American families. In R. VanFleet & L. Guerney, (Eds.), *Casebook of filial therapy* (pp. 417–428). Professional Resource Press.

Guerney, L. F., and Ryan, V. M. (2013). *Group filial therapy: A complete guide to teaching parents to play therapeutically with their children.* Jessica Kingsley.

Hook, J. N., Farrell, J. E., Davis, D. E., DeBlaere, C., Van Tongeren, D. R., & Utsey, S. O. (2016). Cultural humility and racial microaggressions in counseling. *Journal of Counseling Psychology, 63*(3), 269–277. https://doi.org/10.1037/cou0000114

Rosita, W. (2010, April 2). *Reconstructing sovereignty in Alaska.* Cultural Survival. www.culturalsurvival.org/publications/cultural-survival-quarterly/constructing-sovereignty-alaska

SAMHSA (2009). *American Indian and Alaska Native culture card: A guide to build cultural awareness.* https://store.samhsa.gov/sites/default/files/sma08-4354.pdf

Stringer, H. (2018). The healing power of heritage. *Monitor on Psychology, 49*(2). https://www.apa.org/monitor/2018/02/cover-healing-heritage

Topham, G. L., & VanFleet, R. (2011). Filial therapy: A structured and straightforward approach to including young children in family therapy. *Australian and New Zealand Journal of Family Therapy, 32*(2), 144–158.

Topham, G. L., Wampler, K. S., Titus, G., & Rolling, E. (2011). Predicting parent and child outcomes of a filial therapy program. *International Journal of Play Therapy, 20*(2), 79–93. https://doi.org/10.1037/a0023261

VanFleet, R. (1985). *Mothers' perceptions of their families' needs when one of their children has diabetes mellitus: A developmental perspective.* [Unpublished doctoral dissertation, Pennsylvania State University, University Park, Pennsylvania.]

VanFleet, R. (2014). *Filial therapy: Strengthening parent-child relationships through play* (3rd ed.). Professional Resource Press.

VanFleet, R. (2022). *A parent's handbook of filial therapy: Building strong families with play* (3rd ed.). Play Therapy Press.

VanFleet, R., & Guerney, L. (2003). *Casebook of filial therapy.* Play Therapy Press.

CHAPTER 10

Divorced Parents
Child-Parent Relationship Therapy with Parents of a White Child
Dalena Dillman Taylor and Caitlin Frawley

Elijah is a 7-year-old, White, cisgender boy who lives with his mother, Jessica. Elijah's father, Edward, lives nearby in a studio apartment with a new girlfriend. Elijah's parents, Jessica and Edward, divorced in July 2022 after a 10-year marriage. Jessica reported that she and Edward divorced last year because of intense conflict resulting from her occupation as an emergency room nurse during the COVID-19 pandemic. During the pandemic, Jessica was called to work long hours and often needed to isolate from extended family because of her frequent COVID exposures during this time. Edward, an auto mechanic, reported feeling lonely and isolated from the world because of Jessica's occupation as an emergency room nurse. The resulting tension and constant arguments precipitated their divorce. Jessica explained that she is seeking counseling for Elijah because of recent changes in his behaviors at home, including frequent outbursts, rule breaking, and hitting. Also, Elijah is having a difficult time adjusting to his new routine because of a shared custody agreement (split week between mother's and father's apartments). Elijah's father, Edward, also wants to be involved in Elijah's mental health treatment and is willing to meet with the counselor as needed.

For this case study, consider:

1. What are some common problems among children experiencing divorce and their reactions to new routines?
2. How did Elijah's caregivers' careers impact his experiences during the COVID-19 pandemic?
3. What is the rationale for using Child-Parent Relationship Therapy (CPRT) with Elijah's parents?
4. What are some unique ethical and legal issues that must be considered while working with Elijah and his caregivers?

Impact of Divorce on Children

Divorce is a serious concern for mental health professionals working with children and families. Of the 331.4 million individuals living in the United States, children under the age of 18 represent 25% or 73.1 million of these individuals (Ogunuole, Rabe, Roberts, & Caplan, 2021). In the past decade, the number of children living solely with their mother has doubled. Whereas 1% of children live with their father only, 12% of children under the age of 18 live with their mother only (Hemez & Washington, 2021).

The divorce of parents likely impacts children and their behaviors in negative ways, including children having more difficulty paying attention and feeling overwhelmed when compared to peers (Nusinovici et al., 2018). Children tend to be at higher risk for behavioral difficulties even up to one year prior to the divorce of their parents (Strohschein, 2005). These difficulties tend to include externalizing problems (Sillekens & Notten, 2020; Tullius, De Kroon, Almansa, & Reijneveld, 2022), such as disruptive conduct (Amato, 2001), aggressive and rule-breaking behavior (Lansford et al., 2006), and delinquency (Tullius et al., 2022). Children of divorce may also display increased internalizing problems such as anxiety and depression (Bannon, Barle, Mennella, & O'Leary, 2018) and emotional maladjustment (Harland et al., 2002). However, researchers have noted that children did not seem to display cognitive difficulties if the divorce/separation occurred within the first three years of life (Nusinovici et al., 2018). Yet, the implications of divorce can have long-term effects on children that persist into adulthood, such as risk of increased internalizing problems (D'Onofrio, Emery, Maes, Silberg, & Eaves, 2007), lower educational attainment, higher marital disagreements, and poorer parental relationships (Amato & Cheadle, 2005). Timing of the parental divorce can impact outcomes of the children: preteens and teenagers appeared to be at higher risks for antisocial behaviors (Strohschein, 2005) and academic problems (Lansford et al., 2006).

Child-Parent Relationship Therapy

The origins of Child-Parent Relationship Therapy (Landreth & Bratton, 2020) began in 1964 when Bernard and Louise Guerney introduced Filial Therapy, a child mental health intervention that involved training parents to conduct play therapy sessions with their children. Guerney (2000) described a key rationale for the development of filial therapy: children's mental health and behavioral problems are "not the product of pathology of the parent but rather lack of parenting knowledge and skill" (p. 2). That is, caregivers receive several messages about "correct parenting," and sometimes, these messages are not developmentally or relationally appropriate. However, caregivers can learn to become therapeutic change agents for their children through holding special playtimes (in an intentional and specific manner) and becoming more attuned, sensitive, and responsive to their children's inner worlds.

The caregiver-child relationship is the child's most important and cherished bond—therefore, experiencing unearned acceptance, understanding, and attention from a caregiver (rather than a therapist) can be far more therapeutic for a child (Bratton, Ray, Rhine, & Jones, 2005; Guerney, 2000). Therefore, Filial Therapy is constructed to help parents gain more confidence in their parenting skills, understand their children better, and build stronger parent-child relationships (Guerney, 2000). Filial Therapy builds upon the existing relationship between the parent and child to positively influence the child's adjustment to daily challenges and events (Landreth & Bratton, 2020; VanFleet, 2005). In this model, trained play therapists teach parents how to use Child-Centered Play Therapy skills during special playtimes with their children.

With this grounding in the Guerneys' Filial Therapy model, Landreth and Bratton (2020) created the 10-session, manualized model titled Child-Parent Relationship Therapy (CPRT). CPRT is designed as 10 two-hour group caregiver-training sessions that caregivers attend without their child(ren) and is intended for caregivers of children ages 3 to 10 years who may be experiencing emotional or behavioral problems (Landreth & Bratton, 2020). A trained play therapist facilitates the sessions by teaching the caregivers how to use Child-Centered Play Therapy (Landreth, 2012) skills and principles, integrating child development knowledge, and instructing caregivers on the skills to implement in their weekly 30-minute special playtimes with their children. In addition, group leaders provide caregivers supervision and feedback on their video recorded playtimes and encourage other parents to demonstrate support during the supervision process. With this CPRT group process and psychoeducational approach, caregivers learn therapeutic ways of responding to their children to improve the parent-child relationship (Landreth & Bratton, 2020).

Landreth and Bratton (2020) identified a number of studies demonstrating the effectiveness of CPRT with single parents (Bratton & Landreth, 1995), parents from diverse cultures (Ceballos, 2009; Glover & Landreth, 2000; Jang, 2000; Kidron, 2004; Lee & Landreth, 2003; Sheely, 2009; Villarreal, 2008; Yuen et al., 2002), non-offending parents of sexually abused children (Costas & Landreth, 1999), parents of children with chronic illness (Tew et al., 2002), incarcerated parents (Harris & Landreth, 1997; Landreth & Lobaugh, 1998), parents of children with learning difficulties (Kale & Landreth, 1999), parents of children who have witnessed domestic violence (Smith & Landreth, 2003), and divorced parents (Dillman Taylor et al., 2011). In view of these findings, CPRT appears to be an effective treatment modality that addresses the specific needs of families of divorce. In addition, Bratton et al.'s (2005) meta-analysis of 93 play therapy research studies revealed that play therapy by parents (i.e., filial therapy) had the largest effect size of 1.15, meaning it is more effective than play therapy by professionals and more effective than children not receiving treatment.

Case Study Application

With this greater understanding of the impacts of divorce, medical professionals' familial experiences during the pandemic, and CPRT treatment, we can now apply these to our mental health treatment with Elijah and his family. We selected CPRT for Elijah's treatment because: (a) divorce-related stress negatively impacted the parent-child relationship; (b) routine shifts decreased Elijah's feelings of connection and security; (c) Elijah is exhibiting new externalizing behavior problems, which started post-separation; and (d) Jessica and Edward are experiencing high levels of parenting stress, which have direct impacts on the quality of the parent-child relationship (Dillman Taylor, Purswell, Lindo, Jayne, & Fernando, 2011). We opted to use CPRT rather than individual CCPT with Elijah because filial therapy can result in improvements within not only the child, but also the caregiver and the overall parent-child relationship (Bratton et al., 2016). By using CPRT, we supported both Jessica and Edward in becoming therapeutic change agents for their son, Elijah. As co-facilitators, we worked with Jessica and Edward in a group format with other caregivers for 10 weeks. Because the caregiver-child relationship is the primary vehicle for therapeutic change in CPRT, we began treatment with one focus: *supporting Jessica and Edward in strengthening their relationship with Elijah*. Thus, we focused on Elijah and his caregivers' capacities, rather than on a problem within Elijah or his family system.

Initial Intake Session

We met with Jessica and Edward for an initial intake session to gain a better understanding of their present concerns with Elijah's behaviors and reactions to their divorce. We used the *Intake Questionnaire for Child-Parent Relationship Therapy* (Line & Ray, 2023) to guide the intake process. Following Line and Ray's (2023) recommendations, we started the CPRT intake process by providing them with an overview of CPRT and what they could expect during the treatment and group process. With the intention of building trust and providing Jessica and Edward with clear expectations for treatment, we discussed our theory of therapeutic change, as well as expectations related to attending weekly group sessions, facilitating 30-minute special playtimes, and recording sessions for supervision.

After the parents provided their informed consent for CPRT treatment, we transitioned into information gathering and screening protocols. Through following Line and Ray's (2023) intake questionnaire, we learned, in addition to the information provided at the beginning of this chapter, that both Jessica and Edward shared their dedication to working together to support Elijah's mental health and well-being. Regarding mental health history, Edward reported no history of mental health diagnoses, medications, or treatments. Jessica shared that she recently began individual therapy to process vicarious trauma and grief that she endured as an emergency room nurse within a COVID unit.

Based on the information collected during screening, we agreed that Jessica and Edward were appropriate candidates for CPRT treatment. Next, we gathered additional information about Elijah's history. Elijah witnessed his parents argue and often yell at each other during their marital distress period (roughly 1½ to 2 years). However, there was no reported history of intimate partner physical violence or domestic abuse in the household. In addition, the parents reported that there were no previous experiences of child abuse, neglect, maltreatment, or additional adverse childhood experiences. Prior to this time, Elijah had not received mental health diagnoses, therapy/treatments, or medication. Parents indicated that Elijah had significant levels of externalizing problems. During the past year, he started experiencing frequent emotional outbursts that were explosive during times of transition (e.g., routine transition, leaving one parent's house to go to the other parent's home). He had hit his mother during one of his outbursts. He has also started "testing boundaries" and pushing back on household rules through statements such as "mom lets me do that at her house," despite their reported consistent parenting practices and household rules. Jessica and Edward agreed that they sought counseling because they want to help Elijah stay safe, as well as experience relief from his high levels of distress.

Following the intake process, we determined that Jessica and Edward were appropriate candidates for group CPRT with other caregivers and that Elijah's presenting concerns (externalizing problems) and areas of distress (divorce, family transitions) were compatible with the goals and research-evidence outcomes associated with CPRT treatment. In the following sections, we describe Bratton, Landreth, Kellam, and Blackard's (2006) CPRT treatment manual process with Jessica, Edward, and other caregivers in their group.

Treatment Objectives

1. Jessica, Edward, and Elijah will experience stronger parent-child relationships through increased feelings of trust, empathy, and connection.
2. Jessica and Edward will learn to sensitively understand and accept Elijah's emotional world.
3. Jessica and Edward will use Child-Centered skills and principles during 30-minute special playtimes.
4. Elijah will experience growth in feelings of self-worth and self-esteem.
5. Elijah will experience increased adaptive coping and communication capacities and decreased emotional outbursts.

Session 1

During the initial CPRT group session, we aimed to establish a safe space for Jessica, Edward, and the other caregivers in the group so they could share their experiences in a comfortable and nonthreatening manner. In addition, we oriented them to the CPRT group and introduced the main objectives of treatment. We provided an overview of how children communicate their inner world and experiences through their natural language of play. During the session, Edward asked whether he would learn some concrete methods of disciplining his son when he is acting out and behaving inappropriately. He further emphasized his frustrations with the behaviors by stating, "I want to be a good dad, but I sometimes feel like giving up when Elijah gets into one of his rage episodes . . . I just wish I knew something to say or how to discipline him, so this stops before getting too out of control." We validated Edward's frustrations and feelings of being overwhelmed, and asked the group, "Has anyone else in the group experienced frustration with their child's behaviors this week?" Multiple group members shared experiences and discussed similar emotional reactions. During this session, we introduced caregivers to reflective responding skills and how reflective responding will allow the child to lead during special playtimes.

Session 2

For CPRT session 2, our objective was to help the caregivers prepare to facilitate their first special playtime with their children. We reviewed the "Be-With" Attitudes: I am here, I hear you, I understand, and I care (Landreth & Bratton, 2020), and how parents may use and operationalize these principles during their sessions. We discussed how parents will prepare for their special playtimes through (1) gathering toys and materials for play sessions, (2) establishing a consistent and predictable weekly time (e.g., Mondays at 3:30) for play sessions, (3) choosing an appropriate and private setting to conduct play sessions each week. Edward and Jessica discussed times that would work with their schedules on a consistent and predictable basis that would also align with their shared custody schedule. Jessica decided that she would facilitate special playtimes on Mondays at 4:30 p.m., and Edward chose Wednesdays at 6 p.m. Jessica and Edward also discussed shopping for toys together to maintain some consistency in materials, because Elijah often feels frustrated when he is missing toys from the other house.

Session 3

In session 3, we continued our work from the previous session with the objective of preparing Edward, Jessica, and the other group members for their initial home play session with their child this week. We covered the importance of structuring the sessions and environment, allowing the child to take the lead during special playtime, and provided a brief introduction to limit setting with concrete examples. We asked the caregivers to share their feelings and expectations related to conducting their initial home play sessions, and Jessica and Edward shared similar feelings of excitement and worry with other parents in the group. We asked two caregivers to record their sessions the following week based on their previous role plays (i.e., chose two parents who showed greatest potential for success and openness to receiving feedback).

Session 4

During session 4, we focused on checking in with group members about their experiences conducting the initial special playtimes with their children. We ensured that we had enough time to discuss their experiences, review previous skills, and review recordings for the first time. As parents shared their experiences during the initial home play sessions, we encouraged their efforts, validated and normalized reactions, and reflected their feelings. Edward shared that he really enjoyed his playtime with Elijah but asked a few questions by accident. We normalized his use of questions during this initial session by emphasizing the fact that they are learning a new language and way of being with their child. Edward shared that Elijah invited him to play with musical instruments together, and how he felt very connected with Elijah during this play. Jessica shared that she felt some jealousy as Edward discussed his playtime and disappointment that Elijah did not invite her to join in his play. Another caregiver in the group, Tom, let out a sigh of relief, and shared, "I'm glad I'm not the only one . . . when Kate (Tom's wife) played with Jacob, they were doing all kinds of fun things together, and it made me think—she should just do two sessions per week instead of me doing one." Jessica thanked Tom for sharing his experience, and we encouraged Jessica's and Tom's vulnerability in group while pointing out what they did well (e.g.,

TABLE 10.1 JESSICA AND EDWARD: SESSION 4

Transcript	Analysis
J: "Well, I do feel a little embarrassed to show this video. I'm used to getting everything right at work, and I know I didn't here."	Many caregivers experience an incongruence between their ideal self as a "perfect parent" and their experience as a beginner in the new CPRT skill set.
T: "How many other of you may feel the same thing? Yes, this is a common feeling. Let me reassure you that we all want to be supportive and encouraging to you."	As the CPRT group leaders, we provided normalization through group member validation as well as reassurance for all.
E: "Wow. A new bowling set."	Elijah is excited about the new toys.
J: "Yup. It is new."	Jessica was engaged but missed an opportunity to reflect feelings.
T: "Let's pause the video here and start with positive feedback for Jessica. Someone state what she did well." . . . [Tom said, "Your toes followed your nose, and you were engaged with him."] "Yes, I noticed that, too. Jessica your nonverbals really showed your interest. Now, let's think about how you would reflect a feeling here."	We start with positives and encouragement. Then we give a prompt by naming the skill that needed to be demonstrated.
J: "I could have said, 'You are excited about the new bowling set.'"	Jessica self-corrects, indicating her understanding of the skill.
T: "Yes, you got it! Now, I'll rewind the tape, pause it right after he says that, and ask you to say your new response as if you were in the session with him now."	Inviting the parent to say it gives her the opportunity to practice the skill. It also gives the CPRT leader an opportunity for further guidance on matching the child's affect.

allowing the child to take the lead, not inserting themselves into their child's play, using reflective responses). When it came time for selecting a participant for video recording this week, Jessica volunteered because she desired the group's feedback and support.

Session 5

We facilitated session 5 with similar objectives as the previous session by providing support and encouragement as parents continue conducting play sessions. Jessica shared her video recording of her week's play session with Elijah, and we worked to point out what Jessica was doing well during her session, such as her use of reflections of feeling. After pausing the recording, we asked Jessica what she felt most proud of during this session. Jessica shared that she was happy to see her use of reflections and reductions in questions. Also, Jessica shared that she felt more connected and sensitive to Elijah's experiences during this session. She shared that she felt happy when Elijah invited her to play with the musical instruments; however, she also discussed her acceptance of Elijah when he decided he wanted to move on and play more independently.

After reviewing tapes, we reviewed limit-setting procedures to be used during play sessions. We demonstrated limit setting for the parents (along with other skills) and invited the group members to practice limit setting and reflecting together in role-plays. Edward expressed that he was unsure that this method would work with Elijah, especially if he gets upset or distressed during the session. We validated his worries and asked if other group members shared similar concerns about scenarios that are specific to their child. Jessica encouraged Edward to "give it a try" and disclosed that she is similarly nervous about trying out this new way of limit setting.

Session 6

We began session 6 by inviting informal sharing among the caregivers and discussing their experiences during this week's play sessions with their children. Edward shared that he needed to use limit setting during this week's session because Elijah desired to continue his special playtime. Edward shared that he used the A-C-T (i.e., Acknowledge the feeling, Communicate the limit, and Target an alternative) limit-setting approach but stumbled at first because he was avoiding toys being thrown. However, Edward continued setting the limit, and eventually, Elijah was able to transition from the play session. Edward expressed that he was surprised that it worked, but he wanted to "give it his best shot and stick with it" based on Jessica's words of encouragement during last week's session. After reviewing group members' session recordings, we transitioned to discussing age-appropriate choice-giving practices that provide children with opportunities to make positive decisions. The parents practiced choice giving in role-play exercises, and Edward volunteered to share his recording during next week's session.

Session 7

Session 7 began similarly to the previous week, with caregivers sharing their experiences with parenting and facilitating play sessions during the week. When it came time for the supervision component, Edward shared his recording from his special playtime with Elijah. We noted his use of appropriate limit setting, as well as his use of reflective responses and overall connection with Elijah throughout the session. Edward shared, "setting the limit felt easier this time. . . . The small success last week gave me the confidence to continue setting limits and worry less about Elijah doing the wrong thing or not listening. . . . I trust myself more, and I trust Elijah, too."

After discussing others' sessions and providing video feedback, we transitioned into a discussion about self-esteem building responses that parents can use during their play sessions. As we did with the other skills, we demonstrated self-esteem building for the parents to observe. Next, we invited parents to get into role-play pairs and practice self-esteem building responses with each other.

TABLE 10.2. JESSICA AND EDWARD: SESSION 7

Transcript	Analysis
Ed: "In the first part of my video, I messed up the limit setting."	Edward demonstrated understanding of A-C-T and acceptance of his own mistake. This realization can promote empathy for his son.
T: "You already know how you want to improve. You are also accepting of your mistakes, which is encouraging because it helps you increase empathy of Elijah's mistakes throughout the week." [Turns on video]	CPRT leader encourages him and increases his awareness of his own change with potential for change in his relationship with his son by showing empathy when his son makes mistakes.
El: "Watch out, Dad. I'm going to shoot you right between the eyes."	Although he says it in a playful way, he still challenges dad to set a limit. Elijah's play themes of aggression and power illustrate his attempt to gain self-control of his own power.
Ed: "Don't shoot me. You can choose to shoot the bop bag." [Ed responds to watching this part and says], "See, I forgot the A and messed up the C."	Self-awareness and self-correction reveal his learning of the A-C-T skill.
T: "You're teaching yourself just like Elijah will eventually teach himself. I'll back up the tape and pause it so you can say it how you wanted."	Makes a connection between dad's own learning process and his son's learning process to extend empathy.
Ed: "Elijah, I know you are being playful and want to shoot me, but I am not for shooting. You can *choose* to pretend the bop bag is me and shoot that."	Accurately says A-C-T with confidence and pride, revealing his internal locus of evaluation and control.
J: "Way to go, Edward. I'm impressed."	Jessica's trust in Edward as a parent is being restored as she witnesses his skills.

Session 8

For session 8, we continued providing space to discuss parenting experiences and weekly play session experiences, as well as review videos. In terms of new group material, we introduced encouraging skills and differentiated encouragement and praise. We provided an overview of encouragement and how parents can promote their children's self-esteem and self-direction/motivation through encouraging rather than praising. Jessica and Edward both shared their tendency to praise Elijah, and other caregivers discussed similar natural tendencies.

Session 9

During session 9, Edward and Jessica both shared that they noticed significantly fewer outbursts during the day with Elijah. In addition, they agreed that choice giving has been a "game changer," and they notice that Elijah is feeling more empowered to make positive choices with both parents. During this session, we discussed and encouraged the use of A-C-T limit-setting practices outside of the play sessions. Edward and Jessica agreed that this would be helpful for getting on "the same page" and giving Elijah some extra consistency and predictability during this time of change and transition. We further emphasized the power of limit setting and how this approach to setting limits can promote safety within the parent-child relationship.

Session 10

For our final CPRT session, we invited the group members to think about their own personal experiences, growth, and challenges during the previous 9 weeks. Jessica and Edward shared that they feel more connected to Elijah, and that they feel more connected in their co-parenting capacities after learning these new ways of relating with Elijah. We shared our observations of parents' growth in acceptance, empathy, and trust in their children during this treatment process. We encouraged parents to continue their weekly play sessions even after the group ended to maintain gains and their positive connection with their child.

Ethical and Cultural Considerations

Throughout the treatment process, there are several ethical obligations that we needed to consider for Elijah, as well as Jennifer and Edward. First, we made sure to take appropriate time to explain the CPRT treatment process with Jennifer and Edward during our initial intake interview so they could make an informed decision about whether to participate. In addition to reviewing the information on the informed-consent document, we made sure to include information related to (a) what they may expect during CPRT group sessions, (b) time commitment, and (c) monetary costs.

As professional counselors, we followed the American Counseling Association (2014) *Code of Ethics*. Because play therapists represent professionals across mental health professions, we encourage counselors using CPRT to consult their relevant ethics codes, such as the American Psychological Association (APA, 2017) *Ethical Principles of Psychologists and Code of Conduct*, National Association for Social Workers (NASW, 2021) *Code of Ethics*, and the American Association for Marriage and Family Therapy (AAMFT, 2015) *Code of Ethics*. Moreover, all play therapists should consult with the *Play Therapy Best Practices: Clinical, Professional, and Ethical Issues* document available on the APT website (APT, 2022). During screening procedures, clinicians are ethically obligated to consider whether the client(s) goals are compatible with the goals and outcomes associated with treatment groups (ACA, 2014, A.9.a.).

During the intake session, we spent time gathering information to make sure that Elijah's presenting concerns (e.g., attachment-related, externalizing problems, high caregiver stress levels) aligned with CPRT goals (e.g., strengthen attachment bonds) and research-evidence outcomes (e.g., decreased externalizing problems, decreased caregiver stress). We also discussed the limits to confidentiality associated with counseling/therapeutic groupwork, as well as the need to record a session with their child and share during a group session. There are also ethical considerations related to divorce. For example, during our initial intake, we made sure to gather information about Edward and Jessica's legal rights and responsibilities and gathered documentation to ensure guardianship rights related to treatment disclosures and consent (APT, 2022).

In our work with Elijah and his caregivers, we continually reflected on how CPRT treatment would be appropriate for them within cultural contexts, as all treatments are culture bound. Researchers have demonstrated that CPRT is culturally adaptable and effective with racially and ethnically diverse caregivers, including African American families (Sheely-Moore & Bratton, 2010), Chinese American caregivers (Yuen et al., 2002), Native American caregivers (Glover & Landreth, 2000), and Latino/a/x families (Ceballos & Bratton, 2010). The CPRT protocol is flexible, and facilitators can adapt the protocol to ensure that they are delivering culturally responsive treatment. Given Jennifer and Edward's cultural identities as White, middle-class caregivers, we did not identify clear cultural adaptations that needed to be incorporated in treatment. However, familial factors played a large role in how we responded and interacted with these caregivers (e.g., encouraging open dialogue surrounding Elijah's behaviors at each home).

In addition, Jennifer and Edward identified as Christians during the initial intake session. Scholars have noted congruence between Child-Centered principles and Christian bible-based caregiving practices, such as disciplining with love and kindness, modeling acceptance, and promoting children's capacities to make healthy choices (Bornsheuer-Boswell, Garza, & Watts, 2013). To practice cultural humility, we did not make assumptions about the cultural fit of CPRT based on our interview during the intake session. Instead, we sought to gain deeper understandings and appreciations for Jennifer and Edward's cultural identities throughout the therapeutic treatment process.

Conclusion

Divorce can be a challenge because of the many changes that occur within a short period. Divorce coupled with the impact of the COVID-19 pandemic created even more challenges for Elijah, Jennifer, and Edward. Although CPRT is an evidence-based intervention that would be a good fit, Jennifer and Edward still needed an open mind and willingness to engage in the process together. This commitment may not always be apparent or possible for divorced couples. We would encourage counselors to consider a parent's potential for engagement in the process with the other parent in the same group. Could divorced parents you work with, over time, become more open to the CPRT process, or would individual parenting work need to take place first?

In just over 10 weeks, Jennifer and Edward made significant strides toward their goals for their relationship with Elijah and toward co-parenting. Although at times, commitment to the 10 weeks was a struggle, they persevered and found meaning in their special playtimes with Elijah. Both reported a strengthening in the parent-child relationship as well as gaining tools to work together to help Elijah during this transition. Parenting after divorce is not easy; and yet, when parents put in time and effort in a CPRT group, parenting can be very rewarding. These parents made the best of their situation, and Elijah benefited from their efforts.

Sample Case Note

TEXTBOX 10.1. CPRT PROGRESS NOTES: SESSION 1

Parent Name: <u>Edward</u> Case #: _____
Location: <u>PLAY Lab</u> Date: <u>4/6/2022</u>

Mood: ___ Euthymic   ___ Depressed   ___ Angry   ___ Anxious   ___ Fearful
___ Agitated   ___ Apathetic   ___ Elevated   ___ Calm   ___ Cheerful
_x_ Other: <u>Nervous; overwhelmed</u>

Behavior: _x_ Cooperative   ___ Uncooperative   ___ Detached   ___ Agitated
___ Anxious   ___ Relaxed   ___ Hostile   _x_ Open   ___ Hyperactive
___ Defensive   ___ Compulsive   ___ Other: _____

Participation:
Level: _x_ Responsive: (___ Highly   ___ Minimally)   ___ Resistant   ___ Variable
Quality: ___ Unexpected   _x_ Supportive   _x_ Sharing
_x_ Attentive   ___ Intrusive ___   Monopolizing

Topics/Issues Discussed:
Introductions
Overview of CPRT training
Filial training objectives and essential concepts
Reflective responding

Goals of Session:
_x_ Assessment   _x_ Psychoeducation
_x_ Decrease symptoms of emotional outbursts
_x_ Insight/Understanding   _x_ Improve problem solving skills
_x_ Develop coping/social skills   _x_ Improve communication
_x_ Behavior management   _x_ Treatment compliance
Other: _____

Primary Intervention(s) Used: CPRT

Homework/Recommendations:
Notice some physical characteristic about your child you haven't seen before.
Practice reflective responding (complete Feeling Response: Homework Worksheet
   and bring next week).
Practice giving a 30-second burst of attention.

Other Notes: (continue on additional page below if needed)
Edward appeared open and vulnerable to the process as evidenced by tearing up and sharing
moments of doubt in his parenting abilities. He also appeared excited and enthusiastic about the
curriculum as evidenced by his statement that this is just what he needed and it fits with what he
was hoping for.

Resources

For Professionals

American Association for Marriage and Family Therapy. (2015). *Code of Ethics.* https://www.aamft.org/Legal_Ethics/Code_of_Ethics.aspx

American Counseling Association. (2014). *2014 ACA code of ethics.* https://www.counseling.org/docs/default-source/default-document-library/2014-code-of-ethics-finaladdress.pdf

American Psychological Association. (2017). *Ethical Principles of Psychologists and Code of Conduct.* https://www.apa.org/ethics/code/ethics-code-2017.pdf

Association for Play Therapy. (2022). *Play Therapy Best Practices: Clinical, Professional & Ethical Issues.* https://cdn.ymaws.com/www.a4pt.org/resource/resmgr/publications/best_practices.pdf Bratton, S. C., & Landreth, G. L. (2020). *Child-parent relationship therapy (CPRT) treatment manual: An evidence-based 10-session filial therapy model* (2nd ed.). Routledge.

Child-Centered Play Therapy training at https://cpt.unt.edu/ccpt-certification-trainings

Child-Parent Relationship Therapy training at https://cpt.unt.edu/child-parent-relationship-therapy-certification

Landreth, G. L., & Bratton, S. C. (2020). *Child-parent relationship therapy (CPRT): An evidence-based 10-session filial model* (2nd ed.). Routledge.

National Association of Social Workers. (2021). *Code of Ethics.* https://www.socialworkers.org/About/Ethics/Code-of-Ethics

Research Evidence available at http://evidencebasedchildtherapy.com/research/ and https://cpt.unt.edu/researchpublications/meta-analyses

For Parents

Siegel, D. J., & Hartzell, M. (2013). *Parenting from the inside out: How a deeper self-understanding can help you raise children who thrive.* Tarcher Perigee.

Siegel, D., & Payne Bryson, T. (2012). *The whole-brain child: 12 revolutionary strategies to nurture your child's developing mind.* Bantam Books Trade Paperbacks.

Videos through the University of North Texas Center for Play Therapy at https://cpt.unt.edu/cprt-therapistparent-resources

Discussion Questions

1. Prior to beginning CPRT, parents need openness, commitment, and goals that align with the CPRT program. What other considerations would be important to ponder prior to parents/caregivers starting CPRT?
2. Based on the research presented regarding divorce and the potential long-term impact on children, what potential modifications may be needed to CPRT for parents/caregivers who are not as likely to be on the same page as Jennifer and Edward?

3. In CPRT, the curricula do not address problematic behaviors/challenges until session 9, given that the focus is on strengthening the parent-child relationship. In what circumstances would it be necessary to pause the curricula and address behaviors? Or would waiting until session 9 be okay for all behaviors?

References

Amato, P. R. (2001). Children of divorce in the 1990s: An update of the Amato and Keith (1991) meta-analysis. *Journal of Family Psychology, 15*(3), 355–370. doi: 10.1037/0893-3200.15.3.355

Amato, P. R., & Cheadle, J. (2005). The long reach of divorce: Divorce and child well-being across three generations. *Journal of Marriage and Family, 67,* 191–206. doi: 10.1111/j.0022-2445.2005.00014.x

Bannon, S. M., Barle, N., Mennella, M. S., & O'Leary, K. D. (2018). Parental conflict and college student functioning: Impact of child involvement in conflict. *Journal of Divorce & Remarriage, 59*(3), 157–174. https://doi.org/10.10 80/10502556.2017.1402654

Bornsheuer-Boswell, J. N., Garza, Y., & Watts, R. E. (2013). Conservative Christian parents' perceptions of child–parent relationship therapy. *International Journal of Play Therapy, 22*(3), 143.

Bratton, S. C., & Landreth, G. L. (1995). Filial therapy with single parents: Effects on parental acceptance, empathy, and stress. *International Journal of Play Therapy, 4*(1), 61–80. doi: 10.1037/h0089142

Bratton, S. C., Landreth, G. L., Kellam, T., & Blackard, S. R. (2006). *Child-parent relationship therapy (CPRT) treatment manual: A 10-session filial therapy model for training parents.* Routledge/Taylor & Francis Group.

Bratton, S., Ray, D., Rhine, T., & Jones, L. (2005). The efficacy of play therapy with children: A meta-analytic review of the outcome research. *Professional Psychology: Research and Practice, 36*(4), 376–390.

Ceballos, P. (2009). School-based child parent relationship therapy (CPRT) with low income first generation immigrant Hispanic parents: Effects on child behavior and parent-child relationship stress. [Doctoral dissertation, University of North Texas, 2008.] *Dissertation Abstracts International, 69*(08), A.

Ceballos, P. L., & Bratton, S. C. (2010). Empowering Latino families: Effects of a culturally responsive intervention for low-income immigrant Latino parents on children's behaviors and parental stress. *Psychology in the Schools, 47*(8), 761–775. https://doi.org/10.1002/pits.20502

Costas, M., & Landreth, G. (1999). Filial therapy with nonoffending parents of children who have been sexually abused. *International Journal of Play Therapy, 8*(1), 43–66. doi: 10.1037/h0089427

Dillman Taylor, D., Purswell, K., Lindo, N., Jayne, K., & Fernando, D. (2011). The impact of child parent relationship therapy on child behavior and parent-child relationships: An examination of parental divorce. *International Journal of Play Therapy, 20*(3), 124–137. doi: 10.1037/a0024469

D'Onofrio, E. T., Emery, R. E., Maes, H. H., Silberg, J., & Eaves, L. J. (2007). A children of twins study of parental divorce and offspring psychopathology. *Journal of Child Psychology and Psychiatry, 48*(7), 667–675.

Glover, G., & Landreth, G. (2000). Filial therapy with Native Americans on the Flathead Reservation. *International Journal of Play Therapy, 9*(2), 57–80. doi: 10.1037/h0089436

Guerney, B., Jr. (1964). Filial therapy: Description and rationale. *Journal of Consulting Psychology, 28*(4), 304–310. doi: 10.1037/h0041340

Guerney, L. (2000). Filial therapy into the 21st century. *International Journal of Play Therapy, 9*(2), 1–17. doi: 10.1037/h0089433

Harland, P., Reijeveld, S. A., Brugman, E., Verloove-Vanhorick, S. P., & Verhulst, F. C. (2002). Family factors and life events as risk factors for behavioural and emotional problems in children. *European Child & Adolescent Psychiatry, 11*, 176–184.

Harris, Z. L., & Landreth, G. L., (1997). Filial therapy with incarcerated mothers: A five week model. *International Journal of Play Therapy, 6*(2), 53–73. doi: 10.1037/h0089408

Hemez, P., & Washington, C. (2021). Percentage and number of children living with two parents has dropped since 1968. *US Census Bureau.*

Jang, M. (2000). Effectiveness of filial therapy for Korean parents. *International Journal of Play Therapy, 9*(2), 39–56. doi: 10.1177/0011000005283558

Kale, A. L., & Landreth, G. (1999). Filial therapy with parents of children experiencing learning difficulties. *International Journal of Play Therapy, 8*(2), 35–56. doi: 10.1037/h0089430

Kidron, M. (2004). Filial therapy with Israeli parents. [Doctoral dissertation, University of North Texas, 2003.] *Dissertation Abstracts International, A, 64*(12), 4372.

Landreth, G. L. (2012). *Play therapy: The art of the relationship.* Routledge.

Landreth, G. L., & Bratton, S. C. (2020). *Child-parent relationship therapy (CPRT): An evidence-based 10-session filial model* (2nd ed.). Routledge.

Landreth, G., & Lobaugh, A. (1998). Filial therapy with incarcerated fathers: Effects on parental acceptance of child, parental stress, and child adjustment. *Journal of Counseling & Development, 76*, 157–165.

Lansford, J. E., Malone, P. S., Castellino, D. R., Dodge, K. A., Pettit, G. S., & Bates, J. E. (2006). Trajectories of internalizing, externalizing, and grades for children who have and have not experienced their parents' divorce or separation. *Journal of Family Psychology, 20*(2), 292–301. doi: 10.1037/0893-3200.20.2.292

Lee, M., & Landreth, G. (2003). Filial therapy with immigrant Korean parents in the United States. *International Journal of Play Therapy, 12*(2), 67–85. doi: 10.1037/h0088879

Line, A. V., & Ray, D. C. (2023). Intake procedures for child–parent relationship therapy: Moving toward an evidence-based process. *International Journal of Play Therapy, 32*(2), 79–94. https://doi.org/10.1037/pla0000196

Nusinovici, S., Olliac, B., Flamant, C., Müller, J.-B., Olivier, M., Rouger, V., Gascoin, G., Basset, H., Bouvard, C., Rozé, J.-C., & Hanf, M. (2018). Impact of parental separation or divorce on school performance in preterm children: A population-based study. *PLoS ONE, 13*(9), e0202080. doi: 10.1371/journal.pone.0202080

Ogunwole, S. U., Rabe, M. A., Roberts, A. W., & Caplan, Z. (2021). Population under age 18 declined last decade. *US Census Bureau.*

Sheely, A. (2009). School based child parent relationship therapy (CPRT) with low income Black American parents: Effects on children's behaviors and parent-child relationship stress, a pilot study. [Doctoral dissertation, University of North Texas, 2008.] *Dissertation Abstracts International, 69*(08), A.

Sheely-Moore, A. I., & Bratton, S. C. (2010). A strengths-based parenting intervention with low-income African American families. *Professional School Counseling, 13*(3), 175–183. https://doi.org/10.5330/PSC.n.2010-13.175

Sillekens, S., & Notten, N. (2020). Parental divorce and externalizing problem behavior in adulthood: A study on lasting individual, family and peer risk factors for externalizing problem behavior when experiencing a parental divorce. *Deviant Behavior, 41*(1), 1–16. doi: 10.1080/01639625.2018.1519131

Smith, N., & Landreth, G. (2003). Intensive filial therapy with child witnesses of domestic violence: A comparison with individual and sibling group play therapy. *International Journal of Play Therapy, 12*(1), 67–88. doi: 10.1037/h0088872

Strohschein, L. (2005). Parental divorce and child mental health trajectories. *Journal of Marriage and Family, 67*, 1286–1300. doi: 10.1111/j.1741-3737.2005.00217.x

Tew, K., Landreth, G., Joiner, K. D., & Solt, M. D. (2002). Filial therapy with parents of chronically ill children. *International Journal of Play Therapy, 11*(1), 79–100. doi: 10.1037/h0088858

Tullius, J. M., De Kroon, M. L. A., Almansa, J., & Reijneveld, S. A. (2022). Adolescents' mental health problems increase after parental divorce, not before, and persist until adulthood: A longitudinal TRAILS study. *European Child & Adolescent Psychiatry, 31*(6), 969–978. doi: 10.1007/s00787-020-01715-0

VanFleet, R. (2005). *Filial therapy: Strengthening the parent-child relationship* (2nd ed.). Family Enhancement and Play Therapy Center.

Villarreal, C. E. (2008). School-based child parent relationship therapy (CPRT) with Hispanic parents. [Doctoral dissertation, Regent University, 2008.] *Dissertation Abstracts International, 69*(2), A.

Yuen, T., Landreth, G., & Baggerly, J. (2002). Filial therapy with immigrant Chinese families. *International Journal of Play Therapy, 11*(2), 63–90. doi: 10.1037/h0088865

PART II

Adolescents

CHAPTER 11

Depression
Cognitive Behavior Therapy and Expressive Arts Therapy with a Chinese American Adolescent

Yu-Fen Lin and Chi-Sing Li

Jade is a 16-year-old Chinese American cisgender female whose family moved to Texas from Wuhan, China, 20 years ago. Jade was born in 2006 and was raised in Houston, Texas. In March 2020, Jade was finishing middle school and looking forward to starting high school. However, at that time, the COVID-19 pandemic resulted in school closures in the United States. Jade's high school announced that all classes would be held online. As a result, Jade did not step onto her high school campus for an entire year and did not meet her teachers or classmates. She did not get the chance to make new friends from school. Jade's parents started to feel worried and concerned about some of Jade's behaviors. For example, Jade isolated herself in her room, slept all the time, lost her appetite, was not motivated to attend her online classes, and "hated" most of her teachers. At one point, she even called the suicide hotline of her high school at 3 a.m. The following day, her parents received a call from the school counselor about her suicidal ideation. Out of desperation, Jade's parents found a professional counselor to help their daughter. The counseling sessions were set up as virtual sessions, given that it was during the COVID-19 pandemic. The counselor used the client-centered approach, which helped to establish a working relationship with Jade and reduce Jade's initial stress. The counselor later had more success with Jade and helped her overcome her depression through Cognitive Behavioral Therapy (CBT) (Beck & Weishaar, 2018) and expressive arts therapy (Malchiodi, 2005).

For this case study, consider the following:

1. How did the pandemic crisis impact Jade's mental health? Which characteristics of Major Depressive Disorder did Jade experience?
2. Which aspects of CBT and Expressive Arts Therapy were helpful to Jade?
3. How did Jade's cultural background, particularly the collectivist value and Asian family values, impact the treatment approach?

Depression in Adolescents

Adolescence is a significant period of change for many young people and was termed "a period of storm and stress" by G. Stanley Hall due to frequent conflict with parents, mood disruptions, and risk-taking behavior (Stirrups, 2018). Typically, adolescents experience various emotions, including sadness, anxiety, and stress. However, when these feelings persist and interfere with daily life, they may be a sign of depression if symptoms occur for at least two weeks. Depression can significantly impact an adolescent's thoughts, emotions, and behavior and may manifest in a variety of ways. Common symptoms include persistent feelings of sadness or hopelessness, loss of interest in activities they used to enjoy, changes in appetite or weight, difficulty sleeping or sleeping too much, fatigue or loss of energy, difficulty concentrating or making decisions, feelings of worthlessness or guilt, or thoughts of self-harm or suicide (American Academy of Child and Adolescent Psychiatry, 2017). If five of these symptoms occur over the same 2-week period, a diagnosis of Major Depressive Disorder may be met (American Psychiatric Association, 2013).

Adolescents with depression may also experience physical symptoms such as headaches, stomachaches, or other aches and pains (American Academy of Child and Adolescent Psychiatry, 2017). Depression in adolescents can have severe consequences if left untreated. It can impact their academic performance, relationships with peers and family members, and overall quality of life. In some cases, depression can lead to behaviors of self-harm or suicide attempts.

Recent research suggested that Generation Z (Gen Z, born between 1997 and 2013) may be more inclined to depression than Generation X and Y (Parker & Igielnik, 2020). This may be attributed to this generation's heightened stressors and demands, such as academic and career-related pressures, economic instability, social isolation, and the political climate. Moreover, Gen Z is the first generation to grow up surrounded by digital communication. They spend less time in direct face-to-face contact with others, which is one reason why they had the highest-ever generational reports of depression even prior to COVID-19 (Djafarova & Bowes, 2021; Harari, Sela, & Bareket-Bojmel, 2022; Saw, Aggie, & Jeung, 2021). The growing influence of social media platforms could also be a factor in the elevated incidences of depression among Gen Z. Studies have linked social media use to an increased risk of cyberbullying, social isolation, and negative self-comparisons, which can exacerbate depressive symptoms (APA, 2021; Tandoc, Ferrucci, & Duffy, 2015). Recently, the US Surgeon General (2023) warned about the negative impact of social media on adolescents' mental health as follows:

- Social media may perpetuate body dissatisfaction, disordered eating behaviors, social comparison, and low self-esteem, especially among adolescent girls.
- When asked about the impact of social media on their body image: 46% of adolescents ages 13–17 said social media makes them feel worse.

- Roughly two-thirds (64%) of adolescents are "often" or "sometimes" exposed to hate-based content.
- Some social media platforms show suicide- and self-harm-related content including even live depictions of self-harm acts, content which, in certain tragic cases, has been linked to childhood deaths.

COVID-19 and Adolescent Mental Health

The COVID-19 pandemic has significantly impacted the mental health of individuals globally, particularly Asian adolescents. Various studies have revealed an upsurge in depression and anxiety among this demographic due to the pandemic (Duan et al., 2020; Zhang et al., 2021). One factor that has led to an increase in depression among Asian American adolescents is the rise of Asian hate crimes, as Asians were blamed for the pandemic (Ramakrishnan, Wong, Lee, Sadhwani, & Shao, 2021; Asian American Psychological Association, 2021). In addition, the disruption of daily routines and social isolation added to adolescents' stress. Many had to adapt to online learning and had limited opportunities to interact with peers and engage in extracurricular activities. Further, the pandemic brought economic challenges for families, increasing stress levels and potentially exacerbating preexisting mental health conditions (Wu et al., 2021).

Asian Culture and Mental Health Stigma

The stigma surrounding mental health in some Asian cultures may also contribute to depression among adolescents. In such cultures, seeking mental health support can be perceived as a sign of weakness or a failure to uphold familial and societal expectations (Yee, 2021). Therefore, it is crucial to address the mental health concerns of Asian adolescents during their times of stress. Parents and caregivers can provide emotional support and help their children maintain structure and routine. Schools can also provide mental health resources, including virtual counseling and support groups. In addition, increasing awareness and reducing the stigma surrounding mental health in Asian communities is essential. Promoting open and honest conversations about mental health can help reduce barriers to seeking treatment and support (Saw et al., 2021).

Cognitive Behavior Therapy and Expressive Arts Therapy

Although various treatment options are available, Cognitive-Behavioral Therapy (CBT) (Beck & Weishaar, 2018) and Expressive Arts Therapy (Malchiodi, 2005) have been found to be effective in treating depression in adolescents (National Institute of Mental Health, 2017). CBT aims to help adolescents identify negative thought patterns and behaviors that contribute to depression and then guide teens to replace the negative thoughts with more positive, realistic ones

(Tompkins, 2018). On the other hand, Expressive Arts Therapy uses creative processes such as art, music, dance, and drama to help individuals explore and express their emotions in a nonverbal and creative way. This can provide an outlet for emotions that may be difficult to express in words. It can also help adolescents develop a sense of self-awareness and self-expression (Mealer, Cutcliffe, & Gish, 2017).

When used together, CBT and Expressive Arts Therapy can provide a holistic approach to treating depression in adolescents (Mavroveli & Papacharalambous, 2018). Expressive arts therapy can help adolescents become more aware of their emotions and their physical sensations. This increased awareness can complement the cognitive strategies learned in CBT and help them develop greater self-awareness and emotional regulation skills. Empirical evidence has demonstrated the efficacy of Expressive Arts Therapy in reducing depressive symptoms and improving overall mental health in this population. For instance, Timulak and Connelly (2012) reported that Expressive Arts Therapy was effective in reducing depression and enhancing self-esteem among adolescents who were experiencing emotional difficulties. In addition, adolescents with depression may struggle with low self-esteem and confidence. Expressive Arts Therapy can provide them with a sense of accomplishment and mastery, which can boost their self-esteem and confidence (Kaimal, Carroll-Haskins, & Mensinger, 2016).

Expressive Arts Therapy (Malchiodi, 2005) has emerged as a potentially effective intervention for treating depression in adolescents. By incorporating creative arts such as music, dance, drama, and visual arts, this therapeutic approach offers a nonverbal outlet for adolescents to express themselves and process their emotions. The effectiveness of Expressive Arts Therapy can be attributed to several factors (Timulak & Connelly, 2012). First, the nonverbal nature of creative arts can enable adolescents to communicate their feelings in a way that may feel less intimidating than traditional talk therapy. Second, engaging in expressive arts can promote a sense of accomplishment and empowerment, enhancing motivation to continue treatment and work toward recovery. Finally, the sense of ownership that adolescents may experience over the creative process in Expressive Arts Therapy can provide a source of control and self-determination.

In conclusion, Expressive Arts Therapy offers a safe and supportive environment for adolescents to express themselves and process their emotions. Integrating this with CBT can improve mental health and well-being in adolescents. However, further research is needed to better understand the mechanisms underlying Expressive Arts Therapy's therapeutic effects and identify the specific factors contributing to its effectiveness.

Case Study Application

Session 1

My (first author's) counseling goals for the first session with Jade were to inform her about the counseling process, develop rapport, and establish a therapeutic alliance through compassionate listening, validation, and empathy. Being aware of Jade's Asian family background and culture, I tried to create a safe and trusting environment so that she felt comfortable in counseling. I also allowed Jade to take her time to open up and share herself, as she had not used counseling services before. During our telehealth counseling session, Jade was initially unwilling to show herself through the camera. Hence, I invited her to share with me a piece of music that could represent her experience, and she did. I tuned in to her emotions by reflecting on the sadness of the music she selected. Later, she felt more comfortable and could share more about her anxiety and depression. Since the COVID-19 pandemic, Jade indicated that she experienced multiple symptoms of depression, such as sadness, irritability, crying spells, lack of concentration, loss of appetite, and insomnia. Music seemed to be a channel for Jade to express herself and her experience. At the end of the first session, I presented a simple breathing exercise for her to practice, which seemed to help when she felt negative emotions.

I did not immediately set goals with Jade but gave space and time for the process of relationship building. My immediate goal was for her to feel totally at ease, reduce her defensiveness, and gradually trust the therapeutic process. In addition, the breathing technique assisted her in gaining some level of control and regulation of her emotions.

TABLE 11.1. **JADE: SESSION 1**

Transcript	Analysis
T: "I know that this is your first counseling session. So, we'll take our time to get to know each other. You don't need to turn on your camera if you don't feel comfortable. I understand."	Attempt to join with the client and establish safety and trust.
J: "Okay. I don't want to show my face. I'd rather just talk to you."	Adolescents can sometimes be a bit cautious going into a new environment.
Therapist: "I wonder if there is a song or music you can share with me that illustrates where you are now?"	I am introducing to the client a different channel of communication through music.
J: "This is the music I listen to almost daily." [Shares a song]	Music seemed to open the door to the client, which surprised her.
T: "I tune in to the sadness of your music. How does this music reflect your emotions lately?"	The client felt the support and was able to open up more.

Sessions 2 and 3

My goals for the second and third sessions were to continue encouraging Jade to express her experience, thoughts, and emotions freely and strengthen our therapeutic alliance. Through deep listening and unconditional positive regard toward her, I could assess her depression, loneliness, and sadness during the pandemic. Jade also enjoyed painting with watercolors, which is a traditional and esteemed Chinese art form, so part of the session was to discuss her painting and let her tell her story. Through expressive arts and music, Jade found the medium to express herself and gained more awareness of her thoughts, emotions, and behaviors.

During our third therapy session, some of Jade's cognitive distortions, which connected to her depression, were identified. Jade tended to see only the worst possible result of any situation and overgeneralize the outcome. For example, Jade saw her parents watching TV and enjoying each other (event); she jumped to a conclusion that "they don't care about me or need me" (cognitive distortion); she felt neglected, left out, and unloved (emotional consequence); and she locked herself in her room for 24 hours (behavioral consequence). Another example is that Jade did not receive many texts from her friends in school (event); she thought "all my friends hate me because I'm Chinese" (cognitive distortion); she felt abandoned (emotional consequence); and she deleted phone numbers of several friends (behavioral consequence). Based on these two experiences, Jade's thoughts exhibited the cognitive triad of depression that she was unlovable, her world was falling apart, and there was no hope for her future. I offered Jade psychoeducation on the cognitive triangle; helped her understand that her thoughts, emotions, and behaviors affected one another; and helped her develop balanced thoughts of "my parents need time together, and they do spend time with me

TABLE 11.2. JADE: SESSION 3

Transcript	Analysis
T: "Oh, this is beautiful! I appreciate you sharing this water painting with me. Could you share with me what this is about?"	Assisted client in communicating herself through Expressive Arts Therapy.
J: "This is me all alone in my room. And look at what my parents and friends are doing without me."	She illustrated negative emotions of sadness in blue; anger in red; and helplessness in yellow. Her verbal response reveals her belief that others' behavior must result in her isolation.
T: "Now I can see how you have been feeling lately. Thank you for sharing with me and trusting me. I bet you're feeling very lonely even now. I want you to know I'm with you and support you."	Empathized with the client's experience and provided immediate support and care.
J: "I don't think they [parents] love me or even care about me anymore. That is why my emotions are so negative."	Her cognitive distortion of jumping to a conclusion surfaces. She believes her emotions are automatic based on events.
T: "On the one hand, I can see that your emotions are so real to you, and on the other hand, I'm not sure whether it's true that your parents don't love you."	Mildly addressed the issue and educated the client on the cognitive triangle.

daily" as well as "my friends may also be feeling depressed or awkward, and I have a choice to reach out to them."

Case Conceptualization and Treatment Goals

Like many adolescents, Jade's depression was influenced by the COVID-19 pandemic when public schools were closed in the United States. The platform of educational delivery had drastically changed from face-to-face to online education. Consequently, adolescents were isolated in their homes with minimal social interaction. In addition, Asian Americans were blamed for the pandemic and became the targets of many hate crimes. This seriously affected Jade, her family, and the Asian community. The prolonged isolation kept Jade from social interaction with friends, and later she became increasingly withdrawn even from her parents. She had no channel to express her stress, frustration, and sadness, leading to her having cognitive distortions and negative automatic thoughts. Thus, her overwhelming stress led to depression and mental breakdown. The call to the school hotline was Jade's outcry for help. Luckily, her parents responded immediately to the crisis and supported her to seek counseling.

Based on this information and my interaction with her in the first two sessions, Jade and I agreed on the treatment goals to (a) minimize depressive symptoms, frustration, and crying spells and (b) increase effective emotional regulation and communication skills. Treatment objectives were as follows:

1. Assist the client in freely expressing herself to gain insight and self-awareness through Expressive Arts Therapy.
2. Give psychoeducation on the cognitive triangle and help the client identify and understand the relationships of thoughts, feelings, and behaviors.
3. Replace distorted cognitive thoughts with more appropriate and positive thoughts through CBT.
4. Develop effective coping, such as mindfulness techniques, to regulate the client's emotions.
5. Enhance communication skills so that the client can reestablish connections with family members and friends.

Later Sessions

Because the third counseling session was a turning point for Jade, I continued to encourage her to express herself through her water painting. I continued to explain expressive arts and CBT strategies to her. As a result, she began making connections between her depression and her lack of communication with family and friends. With psychoeducation, she understood her cognitive distortions, which impacted and deepened her depression. By using CBT strategies, I was able to help strengthen her cognitive ability so that she could examine her thought process and ultimately dispute her negative and distorted thoughts. The mindfulness techniques helped her regulate her emotions and lower her stress level. As a result, Jade was willing to practice more effective communication skills with her parents and friends to express her needs.

Ethical and Cultural Considerations

Ethical and cultural considerations were imperative in Jade's case for various reasons. First, as Asian Americans, Jade and her parents were reluctant to seek services because Asian Americans historically have viewed counseling as a Western idea. For many traditional Asian Americans, focusing on emotions may cause discomfort, shame, and embarrassment. Therefore, it was ethically essential for me to educate Jade and her parents on the therapeutic process, which typically requires at least 10 sessions. Doing so prevented Jade and her parents from prematurely terminating counseling out of embarrassment.

Second, counselors should be mindful that most Asian Americans come to counseling only when they are in crisis. Given Jade's outcry of suicidal ideation, I needed to clearly explain the limits of confidentiality, which included serious and foreseeable harm to self, among other limits. I explained that I may need to call the police if I believed Jade was going to seriously harm herself. I also needed to develop a safety plan with Jade with a list of places and people to contact when she had suicidal thoughts.

Third, because many people were blaming the COVID-19 pandemic on Asians and Asian Americans, Asian American Pacific Islander (AAPI) hate crimes increased rapidly. This racist dynamic contributed to mental health concerns among many Asian Americans. Counselors need to view clients' symptoms within the societal context and political atmosphere rather than just individual factors. Counselors have an ethical obligation for social advocacy such as joining rallies to increase awareness of AAPI hate crimes, providing critical stress incident debriefings for Asian churches and community centers, and communicating with legislators about stricter laws to protect Asians.

Parent Consultations

Parent consultations in the context of Asian Americans play a significant part in the success of therapy. The problem presented by the individual client is more appropriately viewed as a family challenge in a collectivistic and systemic context. Because the parents play a vital role in assessing and treating the problem, regular parent consultations with the client's consensus would be helpful. The counselor needs to communicate with parents in a culturally responsive way and view parents as a reliable resource for the adolescent client while protecting the privacy of the adolescent within confidential limits.

Conclusion

Jade made incredible progress by participating in CBT and Expressive Arts Therapy. After several sessions, Jade could express her inner world and gain insight and significant awareness of herself and her depression through Expressive Arts Therapy. In addition, she identified her cognitive distortions and replaced her negative and self-defeating thoughts with more positive and reasonable thoughts through Cognitive Behavioral Therapy. As her counselor, I learned that although many Asian parents may hold biases toward counseling, many are willing to step out of their comfort zone to access counseling to support their children, especially in times of crisis. In addition, the fundamental therapeutic skills of empathy, congruence, and nonjudgmental acceptance aided in building an effective therapeutic alliance with Asian clients. Most importantly, I learned to be mindful of the cultural background and the impact of the family system when working with Asian clients. Integrating Expressive Arts and Cognitive Behavioral Therapy helped create a successful outcome for Jade and her family.

Sample Case Notes

Session 1

Subjective: The client reported having anxiety and sadness as she had no social interaction with her friends or schoolmates. She also said that she had no appetite lately, and her energy was low. She reported that she stayed in her room most of the time and was not motivated to even call her friends on the phone.

Objective: Initially, the client was reluctant to turn on the camera during our telehealth counseling session. The client appeared passive and shy, only responding when the counselor asked her questions. However, after about 20 minutes of warmup with her favorite music, the client understood the counseling process better and could speak more.

Assessment: The client's reluctance and shyness seemed to relate to her cultural upbringing in an Asian family. It seemed apparent that the client experienced some level of depression and withdrawal due to a lack of social activities and the impact of the pandemic.

Plan: The main goal of the initial counseling process was to establish a therapeutic alliance with the client and to create a safe and trusting environment for the client to express herself freely.

Session 3

Subjective: The client expressed her perception of her relationships with her parents and friends through water painting. In the painting, she positioned herself in the dark corner of her room, crying while her parents watched TV in the living room and her friends played happily in the playground. The client stated that she felt isolated, abandoned, and unloved. When asked whether her parents cared for and loved her often, the client admitted they did but said they should have played with her instead of watching TV. She blamed her friends for not inviting her to their gathering. However, the client did not express her needs to her parents or friends.

Objective: The client initially had low energy but was willing to turn on the camera to have eye contact with the counselor. While showing the watercolor painting of her family and friends, the client got teary and expressed some sad emotions. The client was able to articulate more negative emotions through her painting activity.

Assessment: The client seemed to have difficulty communicating her needs with her parents and friends. Her depressive symptoms were associated with her cognitive distortions that her parents and friends did not love and care about her as they did not play with her. The drawing activity helped the client to recognize her internal processing.

Plan: Introduce the cognitive triangle and educate the client on relationships among emotions, behavior, and cognition. Encourage the client to communicate her needs.

Resources

For Professionals

American Academy of Child & Adolescent Psychiatry AAPI Resource Library, https://www.aacap.org/AACAP/Families_and_Youth/Resource_Libraries/AAPI_Resources.aspx

American Art Therapy Association, https://arttherapy.org/

International Expressive Arts Therapy Association, https://www.ieata.org

National Asian American Pacific Islander Mental Health Association, https://www.naapimha.org/

National Coalition of Creative Arts Therapies Associations, https://www.nccata.org/

For Adolescents and Parents

Permission to Come Home: Reclaiming Mental Health as Asian Americans by Jenny Wang (2022).

Stigma: Breaking the Asian American Silence on Mental Health by Tanaya Kollipara (2021).

Discussion Questions

1. What issues should a therapist pay attention to when working with an Asian client, particularly after the COVID-19 pandemic?
2. As a therapist, what knowledge and understanding of the Generation Z population could help to build a therapeutic alliance with a Generation Z client?
3. What would be a culturally responsive way to explain Jade's depression, CBT, and Expressive Arts Therapy to her parents?
4. In what situation would you consider family therapy with the adolescent and her parents?

References

American Academy of Child and Adolescent Psychiatry. (2017). *Depression in children and adolescents.* https://www.aacap.org/AACAP/Families_and_Youth/Facts_for_Families/FFF-Guide/The-Depressed-Child-004.aspx

American Psychiatric Association. (2013). *Diagnostic and statistical manual of mental disorders* (5th ed.). https://doi.org/10.1176/appi.books.9780890425596

American Psychological Association. (2021). *Stress in America™ 2020: A national mental health crisis.* https://www.apa.org/news/press/releases/stress/2020/report-october

Asian American Psychological Association. (2021). *Written testimony from the Asian American Psychological Association.* Washington, DC. https://aapaonline.org/wp-content/uploads/2021/03/AAPA-Testimony-to-House-Judiciary-on-3.18.2 021.pdf

Beck, A. T., & Weishaar, M. (2018). Cognitive therapy. In R. J. Corsini & D. Wedding (Eds.), *Current psychotherapies* (11th ed., instr. ed., pp. 237–272). Cengage.

Djafarova, E., & Bowes, T. (2021). "Instagram made me buy it": Generation Z impulse purchases in fashion industry. *Journal of Retailing and Consumer Services, 59.* https://doi.org/10.1016/j.jretconser.2020.102345

Duan, L., Shao, X., Wang, Y., Huang, Y., Miao, J., Yang, X., & Zhu, G. (2020). An investigation of mental health status of children and adolescents in China during the outbreak of COVID-19. *Journal of Affective Disorders, 275,* 112–118. https://doi.org/10.1016/j.jad.2020.06.029

Harari, T. T., Sela, Y., & Bareket-Bojmel, L. (2022). Gen Z during the COVID-19 crisis: A comparative analysis of the differences between Gen Z and Gen X in resilience, values and attitudes. *Current Psychology.* https://doi.org/10.1007/s12144-022-03501-4

Kaimal, G., Carroll-Haskins, K., & Mensinger, J. L. (2016). The effects of art therapy on stress and anxiety in adolescents. *Art Therapy, 33*(2), 74–80.

Malchiodi, C. A. (2005). Expressive therapies: History, theory, and practice. In C. A. Malchiodi (Ed.), *Expressive therapies* (pp. 1–15). Guilford Press.

Mavroveli, S., & Papacharalambous, A. (2018). Cognitive behavioral therapy and expressive writing in the treatment of depressive symptoms among adolescents. *Children and Youth Services Review, 89,* 276–283.

Mealer, L. L., Cutcliffe, J. R., & Gish, K. (2017). Expressive arts therapy for adolescents with depression. *Journal of Creativity in Mental Health, 12*(3), 352–362.

National Institute of Mental Health. (2017). *Depression in children and adolescents.* https://www.nimh.nih.gov/health/topics/depression/index.shtml

Parker, K., & Igielnik, R. (2020). On the cusp of adulthood and facing an uncertain future: What we know about Gen Z so far. https://policycommons.net/

artifacts/616196/on-the-cusp-of-adulthood-and-facing-an-uncertain-future/1 596804/

Ramakrishnan, K., Wong, J., Lee, J., Sadhwani, S., & Shao, S. (2021). *Tip of the iceberg: Estimates of AAPI hate incidents far more extensive than reported.* AAPI Data. http://aapidata.com/blog/tip-iceberg-march2021-survey/

Saw, A., Aggie, J. Y. H., & Jeung, R. (2021). *Stop AAPI Hate mental health report.* https://stopaapihate.org/wp-content/uploads/2021/05/Stop-AAPI-Hate-Mental-Health-Report-210527.pdf

Stirrups, R. (2018). The storm and stress in the adolescent brain. *Lancet Neurology, 17*(5) 404.

Tandoc, E. C., Ferrucci, P., & Duffy, M. (2015). Facebook use, envy, and depression among college students: Is Facebooking depressing? *Computers in Human Behavior, 43*, 139–146.

Timulak, L., & Connelly, C. (2012). A comparison of psychotherapists' and expressive arts therapists' perceptions of adolescents' emotional difficulties and treatment needs. *Arts in Psychotherapy, 39*(1), 10–17.

Tompkins, K. A. (2018). Cognitive-behavioral therapy for depression. *Journal of Psychiatric Practice, 24*(1), 12–20.

US Surgeon General. (2023). *Social media and youth mental health: The U.S. Surgeon General Advisory.* https://www.hhs.gov/surgeongeneral/priorities/youth-mental-health/social-media/index.html

Wu, P., Fang, Y., Guan, Z., Fan, B., Kong, J., Yao, Z., & Hoven, C. W. (2021). The psychological impact of the SARS epidemic on hospital employees in China: Exposure, risk perception, and altruistic acceptance of risk. *Canadian Journal of Psychiatry, 48*(9), 125–130.

Yee, A. (2021). COVID's outsize impact on Asian Americans is being ignored. *Scientific American.* https://www.scientificamerican.com/article/covids-outsize-impact-on-asian-americans-is-being-ignored/

Zhang, X., Yang, H., Zhang, J., Yang, M., Yuan, N., & Liu, J. (2021). Prevalence of and risk factors for depressive and anxiety symptoms in a large sample of Chinese adolescents in the post-COVID-19 era. *Child and Adolescent Psychiatry and Mental Health, 15.* https://doi.org/10.1186/s13034-021-00429-8

CHAPTER 12

Social Anxiety
Mindfulness-Based Cognitive Behavior Therapy with a Pakistani American Adolescent
Yu-Fen Lin and Samuel Bore

Jasmin is a 15-year-old Pakistani American cisgender female. Both of her parents are engineers who came from Islamabad, Pakistan, to the United States in 1998 for college and are devoted Sunni Muslims. Jasmin was born in California, attends public school, and follows some expectations of her Muslim community and family. She wears a hijab and dresses modestly at her parents' request but recently became interested in wearing makeup to fit in with her school friends. She refuses to go to school or other public places without wearing makeup because she is self-conscious about how she appears in front of others. As a result, Jasmin goes to school early to put on makeup without her parents' consent and avoids going out as much as possible because she worries about how others will perceive and judge her. Jasmin's parents prefer for her to present herself with modesty, without makeup. They believe they should educate, shape, discipline, and mold their daughter according to their Muslim teachings and that their daughter should obey them. However, Jasmin wants to assimilate with her peers and express herself fully, which has caused value conflicts and communication problems. She fought with her parents and stopped attending mosque, receiving little emotional support at home. She feels unhappy, lonely, and isolated at school, worrying about how others view her despite having a few friends. At home, Jasmin also feels very anxious around her parents.

For this case study, consider the following:

1. What are common concerns of children experiencing social anxiety, and what are Jasmin's needs? To what extent does being a Muslim in a public school impact Jasmin?
2. What is the rationale for using Mindfulness Cognitive Behavior Therapy with Jasmin?
3. What ethical guidelines and cultural considerations need to be followed for Jasmin?

South Asian Muslim Adolescents

Pakistan is a South Asian country that is predominantly Muslim and has official languages of Urdu and English. As of 2021, approximately 618,000 residents of Pakistani descent were living in the United States (US Census Bureau, 2020). Most Pakistani Americans are well educated and in the middle to upper class in US society. After the September 11, 2001, terrorist attacks, Pakistani Americans experienced increased incidents of discrimination due to Islamophobia (Muslim Matters, 2017).

Muslim high school students frequently perceive themselves as similar to their peers but navigate unique challenges such as difficulty implementing Islamic practices (e.g., prayer) in their school day and coping with Islamophobia (Seward & Khan, 2016). Ahmed (2012) elaborated that "Muslim adolescents . . . are often scrutinized for fear of being the next homegrown terrorists and experience pressures of Islamophobia during an already challenging developmental period" (p. 252). Muslim adolescents in the United States often experience acculturation stress (i.e., internal and external demands from cultural adaptation and negotiation that exceeds personal resources), which can lead to internalizing symptoms such as anxiety (Goforth, Pham, Chun, Castro-Olivo, & Yosai, 2016). Muslim adolescent girls have been found to experience stricter parenting styles than boys out of a desire to protect their modesty, which may contribute to their experience of social anxiety (Peleg, Tzischinsky, & Spivak, 2021).

Social Anxiety

From a developmental perspective, social anxiety is a common mental health issue affecting many adolescents who worry about being judged or evaluated by others. Adolescents can experience excessive fear and self-consciousness in social situations, leading to avoidance and isolation. Adolescents with social anxiety may avoid social situations or struggle to interact with others. The DSM-5 defines social anxiety disorder (SAD) as a persistent and intense fear of social conditions in which others may negatively evaluate the individual (American Psychiatric Association, 2013). Adolescents with social anxiety may struggle to identify and understand their emotions. Social anxiety in adolescents has been linked to psychological inflexibility (Figueiredo, Alves, & Vagos, 2023), perfectionism (Wang et al., 2022), social media (Barry, 2022), racial/ethnic teasing and discrimination (Douglass, Mirpuri, English, & Yip, 2016), and parents' exposure to trauma (Cho, Woods-Jaeger, & Borelli, 2021). Individuals experiencing social anxiety need to seek support and treatment from mental health professionals, which can significantly improve their quality of life.

Mindfulness-Based Cognitive Behavior Therapy

Mindfulness can be defined as paying attention to the present moment (Kabat-Zinn, 2013). Mindfulness-Based Cognitive Behavior Therapy (MB-CBT) is a form of psychotherapy that combines mindfulness practices with cognitive-behavioral therapy techniques. This approach aims to help individuals become more aware of their thoughts, feelings, and bodily sensations in the present moment non-judgmentally while also addressing and challenging negative thought patterns that contribute to social anxiety (Carlton, Sullivan-Toole, Strege, Ollendick, & Richey, 2020). MB-CBT can help adolescents become more attuned to their thoughts and feelings, leading to greater self-awareness and improved emotional regulation. MB-CBT can help adolescents identify maladaptive thinking patterns and develop more realistic and positive perspectives, particularly by challenging negative thoughts that often trigger social anxiety (MacKenzie & Kocovski, 2016).

Mindfulness practices, such as meditation and deep breathing, can help adolescents with social anxiety manage their symptoms and stay focused in the present moment. By practicing mindfulness regularly, adolescents can develop greater self-compassion and acceptance, improving their overall well-being. In addition, MB-CBT can provide adolescents with tools and strategies, such as assertiveness training and role-playing exercises, to help them improve their social skills (Eslami, Rabiei, Afzali, Hamidizadeh, & Masoudi, 2016).

MB-CBT is considered a useful treatment option for Jasmin for the following reasons. First, it can directly address symptoms of social anxiety. Second, it may reduce the intense level of concern. Third, it is well received by anxious adolescent clients who prefer a more interactive approach (Carlton et al., 2020). With the guidance of mental health professionals trained in MB-CBT, adolescents can learn to manage their symptoms and build the skills they need to lead fulfilling and meaningful lives.

Case Application

Based on the information about Pakistani American Muslim adolescents, social anxiety, and MB-CBT treatment approaches, we can now apply them to Jasmin. Her desire for self-expression and assimilation with her peers is typical for teenagers. According to Cognitive Behavioral Therapy (CBT), Jasmin presents with social anxiety symptoms due to a combination of genetic, personality, and environmental factors. Specifically, her social anxiety is exacerbated by an Islamophobic environment; acculturation stress of wanting to be accepted and blend in; social media; psychological inflexibility; genetic predisposition; and her parents' exposure to September 11 trauma and discrimination. Currently, Jasmin's Muslim identity and school experiences play a role in her desire for self-expression, which conflicts with her parents' expectations.

Triggers to Jasmin's social anxiety include her peers' influence to wear makeup, which leads to her self-consciousness and anxiety when not wearing it. Jasmin's conflicts with her parents over makeup and self-expression have created a stressful family environment, leading to anxiety and unhappiness. Jasmin's avoidance of going out without makeup increases her anxiety and self-consciousness, compounded by her negative self-talk and worries about how others view her (Beck, 2011).

Jasmin's parents brought her to counseling due to her intense and frequent arguments with them, "disobedience," isolation in her room when at home, refusal to go out in public without makeup, avoidance of social situations other than school, fear of performance at school, and irritability. Her parents did not realize that these concerns were related to social anxiety.

Session 1

The goal for the first session with Jasmin was to develop a relationship, complete an assessment, explain the MB-CBT approach, and introduce some coping skills to help her begin to feel less anxious without fighting her anxiety but rather learning to ride the anxiety wave. Before the session started, I (first author) ensured that her parents had signed the parental consent in the file. After introductions, I obtained informed assent from Jasmin and discussed limits to confidentiality. This was followed by assessing Jasmin's mental health and well-being by evaluating her emotional, behavioral, and cognitive functioning; recognizing her strengths and weaknesses; and identifying any underlying issues contributing to her current difficulties.

To identify Jasmin's level of anxiety, I administered the Reynolds Children's Manifest Anxiety Scale, 2nd edition (RCMAS-2) (Reynolds & Richmond, 2008). RCMAS-2, a brief self-report inventory, is used to identify the nature and level of anxiety in children from 6 to 19 years. T-scores below 39, from 40 to 60, from 61 to 70, or greater than 71 are categorized as less problematic, no more problematic, moderately problematic, and highly problematic, respectively. Jasmin presented with moderately problematic anxiety with a score of 75 on the RCMAS-2 scale.

At the end of the first session, I asked Jasmin what she wanted to accomplish in therapy. Jasmin and I agreed on the following goal and objectives:
Treatment Goal: Jasmin would manage her anxiety, improve her self-esteem, develop practical communication skills, and develop a sense of self-acceptance.
Treatment Objectives:
1. Decrease anxiety by practicing mindfulness techniques to regulate emotions.
2. Confront fears related to going out without makeup.
3. Increase self-awareness and acceptance of thoughts and emotions.
4. Challenge and reframe negative thoughts and beliefs about herself and her appearance.

After assessing Jasmin's needs, I created a treatment plan with interventions and techniques. My treatment strategies were to introduce MB-CBT methods such as breathing, cognitive restructuring, and exposure therapy to help Jasmin manage her anxiety, challenge negative thoughts, and feel more comfortable without makeup over time.

TABLE 12.1. JASMIN: SESSION 1

Transcript	Analysis
T: "Hi, Jasmin. It's nice to meet you. How are you feeling today?"	Introduction and rapport building.
J: "Hi, I'm feeling a bit nervous but also hopeful."	Clients, especially adolescents, often feel nervous and awkward in the first counseling session.
T: "That's understandable. I'm glad you're here. Can you tell me a bit more about what has been going on for you?"	Supporting the client and assuring her experience is common.
J: "Yeah, it's been tough. I go to school early every day just to put on makeup, and I feel really uncomfortable when I'm not wearing it. I also feel really lonely and isolated at school, even though I have a few friends."	Encouraging the client to express herself and tell her story.
T: "Your loneliness and uncomfortableness sound painful. I can imagine how difficult that would be."	Paraphrasing and reflecting on the client's feelings for understanding and empathy.
J: [Nodding, appears emotional]	The client experiences empathy from accurate reflection of feelings and is emotional.
T: "Mmm." [Silence]	Minimal encouragement and therapeutic silence.
T: "I have some ideas on how to help. Have you heard of mindfulness before?"	Instilling hope. Introducing the mindfulness approach.
J: "No, not really."	
T: "Well, mindfulness is a way of paying attention to the present moment, without judgment or distraction. It can help with anxiety and stress, and can also help you feel more connected to yourself and others."	Explaining the mindfulness approach in simple and age-appropriate language.
J: "Sounds interesting."	Indicates openness to process.
T: "And have you heard about Cognitive Behavior Therapy, or CBT before?"	Introducing the CBT approach.
J: "No."	
T: "Cognitive Behavioral Therapy (CBT) is a therapeutic approach that focuses on the connection between our thoughts, emotions, beliefs, and behavior. Our perceptions and interpretations of events are more significant than the events themselves in determining how we feel and behave."	Explaining the CBT approach in simple and developmental-level language.
J: "That is more interesting . . ."	The client appears fascinated by the explanation of CBT.
J: "I am not sure . . . but maybe paying attention to the present moment and what I am thinking about?"	
T: "You got that right; you pay attention."	I am encouraging the client and continuing to build rapport.
J: [Smiles . . . appears proud of her achievement]	Noticing the client's nonverbals.
T: "You are proud you got it right. Let's start with some deep breathing exercises today. I'll guide you through it. Take a deep breath in through your nose and hold it for a few seconds, then slowly exhale through your mouth. Please do that a few more times as you pay attention to your breath."	Validating the client by reflecting on feelings. Introducing the client to the MB-CBT approach and guiding her through techniques.

Session 2

The goal for the second session was to work with Jasmin to master and practice breathing exercises.

TABLE 12.2. **JASMIN: SESSION 2**

Transcript	Analysis
T: "Hi, Jasmin. How are you doing today, and how have you been since our last session?"	Introducing the session and recapping the last session.
J: "I am doing fine. I've been practicing the breathing exercises you taught me last week."	Client report of practicing the technique.
T: "Okay. You took time to practice what you learned last week. How has the practice gone?"	Validating the client and checking on skill development.
J: "They've been helpful. But I'm still struggling with feeling anxious."	Many clients take time and a lot of practice to master techniques and see change.
T: "I understand. It takes practice to master the technique. Also, it will take time and doing this almost daily. How about we continue working on the skill to help you master it?"	Empathy and encouragement. Set realistic expectations as many adolescents expect instant change after doing exercises once or twice.
J: "Okay."	
T: "Sit comfortably and close your eyes. Begin by bringing your awareness and attention to your toes, and notice any sensations there . . . , then move up to your feet, and notice any sensations there . . . , keep moving up your body and noticing any sensations or tension . . . Don't judge anything. Just notice . . . when you get to the top of your head, take a few deep breaths . . . , and slowly open your eyes."	Practicing for technique comfort and mastery.

Session 3

In the third session, I introduced the cognitive activity of identifying and challenging negative thoughts and beliefs. In addition, I encouraged Jasmin to be aware of body sensations when experiencing anxiety.

During the next sessions, I assisted Jasmin in honing her awareness of her bodily sensations and expressing them to me. We also worked on new methods, such as exposure therapy, to help her feel more comfortable with her natural appearance without makeup. I also motivated Jasmin to challenge herself by going out without makeup more often and to acknowledge and reward her successes.

TABLE 12.3. JASMIN: SESSION 3

Transcript	Analysis
T: "How are you today, and how was last week?"	Checking in with the client.
J: "Things have been good and better."	Client's update
T: "Oh, tell me how the week was good and better."	Giving the client an opportunity to expand on her experience
J: "The mindful exercises have been helpful, and it's easy to perform them."	Client progress details
T: "You are pleased that you are mastering the breathing technique and happy it is helpful."	Reflection of feelings. Validation of client's efforts.
J: "Yes, but I am still struggling with feeling anxious and self-conscious."	The client opens up about her struggles; an indication of a good rapport and trust between the client and therapist.
T: "I am glad they are helping. You feel a little discouraged in still feeling anxious and self-conscious. This is typical to see some progress and want more relief. I can help with that. Which is occurring more?"	Reflection of feelings. Validation that her struggle is common. Encouragement for the client to go deeper.
J: "I think the anxiety is less and the self-consciousness is more."	Demonstrates self-awareness and understands the difference between the two.
T: "I am glad you have been paying attention to your physical sensations, noticing that your anxiety is less. That was one of the techniques we worked on last week. How about we work on a cognitive technique today?"	Paraphrasing and praising the client for effort and introducing a new technique
J: "Okay, sure."	
T: "This technique will help you identify the connection between thoughts, feelings, and behavior. Then we develop a balanced thought."	Explaining the nature of the technique before introduction
J: "Okay."	
T: "Here we go. Just like the last exercise we practiced; I would like you to be as comfortable as you can . . . please think of a situation where you feel self-conscious . . . like when you're at school without makeup. What thoughts come to mind?	Technique details and practice
J: "All the other students are thinking 'look at that ugly girl. Muslims are so weird and never will fit in.'"	Because of the therapeutic rapport, she was honest about her thoughts.
T: "Sounds like an all-or-nothing thought. When you think that, how do you feel and then how do you behave?"	Identify the type of cognitive distortion; introduce the cognitive triangle by drawing a diagram of thoughts leading to feelings and then behavior
J: "I feel self-conscious, lower my eyes so I am only looking at the ground, and avoid talking to anyone."	She connects the cognitive triangle.
T: "If you change the thought to something more balanced like 'I am friendly, smart, kind, and have pretty eyes and a warm smile even when I don't wear makeup' then how would you feel and behave? More self-conscious or less? More withdrawn or less?"	Many adolescents need initial guidance when developing a balanced thought. Later, I will help her challenge the cognitive distortion by examining the evidence and then prompt her to develop her own balanced thoughts.

(continued)

TABLE 12.3. *(CONTINUED)*

Transcript	Analysis
J: "Well, I would feel less self-conscious and less withdrawn. But I still think I look better with makeup."	Adolescents typically admit that the balanced thought would help. However, their validity of cognition is low.
T: "You recognize changing your thought will at least help you achieve your goal of feeling less self-conscious. It is common not to believe it all the way until you practice it several times and see the difference. Would you be willing to practice this balanced thought two times this week—just as an experiment to see what happens?"	Encouraging her recognition of the concept *and* validating her low belief followed by asking for a commitment to try it.

Ethical and Cultural Considerations

I considered several ethical and cultural issues for Jasmin, starting with confidentiality (Haraldsson et al., 2022). Jasmin hesitated to open up, fearing that I would share her information with her parents. From the outset, I assured Jasmin that information shared in counseling sessions is kept confidential, except for the limits of confidentiality. I then explained the limits of confidentiality and the circumstances under which information may be disclosed.

Another ethical consideration was respecting Jasmin's cultural background and her family's Muslim faith (Sue, Zane, Nagayama Hall, & Berger, 2009). Although it was essential to help Jasmin express her desire to wear makeup and feel comfortable, it was also important to avoid imposing other cultural values and beliefs on her and her family. I was mindful of potential cultural biases and maintained cultural sensitivity. As Amari (2021) suggested, I prioritized Jasmin's autonomy and right to self-determination while respecting her parents' role and values. We discussed how Jasmin could balance expressing herself while respecting her parents' wishes and beliefs.

Finally, given that Jasmin is a Pakistani American Muslim adolescent girl, I paid attention to issues of intersectionality (Byrd et al., 2022). I was nonjudgmental and created a safe environment trying to avoid biases and stereotypes for Jasmin to express herself safely. I considered the larger social context, specifically global events and political environment contributing to Islamophobia that was impacting Jasmin's development and mental health (Ahmed, 2012).

Parent and/or Teacher Consultations

Teacher consultation is essential to counseling treatment for children (Vilbas et al., 2021). It is a necessary process with many potential benefits, including supporting and accommodating Jasmin's anxiety and academic difficulties. I consulted Jasmin's teacher and discussed ways of helping Jasmin manage her anxiety in the classroom, such as relaxation techniques like breathing or taking breaks when needed. The meeting was also an opportunity to discuss ways to support Jasmin to promote her success in school and to intervene when racist and Islamophobic remarks were made. In addition, I addressed the teacher's concerns and questions about her behavior and academic performance. On Jasmin's teacher's recommendation, we referred Jasmin to the school's Student Support Team (SST) for additional support and mentoring.

I also met Jasmin's parents and educated them about the benefits of MB-CBT and how it could help them manage anxiety and healthily express themselves. As I did for Jasmin, I assured Jasmin's parents of my respect for their cultural and religious values. To help them understand her treatment process, I explained the rationale behind the treatment approach and goals and addressed their concerns or questions. I addressed scheduling arrangements and transportation to ensure that Jasmin attended her counseling sessions. In addition, I provided Jasmin's parents with a list of parent training community resources.

Conclusion

After implementing MB-CBT, Jasmin made significant progress in her treatment. At the termination of counseling, she could apply MB-CBT techniques to identify and challenge her negative thoughts and beliefs regarding her appearance and interaction with her parents and friends.

Jasmin developed new coping strategies and self-acceptance and reported being more confident and less self-conscious about her appearance. Her relationship and communication with her parents improved. Not only did Jasmin become more autonomous, but she also expressed herself better while respecting the divergent views of her parents. I was sensitive in considering cultural and ethical issues concerning Jasmin and her parents as Pakistani Americans and their Muslim faith. I also facilitated parent and teacher consultations to ensure that Jasmin received appropriate support and understanding at home and school.

Overall, the MB-CBT approach has been effective in helping Jasmin to improve her well-being and relationships and to achieve a greater sense of self-awareness and acceptance. As a therapist, I was mindful of cultural and ethical considerations and tailored the therapy to meet Jasmin's specific needs.

Sample Case Notes

Session 1

Subjective: Jasmin expressed concern about her appearance and interest in wearing makeup. In addition, she reported feeling very anxious about her parents.
Objective: Initially, Jasmin appeared sad and anxious during the session. Her body language was closed off and tense, and she spoke softly and avoided eye contact. However, Jasmin seemed a bit relaxed after the breathing exercise.
Assessment: Jasmin is experiencing value conflicts and communication problems with her parents, contributing to anxiety, social isolation, and low self-esteem. Her fear of judgment and rejection is consistent with a diagnosis of social anxiety

disorder. The pressure to conform to her parents' beliefs and values exacerbates her symptoms. Her grades have started slipping; she has missed several school days due to anxiety and stress.

Plan: Mindfulness-based cognitive therapy will provide Jasmin with skills to manage her anxiety and increase her self-acceptance. She will learn to challenge her negative thoughts about her appearance and develop a more positive self-image.

Resources

For Clients

Butterfly hug, https://www.youtube.com/watch?v=iGGJrqscvtU&t=34s
Creating a mindfulness anxiety plan, https://positive.b-cdn.net/wp-content/uploads/2021/12/Creating-a-Mindfulness-Anxiety-Plan.pdf
Guided box breathing, https://www.youtube.com/watch?v=zq07gbFLCAs&t=148s

For Therapists

Body Scan Meditation guided meditation led by Kabat Zinn, https://www.youtube.com/watch?v=u4gZgnCy5ew

Discussion Questions

1. What attention should a mindfulness-based CBT counselor focus on when working with adolescents dealing with social anxiety?
2. What developmental issues are worth considering in relation to adolescents' social anxiety?
3. Describe some social justice advocacy strategies that counselors could use with Muslim clients.

References

Ahmed, S. (2012). Adolescents and emerging adults. In S. Ahmed & M. M. Amer (Eds.), *Counseling Muslims: Handbook of mental health issues and interventions* (pp. 251–280). Routledge/Taylor & Francis Group.

Amari, N. (2021). Counseling psychology practice as the pursuit of the I-thou relationship. *The Humanistic Psychologist, 48*(4), 410–426. https://doi.org/10.1037/hum0000155

American Psychiatric Association. (2013). *Diagnostic and statistical manual of mental disorders* (5th ed.). https://doi.org/10.1176/appi.books.9780890425596

Barry, K. A. (2022). *Guidance counselor perceptions on the influence of social media on adolescent mental health in affluent middle schools in New Jersey* (Publication No. 28772181). [Doctoral dissertation, Saint Peter's University, 2021.] ProQuest Information & Learning. https://www.proquest.com/open

view/c5cba129142d707a2532cd12531ff920/1?pq-origsite=gscholar&cbl
=18750&diss=y

Beck, J. S. (2011). *Cognitive behavior therapy: Basics and beyond* (2nd ed.). Guilford Press.

Byrd, R., Luke, C., Lorelle, S., Donald, E., Blueford, J., Adams, C., & Hudspeth, E. (2022). Counseling children and adolescents: A call to action. *Journal of Counselor Preparation and Supervision, 16*(1). https://digitalcommons
.sacredheart.edu/jcps/vol16/iss1/2

Carlton, C. N., Sullivan-Toole, H., Strege, M., Ollendick, T. H., & Richey, J. A. (2020). Mindfulness-based interventions for adolescent social anxiety: A unique convergence of factors. *Frontiers in Psychology, 11*. https://doi.org/
10.3389/fpsyg.2020.01783

Cho, B., Woods-Jaeger, B., & Borelli, J. L. (2021). Parenting stress moderates the relation between parental trauma exposure and child anxiety symptoms. *Child Psychiatry and Human Development, 52*(6), 1050–1059. https://doi
.org/10.1007/s10578-020-01087-1

Douglass, S., Mirpuri, S., English, D., & Yip, T. (2016). "They were just making jokes": Ethnic/racial teasing and discrimination among adolescents. *Cultural Diversity and Ethnic Minority Psychology, 22*(1), 69–82. https://doi
.org/10.1037/cdp0000041

Eslami, A. A., Rabiei, L., Afzali, S. M., Hamidizadeh, S., & Masoudi, R. (2016). The effectiveness of assertiveness training on the levels of stress, anxiety, and depression of high school students. *Iran Red Crescent Medical Journal, 18*(1), 300–303. https://doi.org/10.5812/ircmj.21096

Figueiredo, D. V., Alves, F., & Vagos, P. (2023). Psychological inflexibility explains social anxiety over time: A mediation analyses with a clinical adolescent sample. *Current Psychology: A Journal for Diverse Perspectives on Diverse Psychological Issues*. https://doi.org/10.1007/s12144-023-04650-w

Goforth, A. N., Pham, A. V., Chun, H., Castro-Olivo, S. M., & Yosai, E. R. (2016). Association of acculturative stress, Islamic practices, and internalizing symptoms among Arab American adolescents. *School Psychology Quarterly, 31*(2), 198–212. https://doi.org/10.1037/spq0000135.supp (Supplemental)

Haraldsson, J., Pingel, R., Nordgren, L., Johnsson, L., Kristiansson, P., & Tindberg, Y. (2022). Confidentiality matters! Adolescent males' views of primary care in relation to psychosocial health: A structural equation modeling approach. *Scandinavian Journal of Primary Health Care, 40*(4), 438–449. https://doi.org/10.1080/02813432.2022.2144999

Kabat-Zinn J. (2013). *Full Catastrophe Living, Revised Edition: How to Cope with Stress, Pain and Illness Using Mindfulness Meditation*. Hachette.

Khoury, B., Lecomte, T., Fortin, G., Masse, M., Therien, P., Bouchard, V., Chapleau, M. A., & Kabat-Zinn, J. (2013). *Full catastrophe living: Using the wisdom of your body and mind to face stress, pain, and illness*. Bantam Dell.

Lahat, A., Lamm, C., Chronis-Tuscano, A., Pine, D. S., Henderson, H. A., & Fox, N. A. (2014). Early behavioral inhibition and increased error monitoring predict later social phobia symptoms in childhood. *Journal of the American Academy of Child & Adolescent Psychiatry, 53*(4), 447–455.

MacKenzie, M. B., & Kocovski, N. L. (2016). Mindfulness-based cognitive therapy for depression: Trends and developments. *Psychology Research and Behavior Management, 9*, 125–132.

Muslim Matters. (2017). Who is Anila Daulatzai? Students urge boycott of Southwest demanding justice for Muslim professor. https://muslimmatters.org/2017/10/23/who-is-anila-daulatzai-students-urge-boycott-of-southwest-demanding-justice-for-muslim-professor/

Odgers, C. L., & Jensen, M. R. (2020). Annual research review: Adolescent mental health in the digital age: Facts, fears, and future directions. *Journal of Child Psychology and Psychiatry, 61*(3), 336–348.

Paquin, K., & Hofmann, S. G. (2013). Mindfulness-based therapy: A comprehensive meta-analysis. *Clinical Psychology Review, 33*(6), 763–771.

Peleg, O., Tzischinsky, O., & Spivak, L. Z. (2021). Depression and social anxiety mediate the relationship between parenting styles and risk of eating disorders: A study among Arab adolescents. *International Journal of Psychology, 56*, 853–864. https://doi.org/10.1002/ijop.12787

Peterson, T. J. (2018). *The mindfulness workbook for anxiety: The 8-week solution to help you manage anxiety, worry & stress*. Althea Press.

Reynolds, C. R., & Richmond, B. O. (2008). *Revised children's manifest anxiety scale (RCMAS-2): Manual* (2nd ed.). Western Psychological Services.

Rezaei, S., Babapour, J., & Bolhari, J. (2016). The effectiveness of mindfulness-based cognitive therapy on social anxiety disorder in female adolescents. *Iranian Journal of Psychiatry and Clinical Psychology, 22*(3), 214–222.

Semple, R. J., Lee, J., Rosa, D., & Miller, L. F. (2010). A randomized trial of mindfulness-based cognitive therapy for children: Promoting mindful attention to enhance social-emotional resiliency in children. *Journal of Child and Family Studies, 19*(2), 218–229.

Seward, D. X., & Khan, S. (2016). Towards an understanding of Muslim American adolescent high school experiences. *International Journal for the Advancement of Counselling, 38*(1), 1–11. https://doi.org/10.1007/s10447-015-9252-5

Sue, S., Zane, N., Nagayama Hall, G. C., & Berger, L. K. (2009). The case for cultural competency in psychotherapeutic interventions. *Annual Review of Psychology, 60*, 525–548. https://doi.org/10.1146/annurev.psych.60.110707.163651

Twenge, J. M., & Campbell, W. K. (2018). Associations between screen time and lower psychological well-being among children and adolescents: Evidence from a population-based study. *Preventive Medicine Reports, 12*, 271–283.

US Census Bureau. (2020). Pakistani Total Population 2020. https://data.census .gov/table?q=pakistani&g=010XX00US&y=2020

Vilbas, J., & King-Sears, M. E. (2021). An effective elementary school counselor's support of students with disabilities: A case study. *Psychology in Schools, 58*(5) 873–892. https://doi.org/10.1002/pits.22476

Vultaggio, G. (2023). *The most anxious generation: The relationship between Gen Z students, social media, and anxiety*. SUNY Open Access Repository. http://hdl.handle.net/20.500.12648/1916

Wang, Y., Chen, J., Zhang, X., Lin, X., Sun, Y., Wang, N., Wang, J., & Luo, F. (2022). The relationship between perfectionism and social anxiety: A moderated mediation model. *International Journal of Environmental Research and Public Health, 19*(19). https://doi.org/10.3390/ijerph191912934

Wuthrich, V. M., Rapee, R. M., Cunningham, M. J., Lyneham, H. J., & Hudson, J. L. (2012). Randomized controlled trial of group cognitive behavioral therapy for social anxiety disorder with and without mindfulness-based modifications. *Behaviour Research and Therapy, 50*(11), 675–686.

CHAPTER 13

Divorce and Political Extremist Groups
Cognitive Behavior Therapy and Expressive Arts with a White Adolescent

Jennifer N. Baggerly

David is a very intelligent 16-year-old White male who lives with his mother, Debra, and 12-year-old sister, Suzie. David's father, Ed, lives in a nearby apartment with his new girlfriend. During the intake session, Debra said she has been divorced for 1 year. She stated that the divorce was because Ed had become a radical who joined an extremist political group. Yet, she knows that Ed tells people the divorce was because she is a "crazy b—" who misunderstood him. Debra tearfully explained that she is seeking counseling for David because of his depression, isolation from friends, and extreme disrespect as well as outbursts toward his father. Ed does pay child support, so he insists on seeing David according to the standard custody agreement despite David's resistance. Ed does not believe in counseling, so he refused to participate in the intake session.

For this case study, consider:

1. What are common concerns of adolescents experiencing divorce and what were David's needs? What are characteristics of people involved in extremist political groups and how does it impact their children?
2. What is the rationale for using Cognitive Behavior Therapy (CBT) and Expressive Arts with David? What are common strategies?
3. What unique ethical guidelines need to be considered?

Impact of Divorce

Although the United States divorce rate has declined from 944,000 in 2000 to 689,308 in 2021 (Centers for Disease Control, 2022), still 30% of 12- to 17-year-olds do not live with both parents (Anderson, Hemez, & Kreider, 2022). The impact of divorce on adolescents is multifold. Harold and Sellers's (2018) review found interparental conflict such as divorce can result in adolescents' (a) sleep problems of getting to sleep and staying asleep; (b) externalizing symptoms of aggression, conduct problems, and antisocial behavior; (c) internalizing problems

of withdrawal, fearfulness, sadness, low self-esteem, anxiety, depression, and suicidality; (d) academic problems of lower performance; (e) social and interpersonal
relationship problems such as problem solving and wider social competence; (f)
physical health problems of fatigue, abdominal stress, and headaches; and (g)
intergenerational transmission of psychopathology and relationship distress such
as likelihood of partner violence in future romantic relationships.

The extent of impact from interparental conflict depends on the frequency,
intensity, and resolution potential of parental conflict as well as a particular adolescents' quality of parent-child relationship, child temperament, child gender, and
history of exposure to conflict (Harold & Sellers, 2018). These factors influence
adolescents' appraisal of the conflict and subsequent understanding as to why the
conflict occurs (e.g., responsibility and blame) and the adolescent's ability to do
something about it. "Children who blame themselves for parental disagreements
or feel responsible for not helping to end them experience guilt, shame, and sadness" (Harold & Sellers 2018, p. 379).

Tullius, De Kroon, Almansa, and Reijneveld (2021) also found divorce of parents can increase adolescents' risk for depression, anxiety, and substance abuse
(Tullius et al., 2021). In their study of 2,230 US 10- to 12-year-old adolescents,
Tullius and colleagues discovered that externalizing problems (i.e., substance
use and delinquency) and internalizing problems (e.g., depression and anxiety)
increased over 4 years after a parental divorce compared to adolescents who did
not experience a divorce. Some reasons for these increased behavior problems are
linked to socioeconomic effects of moving to an area with more crime and attending a school with lower academic performance. Other reasons are estrangement
from one parent and feelings of guilt. Adolescents are particularly vulnerable to
the impact of divorce due to the plasticity of the adolescent brain and increased
cortical circuitry in response to environmental factors (Tullius et al., 2021). This
critical neurological period makes mental health interventions for adolescents of
divorced parents essential.

Based on this information, I believe the impact of divorce on David includes
his depression, relationship problems with his father, and potential problems in
his future romantic relationships. Because David is the oldest male child, he may
blame himself for not protecting his mother and he may feel powerless over his
ability to "fix" his father. Because David could be at risk for substance use, I will
consider the possibility of needing to screen for any use of weed, alcohol, or other
substances.

Impact of Extremist Groups

In 2021, the Southern Poverty Law Center documented 1,221 hate and antigov-
ernment extremist groups across the United States (Miller & Rivas, 2022). In
2020, there was a substantial increase in US domestic attacks at demonstrations
by violent domestic extremist groups (Doxsee, Jones, Thompson, Halstead, &

Hwan, 2022). Violent domestic extremist groups in the United States can be categorized into four ideologies of violent far-right, violent far-left, religious, and ethnonationalists (Doxsee et al., 2022). Violent far-right groups have extremist ideology such as racial or ethnic supremacy, opposition to government authority, hatred based on sexuality or gender identity, or conspiracy theories that do not correspond to mainstream political parties in the United States. Violent far-left groups have extremist ideology such as opposition to capitalism, support for environmental causes or animal rights, pro-communist, or support for anarchism. Extreme religious terrorist groups are motivated by a faith-based belief system, such as Christianity, Hinduism, Islam, Judaism, or other faiths. Ethnonationalists are motivated by racial, ethnic, or nationalist goals. In each of these groups, violence is most often perpetrated by a single individual or a small network rather than a larger group.

Extremist groups' rhetoric is readily accessible on the internet, where adolescents tend to spend hours of time (Rousseau & Hassan, 2019). The danger for adolescents is that they are still developing their cognitive ability for discerning facts versus opinions, moral judgment, ideology, and identity (Wong, Hall, & Wong Hernandez, 2020). Not all adolescents reach formal operations with the ability to consider various perspectives, systematically test hypotheses, or show hypothetico-deductive reasoning. This makes some adolescents prone to hold idealistic beliefs without considering complexities of problems or contradictions of values. Adolescents can be psychologically vulnerable to extremist groups if they have preexisting mental illness, traumatic experiences, socialization problems, experiences with discrimination, or delinquency (Harpviken, 2020).

In contrast, some adolescents have developed formal operations with the ability to understand why others have certain perspectives, so they are less prone to be swayed by rhetoric of extremist groups. However, typically adolescents have not reached post-formal operations with the ability to understand relativism (e.g., knowing perspectives of truth are based on culture or historical context and are not absolute) (Wong et al., 2022). Therefore, adolescents may understand a different perspective but are insistent that their truth is the right way without the cognitive ability to navigate complexities while maintaining emotional regulation, which results in cognitive distortions, condemnation of others, and emotional cutoff.

Based on this information, because David is very intelligent, he seems to be the latter type of adolescent who has developed formal operations but not post-formal operations. David may understand that his father's extremist group holds ideas that are dangerous and against David's values. However, David's extreme anger and emotional cutoff from his father seem to indicate that David has his own cognitive distortions and needs help navigating cognitive complexities while maintaining emotional regulation.

Treatment Approach

Given David's developmental level, he will benefit from both Cognitive Behavior Therapy (Beck & Weishaar, 2018) and Expressive Arts (Rubin, 2011) for several reasons. First, David has the developmental capacity to analyze his thoughts and develop balanced thinking. Second, his depression and withdrawn stance require a nonverbal engagement to activate his experiences in a nonthreatening manner through expressive arts. Third, he needs coping strategies and conflict management skills to use during interactions with his father.

Cognitive Behavior Therapy

Cognitive Behavioral Therapy is based on the theory that schemas (e.g., core beliefs and basic assumptions about how the world operates) lead to automatic thoughts that determine emotions and behaviors (Beck & Weishaar, 2018). For example, David may have a schema that "I am only secure when my parents get along and stay together" resulting in an automatic negative thought that "it is a catastrophe that my dad got caught up in an extremist political group and divorced my mom." This results in David feeling angry and punishing dad with withdrawn behavior. Common cognitive distortions are (a) arbitrary inference of making conclusions without evidence (e.g., "my dad chats with extremists online, so he must have committed a violent crime"); (b) over-generalization of creating a general rule from one incident (e.g., "all marriages are horrible"); (c) personalization of attributing external events to oneself (e.g., "the divorce was my fault because I could have talked dad out of it"); (d) dichotomous all-or-nothing thinking (e.g., "my relationship with my dad will always be terrible" and "my mom has no responsibility in causing the divorce"); and (e) catastrophizing (e.g., "it is a catastrophe that my dad is in a violent extremist group, and I must have nothing to do with him").

Beck believed these cognitive distortions can contribute to the cognitive triad of depression. A person views (1) self as inadequate and worthless (e.g., "I am worthless because I could not prevent my parent's divorce or control my father's extreme beliefs"); (2) the world is devoid of pleasure (e.g., "No one will want to be my friend when they find out how messed up my dad is, so there is no joy in my life"); and (3) the future is hopeless (e.g., "there is no chance of my future relationship with dad or others being better than the present").

Fortunately, the evidence for CBT efficacy in decreasing depression in adolescents is extensive (Thoma, Pilecki, & McKay, 2015). The role of the CBT counselor is to be a warm, empathic collaborative guide exploring the adolescent's world (Beck & Weishaar, 2018). Together with the client, the counselor gathers information for a functional and cognitive analysis to identify cognitive distortions, examine evidence, develop balanced thoughts, and develop coping strategies. For David, I will use CBT strategies of supportive reflection of emotions and perceptions, relaxation/deep breathing, mindfulness training, psychoeducation about the cognitive triangle and types of cognitive distortions, examination of evidence for cognitions, cognitive reframing to develop balanced thoughts, healthy coping and communication strategies, role-play/behavioral rehearsal, and structured problem solving (Beck & Weishaar, 2018; Phifer, Crowder, Elsenraat, & Hull, 2020). In addition, I will use third-generation CBT strategies from Dialectical Behavior Therapy (Linehan, 2014; Rathus & Miller, 2014) such as mindfulness, emotion regulation, distress tolerance, and interpersonal effectiveness as well as Acceptance and Commitment Therapy (Hayes, Strosahl, & Wilson, 2016; Turrell & Bell, 2016) such as thought defusion, acceptance, connecting with values, and committed action.

Expressive Arts

Expressive arts such as drawing, painting, collages, clay creations, sand tray, music, dance, or drama can promote healing in clients when a therapist guides clients in thoughtful reflection on the process (Malchiodi, 2005; Rubin, 2011). Through expressive arts, adolescents can authentically and effectively express their experiences, perceptions, feelings, and desires without the limits of words (Malchiodi, 2005). D. W. Winnicott was credited with saying "it is only in being creative that the individual discovers the self." This deeper understanding of self can promote self-acceptance, which can improve interpersonal relationships. Recent research shows expressive arts with adolescents helped decrease their stress and anxiety (Lindsey, Robertson, & Lindsey, 2018), increase empathy (Gujing et al., 2019), and increase social competence (Forrest-Bank, Nicotera, Bassett, & Ferrarone, 2016).

Numerous expressive art strategies may be helpful to David. In the first session, I will begin with a sand tray mindfulness activity, asking David to describe how the sand feels and looks without judgment of good or bad but rather curiosity and attentiveness. This practice lays a foundation for him to use this mindfulness skill with people. Then I will ask David to select miniatures to represent each member of his family followed by reflective processing (Homeyer & Sweeney, 2022). This activity helps me identify his perceptions and possibly negative cognitions toward family members.

In a subsequent session, I will ask David to use markers or oil pastels to draw a safe place as a visual reminder that he can self-soothe by visualizing his safe place (Guzman, 2020). I will ask David to select a current song that represents himself now and a song that represents his hopes. This activity can help provide him motivation for the difficult work in therapy. The color-your-life activity (O'Connor, Schaefer, & Braverman, 2015), representing prominent emotions with different colors in an outline of a person (Drewes, 2001), will help David express contrasting emotions he experienced before and after his parents' divorce. I will ask David to create collages of himself and his parents by finding pictures on his phone and online that represent them as a method to help David appreciate their unique characteristics and complexities.

To increase David's sense of power, I will ask him to complete several other art activities such as power affirmation (e.g., writing an affirmation using block letters); strength shield (e.g., drawing a shield and writing his strengths in it); power and protection symbols molded from clay; building boundaries, not walls (e.g., gluing paper around a drawing of self); and bridge drawing of where he wants to go in his relationship with his dad and the obstacles he will have to overcome (Guzman, 2020).

Case Study Application

Treatment Goals

My overall treatment goals for David are to decrease his depressive symptoms and increase healthy coping and communication strategies. My treatment objectives for David are:

1. verbally or artistically expressing his experiences, perceptions, feelings, and desires with eventual emotional regulation by the end of each session;
2. consistent monitoring of automatic thoughts and either replacing with reality-oriented balanced thoughts or committing to value-oriented actions at least once a session;
3. developing a healthy understanding of his parents' divorce as evidenced by believing that it was not his fault and respecting parents' freedom of choice; and
4. demonstrating healthy and effective coping and communication strategies at least once per session.

To accomplish these treatment goals and objectives, I will use the expressive art activities and CBT treatment strategies described above.

Initial Sessions

With this deeper understanding of divorce, political extremist groups, and treatment approaches, we can now apply them to David. My goals for the first session were to develop rapport, assess David's working diagnosis, identify David's treatment goals, facilitate his expression, and provide some beginning coping skills. I prepared by setting out the sand tray and hundreds of miniature items organized into categories (e.g., people, domestic animals, wild animals, cartoon characters, household items, nature, spiritual items, death and scary items, etc.). After introducing myself, obtaining informed assent including limits of confidentiality, I invited David to use the sand tray.

After the sand tray, I asked what he would like to accomplish in our counseling together. We agreed on the treatment goals listed above. I also gave David at least two practical coping strategies for some symptom relief. I explained and demonstrated deep breathing to calm his body and the 5-4-3-2-1 grounding activity (e.g., 5 things he can see; 4 things he can touch; 3 things he can hear; 2 things he can smell; and 1 thing he can taste) to calm his mind. See Session 1 transcript for a summary.

TABLE 13.1. **DAVID: SESSION 1**

Transcript	Analysis
T: "As you can see, I have a sand tray here. I would like to invite you to place your hands into the sand if you would like."	Introduction of a grounding technique. The invitation allows him choice during a time when he believes that he has had little choice.
D: "Okay. This is a little weird."	Adolescents often feel awkward in general and are sometimes surprised by expressive arts.
T: "You feel hesitant, which is common for the first time. You are welcome to go at your own pace or just watch."	Reflection of feeling and normalization helps him feel understood. Giving him a choice facilitates his personal power.
D: "I guess I'll give it a try."	His willingness to engage aids in my assessment of him as a brave young man who is motivated to improve.
T: "How does the sand feel to you? Cool, warm, hot? . . . What do you notice when you look at it closely? Paying attention to describe things without judgment as good or bad is called mindfulness. Have you heard that term before? What do you know about it? Doing this with inanimate objects helps us practice so we can eventually do this with people."	I guide him through a mindfulness activity to lay a foundation of nonjudgmental perspective. My hope is that he will experience me as nonjudgmental and accepting toward him. Eventually I hope he integrates mindfulness so we can apply it to his father and himself.
T: "Now, I would like to invite you to take some time to look through these miniatures and select some that represent each member of your family. Place them in the sand tray as you go along. You can also use items to show how your world looks right now."	I sit quietly as David engages in the activity. When he is finished, I process his creation by saying, "If you would like, you can tell me about your sand tray and what the items represent"; "looking at the position of the items in relation to each other, what do you notice?"; "which family member are you closest to and farthest from?"; "what is each family member thinking and feeling?"; "if you could make your life better, what would you change or add to the sand tray?"; and "what feelings did you become aware of doing this?"
D: "This princess in the cage is my mother. This wild, angry ape is my father. This annoying yappy dog is my sister. I am a big dog trying my best to protect the princess from the ape."	Sand tray miniatures convey David's perceptions of his family members' roles, thoughts, and feelings. It is common for the oldest male to assume a protector role and yet feel ineffective at that role.

For the second session, I asked David to use markers or oil pastels to draw a safe space and helped him internalize the safe space through deep breathing, mindfulness, and visualization. Then I explained the cognitive triangle. Afterward, I used dominos to help him understand the connection between triggers such as his dad's voice, his physiological responses of tense muscles, thoughts, feelings, and behaviors. Finally, I guided David in progressive muscle relaxation. During the third session, we discussed categories of thinking errors such as all or nothing, overgeneralization, personalization, and catastrophizing. To help David apply this, I used an expressive arts technique of searching social media for examples of thinking errors. He was quite enthusiastic about this and found a video of a young child crying because he did not get to eat all the candy to illustrate all-or-nothing thinking. He also found a video of a "Karen" (i.e., an entitled woman loudly complaining about not getting what she ordered) to illustrate catastrophizing.

Middle Sessions

During session 4, David's anger toward his father became intense again.

To reinforce the concept of psychological boundaries, I guide David in the expressive art activity of "building boundaries, not walls" (Guzman, 2020). Throughout the rest of the sessions, I integrate DBT and ACT skills with expressive arts activities.

TABLE 13.2.   **DAVID: SESSION 4**

Transcript	Analysis
D: "My dad is such an idiot. I hate him. How is that for all-or-nothing thinking!"	Intense anger is expected at this point. David feels awkward and hurt so he uses sarcasm as a distractor.
T: "You get an A+ in that! [Therapeutic pause] And it is clear you *are* furious with him. His actions offend you."	In response to his sarcasm, I attempt to add comic relief to honor his need for a momentary break from the intensity. I also stay with his feelings and link them to his perceptions.
D: "Well, what person in their right mind wouldn't be offended by his racist insults and gestures. This weekend, he . . . [describes an incident in which his father openly displayed racism]."	David's voice tone, facial muscles, and arms are tense as he expresses his rage. He seems to accurately perceive his father's actions as racist *and* entangles them in his own sense of self, resulting in a thinking error of personalization and thought fusion.
T: [Deep sigh and shakes head] "Your rage about *his* racism comes from your values of respecting all people."	My deep sigh is intended to show empathy and role model deep breathing. My shaking head is intended to align with his values against racism. My reflection is intended to disentangle his father's racism from David's values.
D: "Yeah. I just don't want to even be associated with him at all. He's embarrassing."	It is common for adolescents to believe everyone is looking at them and judging them. This leads to an entangling thought that David owns his father's values. Consequently, David has all-or-nothing thinking that he must always stay away from his father.
T: "You believe people will assume you are racist as well. Maybe you're concluding that the only way to separate others' misjudgments about you is to stay a thousand miles away from dad. [Therapeutic pause] Let's examine those two thoughts separately. What's the evidence for and against people assuming you are racist? . . . Your own nonverbal unapproving reactions and hanging back for a minute can show others you don't agree. . . . What are ways to establish psychological boundaries with Dad?"	I reflect the two separate thoughts. I invite him into a process of examining evidence and eventually thought defusion. I elicit examples of David being able to separate himself from a good friend's "crazy" idea while still being friends with him. I reaffirm that David is the one that decides his own values and he does not have to allow others' perceptions to fuse him with dad. I introduce the concept of psychological boundaries and interpersonal communication skills of "I statements" and assertively asking for what you need.

Ethical and Cultural Considerations

Ethical considerations were crucial in David's case for several reasons. First, I must inform David's dad that I am seeing David in counseling. Even though the divorce decree gives his mother the right to obtain mental health services for David, I am still legally and ethically obligated to contact his father. I emailed his dad to introduce myself, invited him to schedule a session with me or email me concerns, and explained the overall treatment goals. As expected, David's dad responded to the email that he believes counseling is "BS" but that he will contact his lawyer if there is any trouble. I entered his email into my electronic notes. I reviewed with my colleagues our policies and procedures to ensure that I was following all proper ethical and legal steps.

Second, although I obtained informed consent from David's mother, I must obtain verbal assent from David. I explained that counseling is a professional relationship rather than a social relationship. I explained confidentiality, the limits of confidentiality, and that I intended not to give details of what he says to his parents but that his parents have a legal right to records. Third, because David is a minor, I assumed that my notes will be subpoenaed at some point or at least requested by his dad. I was careful to make sure my notes were clear enough to me but vague enough to maintain David's confidentiality. Fourth, I must carefully consult with colleagues and legal counsel about what may be considered "serious and foreseeable harm" or "duty to warn." In Texas, there are legal limits against duty to warn to protect confidentiality, but counselors can contact police. Therefore, if David disclosed evidence such as an email his dad sent about a planned violent activity, then I would have contacted police.

Parent Consultations

Given these ethical issues, it was crucial for me to have regular parent consultations with David's mom and document due diligence in my communication with his dad. At the end of each session, I gave his mother a brief overview of skills that I had taught David such as deep breathing, progressive muscle relaxation, "I" statements, and psychological boundaries. As I described the skill to the mother, it not only reinforced the skill for David but also taught his mother to use the skills as well. I coached his mother to not demand that David use the skill but rather encourage him to use it by role-modeling the skill for him. I found that focusing parent debriefs on skills learned in session satisfies parents' curiosity about the session and gives them a sense of relief and empowerment. If the father requested information about the sessions, I would focus on skills I had taught David.

In divorce cases, it is common for parents to complain about and disparage the other parent. I manage this by reflecting feelings and perceptions. "You are incredibly angry that his father said that, and you are worried that your son will believe it. I will work on helping your son examine evidence about what is true and what is not. I will help him learn strategies to set boundaries." Sometimes volatile parents will not respond well to children using skills such as "I" state-ments, so I asked David, "What do you think will happen if you tried this with your dad?" David was up front by saying, "I can try it with mom but not with dad, because he will punish me." In this case, I coach David either to not use the skill or modify it in some way. During a parent consultation with his dad, I reframed the skill as important for David to use with peers and asked him to be gentle and encouraging when David practices it at home.

Conclusion

David made remarkable progress in understanding that his parents' divorce and his father's behavior were not his responsibility to "fix." He was able to change automatic negative thoughts into balanced thoughts such as "I prefer that my dad would not believe these things, *and* I am only in control of staying committed to my own values." David experienced empowerment in setting psychological bound-aries with both his mother and father through calming himself and communicat-ing his desires. As a therapist, I learned that David was a resilient adolescent with a bright future in managing his own relationships and being committed to creating a just society.

Sample Case Notes

Session 1

Subjective: Client expressed his perception of family members in the sand tray by illustrating his mother as a "trapped princess," his sister as "an annoying yappy dog," his father as "an angry ape," and himself as "a loyal big dog trying to pro-tect the princess from the ape." Client stated, "I'm not depressed, I'm just pissed and embarrassed of my dad. I just want to chill in my room with video games most of the day."

Objective: Initially, client's posture was slumped over, his speech lacked energy, and his eye contact was minimal. During the sand tray, his speech gained more energy, and he increased eye contact with counselor. After counselor explained and demonstrated coping strategies of deep breathing and 5-4-3-2-1 mindfulness activity, client's body was more relaxed.

Assessment: From a Cognitive Behavior Therapy perspective, David appears to be experiencing depressive symptoms due to thinking errors about himself, his fam-ily, and his future. Expressive arts appear to motivate him to express his thoughts and feelings.

Plan: Counselor will provide expressive arts activity of drawing safe place and introduce concept of the cognitive triangle.

Session 4

Subjective: Client expressed intense anger at his father for a gesture that came across as racist. Client stated that he felt embarrassed by it and was concerned others would view him as racist. Client was able to identify evidence that others would not necessarily assume he was racist. Client described strategies of "I" statements and respectful assertiveness to help establish psychological boundaries.

Objective: At the beginning of the session, client's voice tone, facial muscles, and arms were tense, indicating anger. After discussing psychological boundaries and expressive art activity of "building boundaries, not walls," client's body and face were more relaxed.

Assessment: From a CBT perspective, client had a thinking error of personalization and thought fusion that his father's beliefs were imbedded in him. However, examining evidence, thought defusion, coping strategies, and communication strategies helped David decrease his anger and gain confidence in developing psychological boundaries while still maintaining a respectful relationship with his dad.

Plan: Explain distress tolerance of radical acceptance and interpersonal effectiveness of DEAR MAN (a DBT acronym for Describe, Express, Assert, Reinforce, Mindful, Appear, Negotiate). Expressive arts activity of online collages of himself and his parents.

Resources

For Professionals

CBT Toolbox for Children & Adolescents by Lisa Weed Phifer, Amanda K. Crowder, Tracy Elsenraat, & Robert Hull (2020).

Creative Interventions for Children of Divorce by Linda Lowenstein (2006).

Essential Art Therapy Exercises: Effective Techniques to Manage Anxiety, Depression, and PTSD by Leah Guzman, ATR-BC (2020).

For Adolescents

CBT Workbook for Teens by David Lawson (2021).

Stuff That Sucks: A Teen Guide to Accepting What You Can't Change and Committing to What You Can by Ben Sedley (2017).

Suffer Love by Ashley Herring Black (2016).

For Parents

General Guidelines for Parents to Talk to Children about Mental Health, https://www.mentalhealth.gov/talk/parents-caregivers

How to Talk So Teens Will Listen and Listen So Teens Will Talk by Adele Faber & Elaine Mazlish (2006).

Parenting after Divorce: Resolving Conflicts and Meeting Your Children's Needs by Philip Stahl (2007).

Discussion Questions

1. What were some of David's unique experiences and needs from the overlap of divorce and his father's political extremism?
2. How did combining CBT and Expressive Arts facilitate the achievement of David's treatment goals? Give specific examples.
3. As a therapist, what beliefs, biases, and/or emotions would you need to bracket to effectively work with David and his family?
4. What steps would you take to manage ethical and legal issues related to David's case and family? How would you respond if you received a subpoena for custody dispute?

References

Anderson, L. R., Hemez, P. F., & Kreider, R. M. (2022). *Living arrangements of children: 2019.* Household Economic Studies. www.census.gov/content/dam/Census/library/publications/2022/demo/p70-174.pdf

Beck, A. T., & Weishaar, M. (2018). Cognitive therapy. In R. J. Corsini & D. Wedding (Eds.), *Current psychotherapies* (11th ed., instr. ed., pp. 237–272). Cengage.

Çaksen, H. (2022). The effects of parental divorce on children. *Psychiatriki, 33*(1), 81–82. https://doi.org/10.22365/jpsych.2021.040

Centers for Disease Control. (2022). *Provisional number of marriages and marriage rate: United States, 2000–2021.* www.cdc.gov/nchs/data/dvs/marriage-divorce/national-marriage-divorce-rates-00-21.pdf

Doxsee, C., Jones, S. G., Thompson, J., Halstead, K., & Hwang, G. (2022). *Pushed to extremes: Domestic terrorism amid polarization and protest.* Center for Strategic & International Studies. https://www.csis.org/analysis/pushed-extremes-domestic-terrorism-amid-polarization-and-protest

Drewes, A. A. (2001). The gingerbread person feelings map. In C. E. Schaefer & H. Kaduson (Eds.), *101 more play therapy techniques* (pp. 92–97). Aronson.

Forrest-Bank, S. S., Nicotera, N., Bassett, D. M., & Ferrarone, P. (2016). Effects of an expressive art intervention with urban youth in low-income neighborhoods. *Child & Adolescent Social Work Journal, 33*(5), 429–441. https://doi.org/10.1007/s10560-016-0439-3

Gujing, L., Hui, H., Xin, L., Lirong, Z., Yutong, Y., Guofeng, Y., Jing, L., Shulin, Z., Lei, Y., Cheng, L., & Dezhong, Y. (2019). Increased insular connectivity and enhanced empathic ability associated with dance/music training. *Neural Plasticity, 2019.* https://doi.org/10.1155/2019/9693109

Guzman, L. (2020). *Essential art therapy exercises: Effective techniques to manage anxiety, depression, and PTSD.* Rockridge Press.

Harold, G. T., & Sellers, R. (2018). Annual research review: Interparental conflict and youth psychopathology: An evidence review and practice focused update. *Journal of Child Psychology and Psychiatry, 59*(4), 374–402. https://doi.org/10.1111/jcpp.12893

Harpviken, A. N. (2020). Psychological vulnerabilities and extremism among Western youth: A literature review. *Adolescent Research Review, 5*(1), 1–26. https://doi.org/10.1007/s40894-019-00108-y

Hayes, S. C., Strosahl, K. D., & Wilson, K. G. (2016). *Acceptance and commitment therapy: The process and practice of mindful change* (2nd ed.). Guilford Press.

Homeyer, L. E., & Sweeney, D. S. (2022). *Sandtray therapy: A practical manual* (4th ed.). Routledge.

Lindsey, L., Robertson, P., & Lindsey, B. (2018). Expressive arts and mindfulness: Aiding adolescents in understanding and managing their stress. *Journal of Creativity in Mental Health, 13*(3), 288–297. https://doi.org/10.1080/15401383.2018.1427167

Linehan, M. M. (2014). *DBT Skills Training Manual*. Guilford Press.

Lowenstein, L. (2006). *Creative interventions for children of divorce*. Champion Press.

Malchiodi, C. A. (2005). Expressive therapies: History, theory, and practice. In C. A. Malchiodi (Ed.), *Expressive therapies* (pp. 1–15). Guilford Press.

Miller, C., & Rivas, R. C. (2022). *The year in hate and extremism: 2021*. Southern Poverty Law Center. https://www.splcenter.org/year-hate-extremism-2021

O'Connor, K. J., Schaefer, C. E., & Braverman, L. D. (2015). *Handbook of play therapy* (2nd ed.). Wiley.

Phifer, L. W., Crowder, A. K., Elsenraat, T., & Hull, R. (2020). *CBT toolbox for children & adolescents*. PESI.

Rathus, J. H., & Miller, A. L. (2014). *DBT skills manual for adolescents*. Guilford Press.

Rousseau, C., & Hassan, G. (2019). Current challenges in addressing youth mental health in the context of violent radicalization. *Journal of the American Academy of Child & Adolescent Psychiatry, 58*(8), 747–750. https://doi.org/10.1016/j.jaac.2019.03.031

Rubin, J. A. (2011). *The art of art therapy: What every art therapist needs to know*. Routledge/Taylor & Francis Group.

Sands, A., Thompson, E. J., & Gaysina, D. (2017). Long-term influences of parental divorce on offspring affective disorders: A systematic review and meta-analysis. *Journal of Affective Disorders, 218*, 105–114. https://doi.org/10.1016/j.jad.2017.04.015

Thoma, N., Pilecki, B., & McKay, D. (2015). Contemporary cognitive behavior therapy: A review of theory, history, and evidence. *Psychodynamic Psychiatry, 43*(3), 423–462. https://doi.org/10.1521/pdps.2015.43.3.423

Tullius, J. M., De Kroon, M. L. A., Almansa, J., & Reijneveld, S. A. (2021). Adolescents' mental health problems increase after parental divorce, not before, and persist until adulthood: A longitudinal trails study. *European Child & Adolescent Psychiatry, 31*, 969–978. https://doi.org/10.1007/s00787-020-01715-0

Turrell, S. L., & Bell, M. (2016). *ACT for adolescents: Treating teens and adolescents in individual and group therapy*. Context Press.

Wong, D. W., Hall, K. R., & Wong Hernandez, L. (2020). *Counseling individuals through the lifespan* (2nd ed.). Sage.

CHAPTER 14

Sexual Abuse
Trauma-Focused Cognitive Behavior Therapy and Creative Approaches with a Biracial Adolescent

Felicia R. Neubauer

Ava is a 16-year-old biracial female who lives with her biological mother, Ms. Johnson, and her 14-year-old sister, Alexis. Ava sees her biological father on weekends. He and her mother separated when Ava was 10. Ms. Johnson began dating, and when the COVID-19 lockdown happened, she allowed her paramour to stay with them for financial reasons, as she was not working. During the pandemic, Ava was not allowed to see her father for several months due to his asthma, which was a risk factor for COVID-19. When Ms. Johnson became ill with COVID-19, the paramour went into Ava's room nightly and raped her. When Ava began visiting her father again, she disclosed the child sexual abuse (CSA). Ms. Johnson brought Ava for treatment because of continued anxiety, flashbacks, nightmares, noncompliance, crying frequently, and isolating herself.

For this case study, consider:

1. How did the COVID-19 quarantine impact adolescents who experienced CSA?
2. What should the therapist do if Ava avoids talking about the CSA and only wants to talk about COVID-19?
3. What specific treatment strategies should be provided? What should psychoeducation address? What should the trauma narration focus on?

Child Sexual Abuse

Previous literature (Kendall-Tackett, Williams, & Finkelhor, 1993) describes how CSA has a significant impact on a child's development and can persist into adulthood. Kendall-Tackett et al.'s review of 45 studies on CSA revealed that sexually abused children had more symptoms than non-abused children, with abuse accounting for 15–45% of the variance. The most frequent symptoms of CSA were fears, posttraumatic stress disorder, behavior problems, sexualized behaviors, and poor self-esteem. Akinbode, Pedersen, and Lara-Cinisomo (2020) found that women who experienced CSA during their adolescence had more perinatal depression and anxiety than women who did not experience CSA. Kendall-Tackett et al. (1993) also found that the degree of symptomatology was related to specifics of the CSA, such as if there was penetration, the duration and frequency of the abuse, force, the relationship of the perpetrator to the child, and maternal support. de Arellano et al. (2014) found that the severity of trauma symptoms after CSA can also be related to the child's experience of other childhood traumas, including medical trauma, exposure to domestic violence, terrorism, and natural disasters. The severity and duration of trauma symptoms depend on how quickly effective treatment such as Trauma-Focused Cognitive Behavior Therapy (TF-CBT) is provided to the child (Cohen, Mannarino, & Deblinger, 2006).

CSA during COVID-19

When the COVID-19 lockdowns were initiated in March 2020, a concern was that the combination of increased parental stress, lockdown restrictions that kept family members from having typical breaks, and reduced time children spent with mandated reporters would yield an increase in interpersonal traumas such as CSA. At the same time, Child Protective Service (CPS) professionals were working virtually most of the time due to safety concerns about being exposed to COVID-19. In April 2020, CPS reported that home investigations, the court process, and in-home treatment were at a near standstill (Welch & Haskins, 2020). It was considerably more difficult for the child welfare system to effectively check on the nearly 3.5 million children that they usually contacted (Welch & Haskins, 2020). Also in April 2020, the Rape, Abuse, and Incest National Network (RAINN) reported a 22% increase in monthly calls from minors by the end of March 2020 with 67% identifying their perpetrator as a family member and 79% currently living with that perpetrator (Kamenetz, 2020). According to RAINN, the reports coming in indicated that child sexual abuse was escalating in both frequency and severity.

Description of TF-CBT

TF-CBT (Cohen et al., 2006) is an evidence-based treatment developed by Judith Cohen, MD, Esther Deblinger, PhD, and Anthony Mannarino, PhD, and refined over the past 25 years to help children and adolescents recover from trauma. The TF-CBT model was originally designed and found to be efficacious in treating and reducing symptoms related to child sexual abuse. Later research indicated that TF-CBT was efficacious in treating and reducing symptoms for children who had experienced other traumas as well, including domestic violence, terrorism, and natural disasters (de Arrelano et al., 2014). Twenty-one randomized controlled trials conducted throughout the world document that TF-CBT was superior for improving children's trauma symptoms and responses (TF-CBT, 2023).

TF-CBT is a hierarchical treatment approach with several components including psychoeducation, relaxation, cognitive coping, trauma narrative and processing (i.e., gradual exposure), in-vivo exposure, conjoint parent–child sessions, and enhancing safety skills (Cohen et al., 2006). These components are organized into three phases: stabilization, trauma narration, and integration/consolidation.

Stabilization Phase

The stabilization phase consists of psychoeducation, relaxation skills, affect modulation skills, and cognitive coping skills (PRAC) for adolescents. Caregivers also receive this content as well as parenting skills to respond properly to the trauma and behavioral difficulties. Beginning with psychoeducation, adolescents and caregivers are separately provided information about the specific trauma(s) the adolescent experienced and how TF-CBT can help. They are reassured that not every trauma they experienced will necessarily be a focus of the TF-CBT because the skills will generalize. During psychoeducation, the adolescent and caregiver answer questions about what information they already know about the specific type of trauma they endured. This helps the therapist be able to praise involvement, identify accurate and inaccurate information, and discern possible cognitive distortions. The therapist then adds information and corrects misinformation. This approach is engaging and works well for gradual exposure of the trauma early in treatment.

In the stabilization phase, adolescents also learn and practice relaxation skills, affect modulation skills (e.g., feelings identification, expression, and regulation), and cognitive coping. These skills are taught so that adolescents and caregivers can manage general symptoms as well as trauma symptoms rather than avoiding them. Gradual exposure in which the adolescent and caregiver talk about the CSA occurs in each session.

Parenting and behavior management also begin for the caregiver in this phase. The therapist starts by praising caregivers for seeking services. The therapist gives effective instructions on behavioral management such as exploring functional analysis of behavior, explaining differential attention (e.g., reinforcement and extinction of behaviors), giving 5-minute work chores as consequences for inappropriate behavior, providing positive attention, and demonstrating active listening. These skills are used throughout TF-CBT and hopefully after treatment ends.

The therapist also assesses the caregivers' coping skills as well as teaches them relaxation skills, affect modulation skills, and cognitive coping skills. The therapist encourages caregivers to practice the skills in the session and for homework in between. In contrast to the adolescent's sessions where cognitive coping is addressed in the second phase, caregivers learn cognitive coping and restructuring during the stabilization phase. This helps caregivers begin to change their thoughts and feelings related to their adolescent's trauma so caregivers can give more helpful responses.

When using TF-CBT with adolescents, it is helpful to use playful strategies such as artwork, using the What Do You Know? card game for psychoeducation (Deblinger et al., 2019), and using the Triangle of Life online application for cognitive coping and processing (Mannarino & Cohen, 2014). Bibliotherapy and relevant games can also make treatment more fun.

Trauma Narration Phase

In the trauma narration phase, it can be helpful to read a book related to CSA such as the ones listed in the resources below. Then the therapist invites the adolescent to create her own storybook. The therapist segues into the introduction of the trauma narrative by asking the adolescent to describe herself, her strengths, what she likes about herself and her family, and her interests. She also is asked to name the trauma in some way in the introductory chapter. In subsequent sessions, the adolescent is asked to write chapters on when she disclosed the CSA; details about her CSA; and her thoughts, feelings, and body sensations about it. Depending on how long the CSA occurred, and to what extent, there may be one chapter or several. It can be helpful to develop a table of contents with the adolescent and order the chapters from the least to most anxiety-provoking to develop a gradual exposure hierarchy. If multiple traumas are included, they are worked into the same hierarchy.

A tentative hierarchy for Ava is described in the case example. As long as the caregiver is at the same point in the TF-CBT model, the therapist shares the chapters with the caregivers, without the child present, so the caregiver can share and process their thoughts and feelings about it. If the caregivers aren't at the same point, the caregivers complete the stabilization phase before the therapist shares the chapters.

As the adolescent's narrative concludes, the therapist begins to identify covert and overt/hypothetical cognitive distortions to help the adolescent with cognitive and affective reprocessing. The identification of cognitive distortions occurs through strategies such as Socratic questioning, evidence gathering, the best friend role-play, and psychoeducation. The therapist helps the adolescent reprocess these cognitive distortions, separately from the caregiver. As the distortions are reprocessed successfully, the adolescent adds new thoughts and feelings into the narrative, usually at the end of each chapter. The reprocessed chapters are shared again with the caregivers by the therapist, so there are no surprises. This helps prepare the caregivers for when they attend conjoint sessions where the adolescent shares the trauma narrative.

Integration/Consolidation Phase

The integration/consolidation phase focuses on the final components of TF-CBT, namely in vivo mastery (if needed), conjoint sessions, and enhancing safety skills. (Note: If there are ongoing safety issues related to immediate environment, then safety skills are addressed in the stabilization phase). The therapist helps the adolescent identify concerns and locations for in vivo mastery. For example, if the adolescent is afraid to go down into the basement because that was where the

CSA occurred, then an in vivo plan is developed to desensitize the adolescent to be able to go into the basement and spend time there.

It can be very helpful to plan conjoint portions of sessions along the way. Conjoint sessions set the stage so that the adolescent and caregiver are more comfortable by the time they share the adolescent's trauma narrative. Conjoint sessions also help them both practice stabilization skills. These conjoint sessions reinforce psychoeducation, mutual praise, relaxation skills, sharing feelings, and so forth. It is important that both the adolescent and caregiver prepare for conjoint sessions ahead of time by practicing stabilization skills to prevent retraumatization and to enhance the adolescent's healing.

Regarding the sharing of the trauma narrative, the adolescent and the caregiver should know which portions will be shared that day. If the adolescent has any specifics about how the caregiver should or shouldn't respond, the therapist shares this with the caregiver ahead of time. The adolescent, rather than the therapist, is encouraged to read the narrative to the caregiver. The therapist encourages the caregiver to provide active listening and praise for the adolescent's courage. Afterward, the therapist processes the session with the adolescent and caregiver separately.

Age-appropriate provision of sex education should be discussed ahead of time with the caregiver so that cultural/religious/family preferences are addressed. Personal safety skills should be carefully introduced with the idea that whatever the child did to survive the trauma was the correct response, and the new skills learned are tools for their future toolbox. This is important, so the child's response is not heard as problematic. The therapist can talk about other ways adolescents normally keep themselves safe. The idea of "no-go-tell" is introduced and can be compared to fire drills, which are also behavior rehearsals. It should also be stressed that although it is the adolescent's job to help with their own safety, it is not their *responsibility* but, rather, the perpetrator's not to carry out the CSA in the first place. What-if scenarios as well as role-playing some of these scenarios is done when the adolescent can regulate a heightened level of anxiety or discomfort. When role-playing, it is important not to touch the child and to turn off the phone before practicing calling 911. The therapist emphasizes that if abuse occurs in the future, the adolescent can immediately tell an adult and keep telling until the adolescent gets protection and support. The therapist informs the adolescent that this step of telling, in real life, can be difficult and anxiety-provoking, but she now has the courage and skills to persevere.

Case Study Application

Intake Assessment

An assessment was done with Ava and with Ms. Johnson. Standardized measures were administered to assess Ava's trauma symptoms. Ms. Johnson and Ava both endorsed that Ava had significant symptoms of posttraumatic stress disorder

(PTSD), with some symptoms of depression and anxiety. Ava's PTSD symptoms focused on the CSA by Ms. Johnson's paramour. She did not endorse symptoms related to racial trauma or microaggressions and felt that she had a solid support network in this area. Ava had been a fairly compliant child who did well academically and behaviorally. Now, however, she was often quick to sass her parents when they asked her to do something, and she was sometimes short with teachers. The results of the behavior measure were within norms for her age, but her mother was frustrated with the noncompliance and her negative attitude.

Ms. Johnson reported that she herself was having significant difficulties since Ava disclosed the sexual abuse, although she was supportive and believing. Ms. Johnson reported that she felt bad that Ava not only dealt with the repercussions of their COVID-19 restrictions but was also sexually abused by the man she trusted to take care of Ava while she was sick with COVID-19. She blamed herself for not being aware, acknowledging that she was too sick to do more than sleep for much of her illness. Ms. Johnson also blamed COVID-19 for creating the groundwork for the sexual abuse to take place.

Treatment Goals

Treatment goals were as follows:

1. Increase Ava's understanding about trauma and the CSA and its impact on her.
2. Increase her coping skills through relaxation, affect modulation, and cognitive coping.
3. Discuss and process thoughts and feelings related to the CSA to the point of accurate understanding and restoration.
4. Increase her knowledge about age-appropriate sex education and her personal safety skills.
5. Reduce her noncompliance.

Initial Phase of Treatment: Stabilization and Skill Building

First, I met with Ava and Ms. Johnson to go over the results of the assessment measures and to explain Ava's diagnosis of PTSD. I was careful to explain that TF-CBT has been shown in research studies to reduce PTSD symptoms significantly, so there was every reason to believe Ava's symptoms would be much better at the end of the treatment process. I also discussed the likely length of treatment, instilled hope, and talked about how Ms. Johnson's belief in and support of her daughter were the best predictors of outcome for Ava. Her support combined with evidence-based treatment gave them a lot to be positive about.

I spent the rest of that session and part of the next doing psychoeducation about child sexual abuse and the potential impact of the COVID-19 pandemic on adolescents. This was done with Ava and Ms. Johnson separately. Related to child sexual abuse, the What Do You Know card game was used, because including fun

TABLE 14.1. **AVA: INITIAL PHASE**

Transcript	Analysis
T: "Ava, how do you think other kids felt when they were sexually abused?" A: "I guess sad. Mad." T: "Absolutely they may feel sad or mad. How else might they feel?" A: "Um. Scared." T: "Yes. They may feel scared. What else?" A: "I don't know." T: "Good job! Let me add some others. Kids may feel depressed, betrayed, confused, anxious, even brave, because they got through it and told about it. All feelings about the CSA are okay. How did you feel about it?"	Checking to see how well she can identify the different feelings kids may have when they experienced CSA. Then provided gradual exposure (GE) for her own emotions.
A: "Sad. Angry. Confused. Why would he do that when my mom was so sick with COVID?" T: "Why do you think he did that?"	This is a good place to try to link the CSA and pandemic lockdown and see if she'll tell me her underlying thoughts.
A: "Because Mom had to stay away from us." T: "Yes. CSA usually happens in secret, so the perpetrator doesn't get in trouble. Since back then with COVID-19, your mom had to be quarantined for ten days, it made keeping it a secret more likely. Good job, Ava!"	That's accurate.

activities increases engagement of adolescents (Deblinger et al., 2019). With Ava, the activity was done by going from the general to the specific (gradual exposure), asking her what she knew, and praising her. I provided additional and/or missing information and listened for cognitive distortions. This is described as follows:

In subsequent sessions, I taught Ava relaxation skills of diaphragmatic breathing, square breathing, mindfulness, guided imagery, and progressive muscle relaxation. I helped her identify the skills she enjoyed and encouraged her to use them to manage trauma symptoms in and between sessions. Ava demonstrated to her mother the skill of guided imagery about being at the beach. In a separate session, I taught Ms. Johnson the same skills. I encouraged her to use them for herself as well as help Ava practice them if she needed help.

Building on this, I talked to them separately about affect modulation, including feelings identification, expression, and modulation skills. Ava did not have significant difficulties with affect modulation, and this was all she needed. However, it should be noted that some adolescents do have significant difficulties and need to spend more time in this component. I checked in with Ava about affect modulation skills in subsequent sessions and worked on this component with Ms. Johnson.

I also talked with Ava and Ms. Johnson separately about cognitive coping and taught them the cognitive triangle (triad). This was done slightly differently for the adolescent and caregiver, as previously noted. They learned common types of cognitive distortions and practiced cognitive processing of general thoughts and examples. I elicited thoughts, feelings, and reactions from Ms. Johnson about the

CSA of her daughter, and used strategies such as Socratic questioning, evidence gathering, and psychoeducation for her to learn to reprocess.

Middle Phase of Treatment: Trauma Narration and Cognitive Processing

In the middle phase of treatment, I talked about trauma narration and normalized anticipatory anxiety about it. I stated that many adolescents reported how helpful it was to talk about their traumatic experiences in detail and to process them. I read a book (i.e., *Please Tell*) with Ava about CSA, noting that it was a bit young for her age. Then I worked on a table of contents with Ava for her own book of traumatic experiences. I started with the introduction and ended with the conclusion. We ordered the traumatic experiences from easiest to most anxiety-provoking. Ava, with input from me, included chapters on her disclosure of sexual abuse; when her mother became ill with the virus and had to isolate, which led to the paramour being in more of a caretaking role; and the first, last, and most difficult time he sexually abused her. Ava chose to draw pictures for each of the chapters.

As discussed above, if Ava wanted to talk only about the pandemic and avoid talking about the CSA, I would need to segue to the CSA anyway and not collude with Ava's avoidance. I would need to reinforce relaxation, affect modulation, and cognitive coping (PRAC) skills. I would ensure that the trauma narration includes the quarantine but would focus on the CSA.

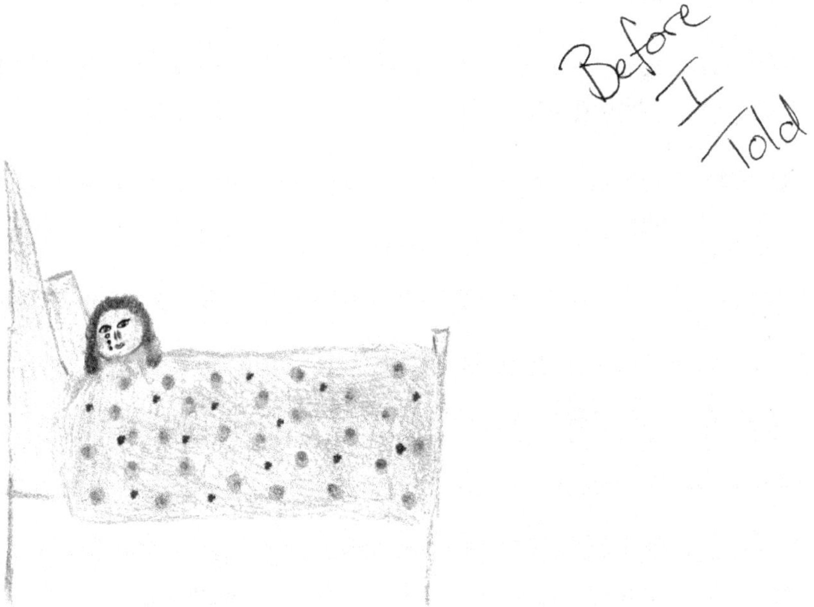

Figure 14.1. "Before I Told" Drawing courtesy of Felicia Neubauer, based on client(s)' representations.

In preparation for this phase, I talked to Ms. Johnson to remind her that this is the part of treatment that increases anxiety, and we needed to work together to help Ava not avoid treatment and to discuss her own avoidance if it arose. I also continued to work with Ms. Johnson on her own skills and behavior management. Once trauma narration began, I met with Ava first to review homework, including skill practice, and elicit the trauma narrative chapter for the session. First, I elicited an introduction; I wrote down everything Ava said and then read it back to her for additional gradual exposure and clarification to make any corrections. Then I shared the chapter with Ms. Johnson, without Ava present, so that Ms. Johnson could process it.

In the following session, I elicited a chapter that was identified by Ava as easiest, which was when her mother became ill, followed by the disclosure and first experience of CSA. These and the remaining chapters were elicited in the order described above. After each chapter was written, I shared it with Ms. Johnson by herself so she could process the information.

Once the trauma narration was completely elicited, I worked with Ava to use strategies including psychoeducation, evidence gathering, and Socratic questioning to process her current and previous thoughts. I helped Ava facilitate more appropriate thinking and better feeling about the trauma experiences. This is shown as follows:

TABLE 14.2.   AVA: MIDDLE PHASE

Transcript	Analysis
T: "Let's look at some of the thoughts you have identified in here. You said if the pandemic didn't happen and your mom didn't get sick, the CSA wouldn't have happened." A: "Yes. If COVID didn't happen, he wouldn't have been living with us, my mom wouldn't have been ill, and he wouldn't have gotten to me to sexually abuse me." T: "That sounds like it could be true. However, do you think all kids quarantined during the pandemic were sexually abused?"	There is some validity to that possibility or at least the timing. Let's see if we can go deeper.
A: "Probably not." T: "Yes. So, what do you think made the difference?" A: "I guess most people wouldn't think about doing CSA, so it didn't happen to the kids around them." T: "Exactly right, Ava. Great job. So, what made the CSA happen then?"	Let's see if she can use logic to dispute and reprocess her own cognitive distortion.
A: "The circumstances were caused by COVID, but it was because he thought about it and acted on it that the CSA happened."	Awesome job, Ava! Praising the cognitive restructuring, this is a much more accurate thought; cognitive processing is working.

As the chapters were reprocessed, I shared them with Ms. Johnson again. When the entire trauma narration was reprocessed, it was put in order, and then I worked with Ava and Ms. Johnson to prepare them for the conjoint sessions where Ava would share the trauma narration directly with her mother. This included having them identify which coping strategies they would use if needed, having Ava give input into how she wanted her mother to respond, and having Ms. Johnson practice her responses. The conjoint sessions were then held to prepare them, share the narration, and talk with each to process the experience.

The remaining components of the TF-CBT, such as age-appropriate sex education, were completed in subsequent sessions. I spoke with Ms. Johnson to discuss the subject matter with her and to encourage her to do the sex education with Ava herself, so she knew exactly what was being said and so she could share her values and beliefs. In preparation for the sex education discussion with Ava, I gave Ms. Johnson a book (*What's Happening to My Body: Book for Girls*, Madaras, 2007) to review and use. Although many caregivers prefer that the therapist discuss the sex education directly with their adolescent, Ms. Johnson did talk with Ava herself. Ava did not need to do in vivo exposure, so that is not included here.

In the final component, which overlapped with conjoint sessions, I explained to Ava that everything she did during the trauma was the right thing, because she survived it, and the skills she learned are additional tools for her toolbox. This is important so Ava did not feel that I thought she responded "wrongly" at the time. Then what-if situations were discussed and role plays were done where she practiced the concepts of personal safety skills, including yelling no, getting away, telling an adult, and continuing to tell until someone believes and helps her.

Ending Treatment

During the final session, Ava and Ms. Johnson completed the same standardized measures for posttreatment results, which showed that Ava had significantly fewer trauma symptoms and no longer met full criteria for a posttraumatic stress diagnosis. These results were shared with Ava and her mother. I gave Ava her certificate of completion. We shared cupcakes together and discussed the importance of continuing to use her treatment skills. I stressed that if Ava has thoughts or feelings about her traumatic experiences, she should continue to talk to her mother about it, and they could call for booster sessions if needed.

Ethical and Cultural Considerations

For racially and ethnically diverse clients, the therapist needs to assess for racial trauma in addition to the CSA. Ava, as a biracial adolescent, felt like she was not exactly like her African American father or her Caucasian mother. However, she had support from her father and community to process racism, so Ava reported that racial trauma was not a concern for her.

The therapist also needs to assess whether adolescents have significant trauma symptoms related to the impact of COVID-19. TF-CBT skills can generalize to manage many traumas. Ava processed her COVID-related concerns with the skills she learned in TF-CBT.

In cases of abuse, the therapist needs to ensure that abuse was reported to authorities and obtain the report number for case records. If the abuse was not properly reported, then the therapist needs to contact police and/or their local Child Protective Services. Finally, therapists need to be aware that they may be called into court to testify. Therefore, every effort needs to be made to keep accurate and timely records as well as review state rules and regulations. In cases of divorce, therapists need to read the most recent divorce decree to determine which person has rights to obtain mental health services. The therapist needs to inform all parents or caregivers of the treatment being provided and offer to meet with them as needed.

Parent Consultations

As described above, I provided parent consultation and guidance throughout TF-CBT to Ava's mother, Ms. Johnson. I invited Ava's father to join the process. He declined to do so on a regular basis due to distance and time constraints. However, he was willing to engage in a few telehealth sessions in which I informed him of treatment goals and strategies, common symptoms of CSA, Ava's progress, and parenting strategies to facilitate her coping skills. Although Ava's father experienced intense guilt and anger regarding her CSA, he declined to seek his own counseling mostly due to stigma. Therefore, I normalized his feelings, coached him on the same coping skills I was teaching Ava, and provided him parenting resources as shown below.

Conclusion

Ava and her mother appeared to benefit from TF-CBT. Standardized measures, anecdotal information, as well as my observations, showed significant treatment progress and symptom reduction. The willingness of Ava and Ms. Johnson to work on and implement the components was instrumental in Ava's symptom reduction. Implementation of behavior management reduced Ava's noncompliance. Ava was able to process the CSA and the impact of her mother's illness. Ms. Johnson was able to reduce her self-blame and to be instrumental in her daughter's symptom reduction. Both Ava and Ms. Johnson learned how resilient they are. Despite being guardedly confident in the beginning of treatment during COVID-19, I learned that the TF-CBT worked well related to the impact of COVID-19.

Sample Case Notes

Session 1

Ava was accompanied to the individual treatment session by her mother. Met with Ms. Johnson, who reported a better week and that Ava was less stressed. Relaxation homework was reviewed with each separately, and both reported using them and found them helpful. Ms. Johnson learned the cognitive triangle, and homework was assigned for her to practice during the week. The cognitive triangle was introduced to Ava, and read and discussed part of a storybook about changing negative thinking to positive thinking. Ava was given homework to continue to practice relaxation skills and to use the cognitive coping skills related to some peer difficulties.

Resources

For Professionals

Helping the Traumatized Child: A Workbook for Therapists (Helpful Materials to Support Therapists Using TFCBT: Trauma-Focused Cognitive Behavioral Therapy) by George Sachs (2015).

NCTSN. *Secondary Traumatic Stress in Professionals Treating Child Sexual Abuse*, https://www.nctsn.org/resources/secondary-traumatic-stress-professionals -treating-child-sexual-abuse

TF-CBT Web 2.0: A course for Trauma-Focused Cognitive Behavioral Therapy, https://tfcbt2.musc.edu/

For Children and Adolescents

Hush: Moving from Silence to Healing after Childhood Sexual Abuse by Nicole Braddock Bromley (2007).

The Hyena Who Lost Her Laugh: A Story about Changing Your Negative Thinking by Jessica Lamb-Shapiro (2000).

It's Not Your Fault by Lindsay Kreps (2020).

Please Tell: A Child's Story about Sexual Abuse by Jessie (1991).

What's Happening to My Body by Lynda Madaras (2007).

For Parents

Healing the Harm Done: A Parent's Guide to Helping Your Child Overcome the Effects of Sexual Abuse (English and Spanish edition) by Jennifer Y. Levy-Peck (2009).

NCTSN. *Creating Supportive Environments When Scary Things Happen*, https:// www.nctsn.org/resources/creating-supportive-environments-when-scary -things-happen

NCTSN. *Teen Sexual Assault: Information for Parents*, https://www.nctsn.org/resources/teen-sexual-assault-information-parents

Discussion Questions

1. What behaviors might be noticed in an adolescent that might concern a parent about possible trauma?
2. If Ava had refused to go into detail in the trauma narrative, how could the therapist have helped her work through avoidance?
3. If Ava's father had also wanted to participate in the TF-CBT, how might the therapist work with separated parents?
4. How did the therapist work with Ava to identify a table of contents and subsequent hierarchy for trauma narration?

References

Akinbode, T. D., Pedersen, C., & Lara-Cinisomo, S. (2020). The price of pre-adolescent abuse: Effects of sexual abuse on perinatal depression and anxiety. *Maternal and Child Health Journal, 25*, 1083–1093. https://doi.org/10.1007/s10995-020-03088-x

Cohen, J. A., Mannarino, A. P., & Deblinger, E. (2006). *Treating trauma and traumatic grief in children and adolescents*. Guilford Press.

de Arellano, M. A. R., Lyman, D. R., Jobe-Shields, L., George, P., Dougherty, R. H., Daniels, A. S., Ghose, S. S., Huang, L., & Delphin-Rittmon, M. E. (2014). Trauma-focused cognitive-behavioral therapy for children and adolescents: Assessing the evidence. *Psychiatric Services, 65*(5), 591–602. https://doi.org/10.1176/appi.ps.201300255

Deblinger, E., Neubauer, F., Runyon, M., Baker, D., Sirois-Geddie, A., Marquez, Y. I., & Pollio, E. (2019). *What do you know? A therapeutic card game about childhood trauma, sex education, and personal safety* (2nd ed.). CARES Institute, Rowan Medicine.

Kamenetz, A. (2020). *Child sexual abuse reports are on the rise amid lockdown orders*. NPR. https://www.npr.org/sections/coronavirus-live-updates/2020/04/28/847251985/child-sexual-abuse-reports-are-on-the-rise-amid-lockdown-orders

Kendall-Tackett, K. A., Williams, L. M., & Finkelhor, D. (1993). Impact of sexual abuse on children: A review and synthesis of recent empirical studies. *Psychological Bulletin, 113*(1), 164–180. https://doi.org/10.1037/0033-2909.113.1.164

Mannarino, A., & Cohen, J. (2014). *TF-CBT triangle of life app*. https://tfcbt.org/tf-cbt-triangle-of-life/

TF-CBT. (2023). *About trauma-focused cognitive behavior therapy (TF-CBT)*. http://Tfcbt.org

Welch, M., & Haskins, R. (2020, April 30). *What COVID-19 means for America's child welfare system.* Brookings. https://www.brookings.edu/articles/what-covid-19-means-for-americas-child-welfare-system/

CHAPTER 15

Self-Harm
Dialectical Behavior Therapy with an African American Adolescent
Anelie Etienne and Domonique Messing

Ashly Johnson is a 14-year-old African American female. Ashly lives with her mother, Amber Johnson, a 34-year-old African American woman, and three younger half siblings, James Johnson, 10, Kevin Johnson, 7, and Nicole Miller, 5. Ashly's mother's boyfriend, Robert Miller, is a 39-year-old Caucasian man and is the father of Nicole, and he resides in the home. Ashly's father, Levi Smith, is a 35-year-old African American man who lives three towns over with his girlfriend, Sarah King, who is African American, and Ashly's half sister Leah Smith, who is 6. Ashly and her father have a strained relationship, in part because he is unable to consistently spend time with Ashly. Mr. Smith works a factory job with no paid time off and relies on his girlfriend for transportation. Ashley's mother and her boyfriend (Mr. Miller) have a contentious relationship, often having verbal arguments and one reported physical fight occurring during Ms. Johnson's pregnancy with Nicole. Ashly frequently stayed with a friend, who lived up the street, to escape the tension and fights at home. Until recently, the family lived in a predominantly African American neighborhood.

Mr. Miller recently won a lawsuit against his former construction employer and decided to move the family to a more affluent, predominantly Caucasian neighborhood. As a result, Ashly changed schools and struggled to make new friends. Ashly reports that "the neighbors are mean, and I feel like an outsider at school." Ashly shared that at school "a group of girls called me nig—and monkey." Ashly is ostracized by her peers, and her grades have begun to decline. Ashly has told her mother, "I feel sad all the time." Ashly wants to move back to her old neighborhood and frequently shares this with her mother. However, Ms. Johnson is unable to afford rent without Mr. Miller. Ashly's father expressed that he is unable to care for her financially and that she must stay with her mother. Ms. Johnson recently noticed cuts on Ashly's right arm. Ms. Johnson is seeking counseling services for Ashly due to her cutting, experience of racism, isolation, and declining grades.

For this case study, consider:

1. What are the common concerns for African American adolescents who experience hate speech? What has contributed to Ashly's behavior of self-harm?
2. What is the rationale for using Dialectical Behavior Therapy (DBT) with Ashly?
3. What ethical guidelines need to be considered?

Hate Speech: A Form of Bullying

For this case study, we will consider hate speech as a form of bullying and will evaluate the prevalence of self-injurious behaviors in adolescents who experience symptoms resulting from hate speech. This information will help us understand the impact of racially motivated behaviors, particularly in adolescents, and the methodology to treat the symptoms effectively.

Many people believe teasing is a common aspect of the coming-of-age process that most children face. However, some believe there is a threshold between harmless teasing and behavior that seems more sinister. With racial tensions rising, hate speech is becoming more common and its impacts more apparent. Kansok-Dusche and colleagues' (2022) study noted that an exclusive definition did not exist for hate speech. However, it was generally described as an aggressive or violent interaction rooted in prejudice, based on nationality, race, ethnicity, or sexual orientation with malicious intent (Kansok-Dusche et al., 2022).

Although the literature reveals gaps in the research about hate speech, the experience of African American youth and the impact of race-related trauma are undeniable. African American girls simultaneously manage the physiological, psychological, and psychosocial challenges of adolescence, race, and gender. They may also face other uncontrollable components such as family income. Socio-economic status is a major factor in the prevalence of hate speech, with lower-income families being more likely to experience hate speech when compared to their more affluent counterparts (Kansok-Dusche et al., 2022).

The experience of hate speech during an African American girl's journey through her developmental stages can pose additional strains on her mental health, as well as negatively impact her behavior and school performance (Evans, 2019). Children lack the emotional intelligence to cope with the trauma imposed on them when they experience race-related stress, and consequently maladaptive behaviors form (Kansok-Dusche et al., 2022). Unfortunately, studies have shown that when challenging behaviors occur in school, African American girls receive harsher discipline compared to their White counterparts (Evans, 2019). Often, this form of systemic racism is one of many examples of the intersectionality of race and institutions that they may encounter on their path through life as an African American girl.

According to a longitudinal study over 10 years, the Centers for Disease Control and Prevention (2023) reported that three out of five high school–age girls experience chronic feelings of sadness and hopelessness, with a record high in 2021. Although sadness and hopelessness may increase for all female high-school students, African Americans were more likely to have attempted suicide and more likely to miss school because they felt unsafe (Centers for Disease Control and Prevention, 2023). More than 90% of African American youth over the age of 8 years old will be exposed to racial discrimination, which will have an adverse impact on their self-esteem, disposition, and interpersonal skills, and significantly reduce their ability to perform academically (Williams, 2020).

Non-Suicidal Self-Injury

Non-suicidal self-injury (NSSI) is defined as "purposeful, self-inflicted destruction of one's own body that is neither socially endorsed (e.g., piercing, tattooing, scarification) nor deliberately intended to lead to death" (Rojas-Velasquez, Pluhar, Burns, & Burton, 2021, p. 368). The rate of self-injurious behaviors among adolescents is between 17 and 60% (Rojas-Velasquez et al., 2021). Of those who engage in these behaviors, 90% of them use it to cope with difficult and unpleasant feelings (Rojas-Velasquez et al., 2021). Literature on NSSI has been dominated by studies primarily focused on middle- to upper-class young Caucasian women. African Americans and other ethnic communities are underrepresented in the NSSI literature (Rojas-Velasquez et al., 2021). This gap in the literature may lead practitioners to believe that fewer disparities exist across different ethnicities; however, African American youth experience race-related stressors that create significant long-lasting mental health outcomes (Williams, 2020). Risk factors for African American youth include emotional dysregulation, difficult social and familial relationship, poor coping skills, and coexisting mental health conditions (Rojas-Velasquez et al., 2021).

Studies have established that people who engage in self-injurious behaviors are much more likely to attempt suicide, especially female adolescents (Kothgassner et al., 2021). The number of African American female adolescents who engage in self-injurious behaviors or attempted suicide has recently increased (Centers for Disease Control and Prevention, 2023). This increase is understandable given that many African American female adolescents may have experienced hate speech and have lacked the tools to manage the distressing emotions. African American girls who engaged in self-injurious behaviors within the context of hate speech need an evidence-based intervention to recover.

Dialectical Behavioral Therapy

Dialectical Behavior Therapy (DBT), created by Marsha Linehan (2015), was initially designed for the treatment of borderline personality disorder. It was later adapted to address a variety of mental health concerns (Lenz, Del Conte, Hollenbaugh, & Callendar, 2016). DBT has skills that can assist a client in managing intense and overwhelming emotions. Dialectic philosophy has three core beliefs:

everything is interconnected, change is constant and inevitable, and opposites can be integrated to get closer to the truth (Lenz et al., 2016).

DBT uses four skill sets to assist clients in overcoming their current mental health struggles: mindfulness, distress tolerance, interpersonal effectiveness, and emotional regulation. The mindfulness models were adapted from Eastern meditation practices. This technique teaches a client to become more aware of the present moment (Lenz et al., 2016). The client learns to focus on a single thing without judgment of self or others. The distress tolerance model teaches clients to accept things over which they do not have control, as well as problem solve and improve their mood. Distress tolerance teaches clients to tolerate uncertainty in life and manage the painful feelings that result. Interpersonal effectiveness teaches self-advocacy, boundaries, and the ability to say no. Emotional regulation will help them understand that emotions are not permanent, and feelings can be fleeting (Lenz et al., 2016).

DBT treatment procedures and strategies that will be helpful to Ashly with self-harm and bullying are mindfulness, distress tolerance, interpersonal effectiveness, and emotional regulation. Given Ashly's developmental level, she will benefit from DBT and has the developmental capacity to understand, learn, and apply the skills of DBT. Ashly has entered Piaget's formal operations stage; she is able to engage in abstract and hypothetical reasoning. In this stage of development, Ashly will be able to review her progress, continually reevaluate her goals, and understand and apply metaphors to her current life circumstances (Miller, 2011).

Distress tolerance skills will teach Ashly to tolerate her strong emotions without using the maladaptive coping skill of self-harming. Self-harming by cutting is an impulsive behavior based on strong emotions. Interpersonal effectiveness will focus on building Ashly's interpersonal communication skills so she can express her needs instead of burying them. Self-injury often occurs because a youth struggles with communication. Ashly resorts to self-injury instead of talking about what she is going through. She will develop control over her emotions and, through emotional regulation, eliminate the impulse to react with a negative coping skill whenever strong emotions come up. Mindfulness will aid Ashly in recognizing her thoughts and feelings while accepting them without judgment. Learning mindfulness will assist Ashly in interrupting her strong emotions and allow her to pause long enough to implement positive coping skills instead of acting on the impulse to cut.

According to Erikson (1950), peers and academic success greatly influence Ashly's self-esteem. Connecting with peers is extremely important in this stage of Ashly's life. The lack of positive peer connection, academic failure, and race-related stress lead to low self-esteem and maladaptive behaviors (Miller, 2011). Ashly's depression, race-related stress, and self-harm require a treatment modality that helps her develop practical cognitive and behavioral coping skills. DBT provides a therapeutic approach that will assist Ashly in moving from a dysregulated to a regulated mind.

Case Study Application

In considering the different factors that make up Ashly's case, I (DM) decided to use two models to help guide my understanding of Ashly: DBT and the RESPECT-FUL model of counseling. The RESPECTFUL acronym refers to Religious/spiritual identity; Economic class; Sexual identity; Psychological maturity; Ethnic/racial identity; Chronological/developmental challenges; Traumatic experiences; Family background; Unique physical characteristics; and Location of residence and language (D'Andrea & Daniels, 2001). As previously stated, DBT provides technical skills that teach clients how to replace maladaptive behaviors and manage difficult emotions. This modality has been effective for adolescents engaging in self-harm and suicidal ideations (Kothgassner et al., 2021). The success was attributed to the holistic approach of integrating the family into the treatment process (Kothgassner et al., 2021).

The RESPECTFUL model helps me consider Ashly's multidimensional background to guide the therapeutic intervention. First, I consider Ashly's spiritual and religious background. Ashly and her mother both report they are of Christian faith. However, they do not attend church regularly. Ashly has reported concerns about "disappointing God because I cut." Next, I consider Ashly's economic class and background (LeBeauf, Smaby, & Maddux, 2009). Ashly is of a lower socio-economic status. The family's socioeconomic status has impacted the resources to which they have access. Ashly's mom reports housing insecurity without the support of her boyfriend. It is possible that Ashly, her siblings, and her mother are also dependent on her mom's boyfriend for other basic needs such as food and clothing (LeBeauf et al., 2009).

Ashly identifies as a cisgender heterosexual female. Ashly's gender identity does not significantly impact her life negatively or positively. Ashly is a 14-year-old African American female who feels increasingly isolated in her new predominantly White neighborhood and school. She believes she has no control over her current living situation and must "deal because I have nowhere else to go." Ashly relates most to her mother's side of the family. She reports having a stronger sibling bond with her mother's children than with her father's daughter. Ashly is very close to her extended family, particularly her first cousins.

Treatment Goals

Ashly's treatment goals were developed with the family. The family and I explored where we should begin. Ashly stated, "I don't really know what depression is or why I feel this way." When developing treatment goals, I combine the client's language with my clinical understanding. Therefore, Ashly's initial treatment goal is "Ashly will be able to understand her depression better." Ashly stated, "I want to be able to know why I am feeling this way." Ashly's initial objective is "Ashly will learn emotional vocabulary in individual weekly sessions to better describe what she is feeling."

During the initial assessment, a safety plan was developed due to Ashly's history of cutting. The family and I reviewed Ashly's protective factors, which she identified as "support from my cousins, going for walks, drawing, and sometimes reading." We identified her triggers, which she stated are "mom not listening, not being able to see my cousins, and tension at home." We also identified which adults Ashly views as supportive. Ashly identified an art teacher (at her former school), her older cousin, and sometimes her mother. We also reviewed 24-hour emergency community resources when my therapy office is closed.

Treatment Process

My goal for the first session was to begin building rapport with Ashly, explore confidentiality and its limits, and explain what DBT is and how I believe it could help her overcome her current mental health struggles. I prepared my office by turning off the overhead lights and turning on the lamp on my desk. I also put fidgets out for Ashly to use if she became nervous or needed a distraction. After introducing myself and giving Ashly three fun facts about me, I asked Ashly to do the same. I then explained to Ashly what Dialectical Behavior Therapy is and how I believed the different skills could help her. I recommended that we start with distress tolerance skills. I invited Ashly to engage in a distress tolerance activity called Pros and Cons to examine the pros and cons of having drama and stress and not having it. See table 15.2 and figure 15.1, Activity from sessions 1 and 2 (Moonshine, 2008).

TABLE 15.1.   **DISTRESS TOLERANCE SKILLS: PROS AND CONS**

Pros of Cutting	Cons of Cutting
• Changes the pain from my heart to my body • I'm in control. I say when it happens. • My dad comes to see me when I cut.	• Leaves marks and scratches/scars • It makes my mom scared. • Cutting doesn't make dad come see me more.
Cons of Not Caring about School	**Pros of Not Caring about School**
• All the attention from adults . . . annoying • I might fail ninth grade. • I have to make up all the schoolwork I did not do.	• I'm in therapy. • Summer school might be an option; also, it can be less stressful than regular school. • I've been given extra time to make up my schoolwork.

TABLE 15.2. ASHLY: SESSION 1

Transcript	Analysis
T: "As I said before, distress tolerance is about learning to deal with frustration and being able to deal with stress, drama, and crisis in a healthy way."	Reinforcing what distress tolerance is and how it can help Ashly in her everyday life will assist in promoting a sense of self-efficacy.
A: "Okay, yeah, I remember you saying that. Not really sure how to do that."	Adolescents often feel unsure about learning new ways of doing things.
T: "We will build your skills by learning different strategies."	Reassuring Ashly that I will be there to help her learn and build her new skills.
A: "So, you want me to do this work sheet? It seems stupid and a lot like schoolwork."	Adolescents often try to make sense of new experiences by comparing them to places or situations that seem similar.
T: "Yes, I would like you to complete the worksheet. I know it seems like schoolwork, and I believe it will be helpful."	Normalizing and reassuring Ashly that her thoughts are common.
A: "Can we do it together?"	Partnering is an excellent way to help adolescents overcome any worries or concerns they may have.
T: "Sure, you let me know when you would like my help."	Giving adolescents a sense of control can help them feel secure and safe in new situations.

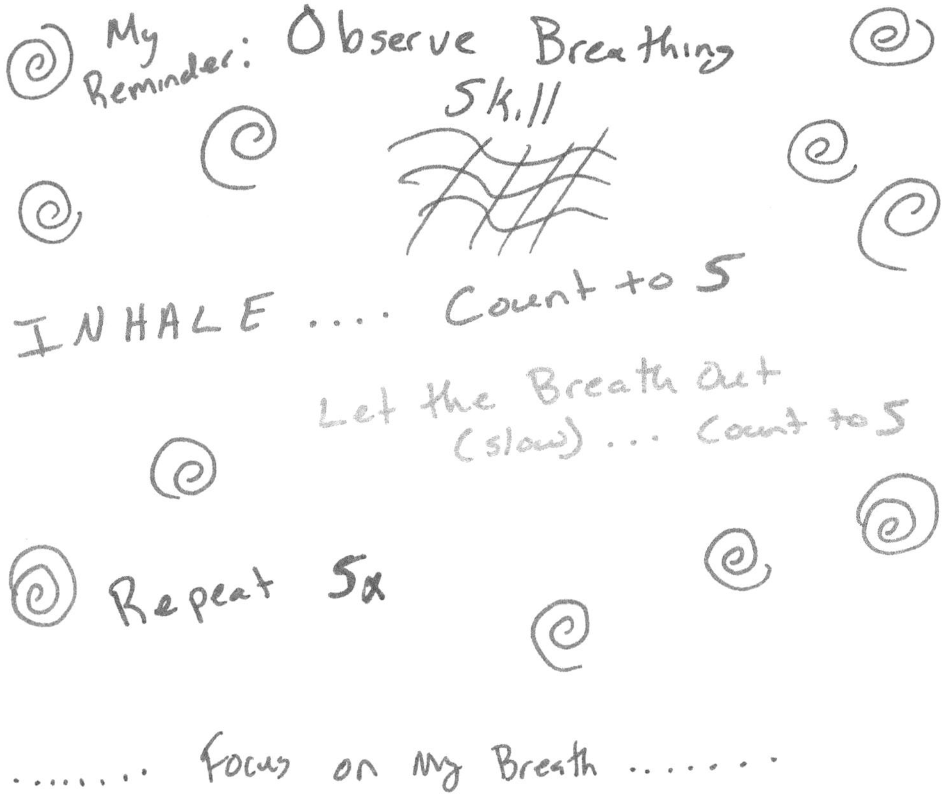

Figure 15.1. Activity. Figure courtesy of Domonique Messing based on client's representation.

My goal for Ashly's second session was to continue exploring distress tolerance and build on the skills learned from the Pros and Cons work sheet. This week I wanted to provide Ashly with a skill she can use outside of the session to aid her during stressful or difficult situations. I explained to Ashly that observe breathing is a breathing technique that would help ground her, keep her focused on the present moment, and distract her from the stressful situation.

TABLE 15.3.   **ASHLY: SESSION 2**

Transcript	Analysis
T: "Ashly, I want to invite you to try a breathing exercise that will help calm you when stressed or in difficult situations."	Inviting Ashly instead of telling her, to give her agency during our session time.
A: "Ms., I don't think breathing will help me when I'm stressed."	Adolescents are often skeptical of new skills and information.
T: "I know it's not something you would usually use when stressed. Are you willing to see what it is about?"	Validating that what I am asking Ashly to do is new and outside of her comfort zone, and again inviting her to try the activity
A: "Ugh, I guess, Ms., but you have to do it too."	It's often easier for adolescents to engage in a new task if they have a partner.
T: "Inhale while counting to five slowly. Let the breath out while counting to five slowly." [Repeat five times.]	Guiding Ashly through the activity while fulfilling her request to do it together. This helps Ashly feel less awkward.
A: "Ms., I can't just stop and do that when something is making me stressed."	Expressing doubt and worry about her own ability to use observe breathing as a coping skill in everyday life
T: "Right now, you see it as impractical. I believe as we practice this together, it will eventually become second nature. Are you willing to practice this with me in session when I prompt you?"	Reflecting her perception. Adding hope that she can learn. Asking for her willingness to engage in just one small step during session [I prompt her to practice it about every 10 minutes the rest of the session and subsequent sessions].

Ethical and Cultural Considerations

Race is a sensitive topic for many people. Therefore, when engaging in race-related conversations, feelings of discomfort may arise. However, in therapeutic relationships, uncomfortable conversations are frequent and expected. A therapist must be nonjudgmental; otherwise, it may impede treatment success. Thus, maintaining self-awareness and using supervision can be helpful.

As an African American therapist, it was ethically important for me to manage my own biases and experiences of microaggressions, especially when working with a client who has similar life experiences. Supervision can be used to address a therapist's thoughts and feelings that arise when addressing sensitive topics. A goal of supervision can be "confronting and exploring emotionally charged subject matter while maintaining an atmosphere of compassion and empathy for the anxiety, pain, ambivalence, and anger that can accompany topics of race" (Harrell, 2014, p. 85). It is highly recommended that therapists use supervision to explore race-related experiences that may be unintentionally triggered while counseling a client so that therapists can maintain a nonjudgmental attitude toward everyone.

Parent Consultations

The first parent consultation meeting was with Ms. Johnson. Mr. Smith was scheduled to join this session; however, he was unable to attend. Mr. Smith did not provide a reason for his absence. I informed Ms. Johnson that parent consultations are essential to the therapeutic process because they allow me to support her while she supports Ashly. I explained that these meetings are an opportunity for her to express her concerns, receive validation, and learn the strategies Ashly was learning in her sessions. Ms. Johnson expressed concern, stating, "I don't know if I will always have time to make these meetings because I have other kids with a lot going on." Ms. Johnson explored other options for meeting with me, including online virtual and phone sessions. During parent consultation, Ms. Johnson and I reviewed and practiced the skills Ashly had been working on in the session.

Conclusion

Throughout treatment, Ashly gained numerous DBT coping skills to assist her in managing her depressive symptoms and self-harm behavior. Ashly identified DBT coping skills that could aid her in stressful situations, even though she reported not implementing them consistently. Ashly and her family reported that she no longer cut herself. Ashly identified one peer with whom she has become "good friends." Ashly continued to be open to learning more DBT skills to manage her mental health symptoms better and remained in ongoing individual therapy as needed.

Sample Case Notes

Session 1

Subjective: The client expressed uncertainty about beginning the therapeutic process, specifically using DBT. She expressed that the initial activity felt "like schoolwork" and was hesitant to write down her thoughts. The client acknowledged her depression symptoms; she stated, "Sometimes it's too much, and I just want to relieve the pain."

Objective: At the start of the session, client was quiet and only engaged this therapist when prompted. The client used fidgets during the session. The client visibly relaxed when this therapist also agreed to complete a Pros and Cons work sheet. This therapist and client explored how understanding the pros and cons of a situation can assist the client in problem solving and finding ways to cope and manage stress or drama.

Assessment: From a Dialectical Behavior Therapy perspective, Ashly appears to be experiencing symptoms of depression and self-harm due to stressors in the home, experiencing hate speech at school, moving to a predominantly White neighborhood, not experiencing validation, and lacking coping skills.

Plan: This therapist will teach concepts of DBT and use different worksheets and activities to reinforce problem solving and effective ways for Ashly to cope with current life stressors and crises.

Resources

For Professionals

Dialectical Behavior Therapy: Volume 1—The Therapist's Guidebook, https://a
.co/d/4MxCg7b

Dialectical Behavior Therapy: Volume 2—Companion Worksheets, spiral-bound,
https://a.co/d/57t4P2t

For Teens

*The DBT Skills Workbook for Teens: A Fun Guide to Manage Anxiety and Stress,
Understand Your Emotions and Learn Effective Communication Skills (Life .
. . Health and Wellness Books for Teenagers)*, https://a.co/d/6VJDH8c

For Parents

*DBT Skills Workbook for Parents of Teens—A Proven Strategy for Understand-
ing and Parenting Adolescents Who Suffer from Intense Emotions, Anger, and
Anxiety*, https://a.co/d/0dlDJKI

Discussion Questions

1. What contributing factors exacerbated Ashly's depression symptoms?
2. As a therapist, how would you prepare to talk to your client about race or racism?
3. As a therapist, how would you prepare yourself to deal with potential triggers from the case that could create therapy-interfering behaviors?

References

Centers for Disease Control and Prevention. (2023). *CDC's youth risk behavior survey data summary & trends reports, 2011–2021.*

D'Andrea, M., & Daniels, J. (2001). RESPECTFUL counseling: An integrative model for counselors. In D. Pope-Davis & H. Coleman (Eds.), *The interface of class, culture and gender in counseling* (pp. 417–466). Sage.

Erikson, E. H. (1950). *Childhood and society.* Norton.

Evans, K. (2019). The invisibility of Black girls in education. *Relational Child & Youth Care Practice, 32*(1), 77–90.

Harrell, S. (2014). Compassionate confrontation and empathic exploration: The integration of race-related narratives in clinical supervision. *Multiculturalism and Diversity in Clinical Supervision: A Competency-Based Approach*, 83–110. http://dx.doi.org/10.1037/14370-004

Kansok-Dusche, J., Ballaschk, C., Krause, N., Zeißig, A., Seemann-Herz, L., Wachs, S., & Bilz, L. (2022). A systematic review on hate speech among children and adolescents: definitions, prevalence, and overlap with related phenomena. *Trauma, Violence, & Abuse.* https://doi.org/10.1177_15248380221108070

Kothgassner, O. D., Goreis, A., Robinson, K., Huscsava, M. M., Schmahl, C., & Plener, P. L. (2021). Efficacy of dialectical behavior therapy for adolescent self-harm and suicidal ideation: A systematic review and meta-analysis. *Psychological Medicine, 51*, 1057–1067. https://doi.org/10.1017/S0033291721001355

LeBeauf, I., Smaby, M., & Maddux, C. (2009). Adapting counseling skills for multicultural and diverse clients. In G. R. Walz, J. C., Bleuer, & R. K. Yep (Eds.), *Compelling counseling interventions: VISTAS 2009* (pp. 33–42). American Counseling Association.

Lenz, S. A., Del Conte, G., Hollenbaugh, M. K., & Callendar, K. (2016). Emotional regulation and interpersonal effectiveness as mechanisms of change for treatment outcomes within a DBT program for adolescents. *Counseling Outcome Research and Evaluation*, 73–85. https://doi.org/10.1177/2150137816642439

Linehan, M. M. (2015). *DBT® skills training manual* (2nd ed.). Guilford Press.

Miller, P. H. (2011). *Theories of developmental psychology.* Worth.

Moonshine, C. (2008). *Acquiring competency and achieving proficiency with dialectical behavior therapy.* Pesi.

Rojas-Velasquez, D. A., Pluhar, E. I., Burns, P. A., & Burton, E. T. (2021). Non-suicidal self-injury among African American and Hispanic adolescents and young adults: A systematic review. *Prevention Science, 22,* 367–377. https://doi.org/10.1007/s11121-020-01147-x

Williams, M. T. (2020). Microaggressions: Clarification, evidence, and impact. *Perspectives on Psychological Science, 15*(1), 3–26. https://doi.org/10.1177/1745691619827499

CHAPTER 16

Tourette Syndrome and Risk of Exploitation
Equine Assisted Family Play Therapy with a White Adolescent
Tracie Faa-Thompson

Jenny is a 16-year-old White adolescent female. She moved into our area of England about a year before she and her family commenced therapy. She lives with her mother and her younger sister. The family moved to be near their maternal grandmother and her partner after Jenny experienced bullying due to her Tourette syndrome. Jenny attended the local high school about 20 miles from where she lived until the school closed due to the COVID-19 pandemic. When the lockdown ended, she returned to school. Unfortunately, the stress of being back in school was too much for her, and she was unable to control her Tourette syndrome of vocal and motor tics. Her Tourette syndrome presented as her running down the school corridors past classrooms banging on doors and windows while making threats. This was taken very seriously by school personnel, and she was excluded from school with the caveat that she was not to return until she was "better." Since her mother's parenting style was permissive, her mother struggled to set boundaries or sanctions when Jenny's behavior was unacceptable, which put Jenny at risk for exploitation.

For this case study, consider:

1. How did the combination of Tourette's, risk of exploitation, and the COVID-19 pandemic impact Jenny and her family?
2. What were the benefits of using Equine Assisted Family Play Therapy™ (EAFPT) with Jenny?
3. What procedures in EAFPT were particularly helpful to Jenny?

Tourette Syndrome

Tourette syndrome (TS) is a complex neurological disorder characterized by repetitive, sudden, uncontrolled (involuntary) movements and sounds called tics

(Genetic and Rare Diseases Information Center, n.d.). TS is caused by a variety of genetic and environmental factors. It is estimated that 1% of the population has TS. It affects one schoolchild in every hundred and is more common among boys. More than 300,000 children and adults are living with TS in the United Kingdom (Tourettes Action, 2023) and 1.4 million in the United States (Centers for Disease Control and Prevention [CDC], 2022).

The key features of TS are involuntary motor and/or vocal tics, which must be present for at least 12 months to meet the diagnostic criteria. Motor tics are movements of the body such as blinking, mouth or nose twitches, shrugging the shoulders, or jerking an arm. Vocal tics are sounds that a person makes such as humming, clearing the throat, sniffing, or yelling out a word or phrase, which may include curse words. Simple tics involve just a few parts of the body whereas complex tics involve several different parts of the body in a repeated pattern such as bobbing the head while jerking an arm and then jumping up (CDC, 2022). About 85% of people with TS will also experience co-occurring conditions and features, which might include Attention-Deficit/Hyperactivity Disorder (ADHD), Obsessive Compulsive Disorder (OCD), and Anxiety (Tourettes Action, 2023).

Risk of Sexual Exploitation

The World Health Organization (WHO, n.d.) defines sexual exploitation as actual or attempted abuse of a position of vulnerability, power, or trust for sexual purposes (WHO, n.d., p. 2). The prevalence of sexual exploitation ranges from 15 to 25% among females and 5 to 15% among males in the general US population (Finkelhor, Turner, Shattuck, & Hamby, 2015). Adolescents with disabilities are particularly vulnerable to sexual exploitation due to the social power differential and lack of knowledge about healthy sexual relationships (Treacy, Taylor, & Abernathy, 2018).

Sexual exploitation disrupts adolescents' emotional regulation as well as cognitive and affect integration (Linde-Krieger et al., 2021). Howe (2005) contended that sexual exploitation impairs adolescents' ability to regulate and make sense of their emotions and levels of arousal. Sexually exploited adolescents often present with pseudo mature behavior, meaning a false appearance of independence and indiscriminate affection to any person who takes an interest (Martin & Beesley, 1977). They may have inappropriate and heightened sexualized behavior toward peers (Trickett, 1997). Consequently, their sexually labile behavior can result in adolescents experiencing further exploitation, social confusion, and peer rejection after engaging in sexual activity. Due to these dire consequences, adolescents with disabilities need interventions to protect them from the risk of sexual exploitation.

Needed Interventions

Play therapy is an intervention that gives children the needed space to come to terms with the stress and multiple losses experienced by a child who has been bullied and at risk for sexual exploitation (Cattanach, 1992). Cattanach advised that it is important to assist children to repossess their bodies and find an identity other than one bound up in their past. Adolescents who have been sexually exploited may struggle with the idea of traditional play therapy and may feel it is too "childish" for them. However, an outdoor setting for play therapy may intrigue adolescents.

Beyond the four walls, being outdoors allows "the therapist to hold an internal psychological frame around the work with the client . . . trusting in their own confidence and competence" (Jordan, 2015, p. 93). A sense of "competent therapist self" is a key to feeling able to move away from the "geographical" concept of walls and toward an understanding of "symbolic" walls, created by the therapeutic relationship. Because feelings of psychological safety are dependent on feelings of physical safety, Fearn (2014) suggested that in outdoor play therapy "There is a balance to be struck between children's vital need for risk and challenge and adult concerns for their safety" (p. 117). Fearn goes on to note, "In most cases, children can be trusted to learn to assess and take manageable risk for themselves and it is vital for the development of self-other awareness that they do so" (p. 117).

Adolescents who have been bullied and sexually exploited need assistance with body boundaries to identify safe and unsafe touch. They also need actual experience with safe touch in which they are in control of touch and touching. Horses are large, sensitive creatures that are also very touch sensitive and will let their feelings be felt immediately if they are touched or approached in ways they do not like. Horses can provide the safe touch and trusting relationship that adolescents who experienced bullying and exploitation so desperately need. The lovability conveyed from the horse to adolescents may help build their self-esteem (Gilligan, 2001). Therefore, combining horses with outdoor play therapy for adolescents who experienced bullying and exploitation is a powerful intervention.

Animal-Assisted Play Therapy

Animal Assisted Play Therapy™ (AAPT) is a multidisciplinary therapeutic approach that includes interested animals, such as horses, in the practice of play therapy and other therapeutic or educational interventions (VanFleet & Faa-Thompson, 2017). AAPT requires substantial training of the practitioners who employ it. It can be appropriate for all ages of clients, and it can be used with individuals, families, and groups. It also can be applied within a wide range of therapy orientations and modalities, both nondirective and directive. AAPT represents the full integration of the fields of play therapy, attachment and relationship theories, animal behavior, ethology, animal-assisted interventions, and animal welfare.

AAPT is defined as

the integrated involvement of animals in the context of play therapy, in which appropriately trained therapists and animals engage with clients primarily through systematic playful interventions, with the goal of improving clients' developmental and psychosocial health, while simultaneously ensuring the animals' well-being and voluntary engagement. Play and playfulness are essential ingredients of the interactions and the relationship. (p. 17)

In AAPT, a strong emphasis is on animal welfare, in which the animal must enjoy and not merely tolerate most interactions. The therapist-animal relationship is a metaphor for the therapeutic relationship between the therapist and client(s). The focus of client-animal relationship through play is in service of therapeutic goals (Faa-Thompson, 2022).

Case Study Application

Treatment Goals and Objectives

When thinking about treatment goals and objectives, it is useful to think about whose goal is it and what's the motivation. For Jenny's school, their goal was to "fix" her so that she would be able to return to school and resume her studies. They wanted Jenny "fixed" but were unable to describe what "fixed" would look like. For Jenny's family, their goal was for her to stop presenting with challenging behaviors. What about Jenny? At the beginning of sessions, she was unsure, confused, and believed it was all her fault. She was trying hard to meet everyone's expectations of what "fixed" looked like.

In our Equine Assisted Family Play Therapy (EAFPT) program, we have a loose outline when discussing goals and expressed outcomes with the family and other interested parties. Sometimes goals are very clear, and sometimes they can be "softer" outcomes. However, it's important that we do not follow a set formula. In the 30+ years I have been working in the field of Equine Assisted Psychotherapy, I have read many treatment manuals of varying numbers of sessions in set programs that outline what should be included in each session. Although some of the activities may be useful to include in sessions, in my experience it is important to have the confidence, expertise, and knowledge to be flexible in our approach. As we work outdoors on grass in the horse's natural environment and live in Northern England, sometimes we can have all four seasons in one session because the natural environment plays a big part in which activities we choose. Session content also depends on the mood of the horses, if they choose to attend the sessions, and the moods of the clients when they arrive. We must work with what presents to us on that given day from all those included in the process.

With respect to Jenny and her family's goals, we agreed on the outcomes of Jenny feeling and being safe (two different things), more family cohesion, clear communications, and boundary setting. The stated goal of getting Jenny back to school was just too far when we started and probably would have set her up to fail. Without the feeling of safety and family support, Jenny could not even begin to think about what a return to school would look like. Often in our work, clients and referrers are set on outcomes that are unachievable and miss too many steps. We tend to strip everything back, take small steps, and build strong foundations that we can revert to when challenges are too difficult.

The treatment plan focused on the fun that the family was having together while not ignoring the issues they were facing. We looked at goals for the family as well as Jenny, so that Jenny was not viewed as "the problem needing to be fixed." We found common ground. We did this by emphasizing that like horse herds, "Families come in all shapes and sizes"; "Families are all unique"; and "You can choose your friends, but you cannot choose your family."

The Treatment Process

In our EAFPT program, we follow the diamond model comprising one equine expert, the horses, therapist, and clients. We use the Equine Assisted Growth and Learning Association (EAGALA, 2018) model, which we feel is the safest and most ethical model because it includes a horse expert to observe and keep the horses safe and a human therapist who is qualified and professionally registered to work with the client group. (Note: In the United States, this will be termed licensed counselor, social worker, or psychologist.) It's very difficult if you are a lone therapist to split your attention between horse and human, making the process potentially unsafe for all.

The horses at Turn About Pegasus (TAP), my Equine Assisted Family Play Therapy program, consist of a small band of mixed-breed horses who live together in large fields of 20+ acres. The horses are playful and work at liberty. This setting is also our home, so the horses are not brought to sessions. When clients arrive, we open the field gate, and we invite the horses to join us in sessions if they choose. At TAP, most of our family work is with blended and adopted families as well as kinship carers (foster families), so our focus is on attachment, relationship, and resilience.

Overview and Beginning Sessions

We provided a total of ten 90-minute sessions of EAFPT with Jenny, her mother and grandmother, and however many of the horses wished to be involved. In the beginning sessions, we provided psychoeducation about equine behavior and communication in herds. Boundaries and clear communication were the overriding theme. We focused on relationships and what worked well rather than what was not working.

A fundamental goal was assisting Jenny to keep herself safe, so we emphasized "safe touch" with the horses. At the end of every session, we said thank you to the horses by grooming them in ways they liked to be groomed, observing the invites to groom from the horses and responding to invites. We call this "listen with your eyes" to the horses. They are loose and are not switched off or resigned to being touched by humans with little choice. Rather, they will invite and gesture with their nose the parts of their bodies they like to be touched. They are very expressive about parts of their body that they do not like to be touched. Jenny learned to "listen with her eyes" and to notice when her grooming was pleasurable for the horses or not. We used these grooming opportunities to discuss human-to-human touch and consent. We encouraged Jenny to think of how she could respond in the future to unwanted human touch.

Sessions 5 through 7—Barriers Activity

In session 5, we began the barriers activity. We invited the family to use the equipment in the arena to build themselves a fortress to keep themselves safe from outside influences that could cause them harm. Before we did this, we invited them to label the horses (metaphorically, not actually put labels on them) as things that erode your good self-esteem. An issue that often comes up after a few sessions is that clients make a connection with the horses, and they do not want to label them as anything negative. This is to be celebrated as they develop a positive relationship and empathy for the horses. However, for the purposes of this activity, the family was able to label the three horses present as Bullies, Put Downs, and Abusers.

The family worked at building their first barrier, but there was little communication or planning between them. They made a barrier without much thought or effort right in the middle of the field instead of using a natural wall as a barrier. Once ensconced in their fortress, we gave them each a bucket of horse treats that represented their self-esteem. We asked them to hold onto it for 5 minutes (5 minutes is our maximum time to avoid the horses getting frustrated). The horses on seeing the food broke through their fortress in less than a minute to get to the treats. We rescued the treats and debriefed them. Everyone was laughing.

We asked Jenny's family what had happened. They said their fortress was not strong enough and that it might work better if they worked together. They tried again, this time trying to make it stronger by adding more to it but with no real plan. They ran out of time so had to dismantle the fort and begin again in the next session. The same thing happened at the next session, but it took more time for the fort to be breached. During these times I was reflecting on what was happening and stating things such as, "Oh no, the bully is getting under the barrier. What can you do?" and "Here comes the abuser. He's trying to break through at the side. Who is going to protect your self-esteem?" I kept the narrative coming in an upbeat voice, and the whole family was laughing. Jenny and mum and grandmother put their *self-esteem* together and took turns protecting their fortress. The second time they managed 4 minutes and realized that if they worked together and helped each other, they were stronger together.

In session 7, mum took charge of the fortress, and the whole family discussed how they were going to build it stronger by learning from their first three attempts. Mum directed how it would look and gave rationales for why in discussion with her own mum and Jenny. They spent a long time getting everything just right and even made seats for each other to sit on. They sat close to one another in a triangle with their backs resting against each other and rested their "self-esteem" on their laps. This fortress had an inner and outer ring that was much larger than the two before, so the horses couldn't reach over as it was more interwoven. This time the barrier held strong.

We debriefed with the family about what they had learned in the sessions. They were able to say that when they worked together and stopped trying to control everything, things worked out well. Mum stated that she felt proud of herself that she could take charge as she was always the one to back down. Grandmother was able to state that she felt relieved that she didn't have to be the one always coming up with solutions. Jenny stated that she was pleased that her mother could keep her safe. We do not go into long debriefs in EAFPT as then it would become a talking therapy and defeat the whole purpose.

Session 8

Below is a short transcript of the beginning of session 8. Mum, grandmother, and Jenny had arrived, and all three are smiling broadly.

A check-in, as described above, is important at the start of each session because it reveals the processing that has occurred in the family between sessions.

TABLE 16.1. **JENNY: SESSION 8**

Transcript	Analysis
T F-T: "Good morning. I'm noticing three smiling faces. I'm wondering if there is any particular reason for the smiling faces?" [Jenny and mum share a glance.]	Role-modeling the power of tuning into and stating observed facial expressions. Rather than requiring a response, I invite a response with "I'm wondering."
J: "Yes, Mum confiscated my phone last night, and I won't get it back for a week, and I'm grounded."	Mum had set a boundary and clearly communicated the consequences.
T F-T: "Wow, your mum took your phone from you, and you are grounded, and you are happy about that?"	I was genuinely astonished, as I never expected those words from a teenage girl. Expressing genuineness facilitates safety and a strong therapeutic bond.
J: "Yes, because now I know she can keep me safe. Before she would always give in. Now she doesn't. I now know I am loved by my mum."	Jenny's verbalization reinforces the positive change she experiences in her mom and herself.
T F-T: "Mum, hearing what Jenny has just said, I wonder how you might be feeling?"	Inviting mum's verbalization provides confirmation, role-models communication, and facilitates connection.
Mum: "Proud and confident and relieved that I can keep Jenny safe."	Mum's verbalization reinforces her experiences and reveals achievement of one of the overall goals for therapy, Jenny's safety.

(continued)

TABLE 16.1. *(CONTINUED)*

Transcript	Analysis
T F-T: "So you feel proud you can keep Jenny safe, and Jenny feels safe. That must be so fantastic for you both to feel like that. I am astonished, though, as I never ever thought I would hear those words from a teenage girl in relation to her phone or being grounded." [Laughter all around. Two weeks prior, grandmother had a breast cancer scare, so I turned to her next.] "Grandmother, hearing all this, I'm wondering what your thoughts are?"	My response and humor help me celebrate with them. This reaffirms the strength of our therapeutic relationship. Intentionally addressing grandmother honors her role in the family.
Grandmother: "Relief that no matter what happens to me, I know that Jenny will be kept safe by her mother and that her mother is now so much more confident, which fills me with joy." [Spontaneous family hug and a misty eye all around, including therapy team]	Affirmation from grandmother to mother strengthened their bond and increased mother's confidence even more. Hugs from the entire therapy team role-modeled safe touch, which became Jenny's internal working model of safe relationships.

Ending Sessions and Learnings

The last two sessions were focused on strengthening that trust and bond within the family. Jenny came to our sessions initially because she was told to, and the goal was to get her back into school. She felt like it was all her fault and was terrified of her Tourette's. She had little interest in horses. However, Jenny quickly found a connection with the horses and wanted to learn about equine ethology and behavior as well as the human-animal bond, which were gently weaved into and integral to all our sessions. Jenny and her family decided that she wouldn't be going back to school. (Although the school wouldn't have her back, Jenny's decision illustrated her self-determination.) Instead, Jenny was accepted at the local equine college. After three years, Jenny successfully completed her higher-level diploma in equine studies.

Her relationship with her mother and grandmother continued to be strong with the grandmother taking on the role of grandmother and not having to step in and mother maintaining her authoritative parenting style. Jenny no longer was a victim of unequal relationships and made many friends of all genders.

Interestingly for us, during Jenny's EAFPT sessions, even when sessions were tough for her, she never displayed any motor or vocal tics. Of course, her Tourette's had not disappeared but, rather, there was something about the interaction with the horses and the therapy team that did not set off her Tourette's. We noticed this but did not draw attention to this fact so as not to cause stress, which could have made her tics more likely. Not drawing attention to her lack of tics was especially important because Jenny had been accused by others of putting it on despite having had a Tourette's diagnosis since she was 5. Whether to draw attention to or leave something out that has happened or not during EAFPT sessions is always a choice for the therapy team. This therapeutic choice emphasizes the importance of extensively qualified therapy team members who can provide a valid rationale for their modality of intervention in each session. A manualized formulaic approach relies on the manual's guidance rather than the expertise of the therapists.

Ethical and Cultural Considerations

To date, the whole industry of Equine Assisted Therapy is unregulated, which means that anyone can call themselves an equine-assisted therapist and indeed some do. The internet is liberally littered with impressive websites offering a whole range of animal-assisted therapies with myriad client groups. On closer inspection and wading through the list of trainings, you might find that the "therapists" are not trained in working with the client population they are engaging with, nor do they have any equine credentials.

It is important to follow EAGALA ethics and have advanced training in equine-assisted therapy. Both my co-therapist and I are qualified human therapists and equine specialists at the MA/MSc level. At the heart of our work is animal sentience and enjoyment. If the animals do not feel safe and do not enjoy the interactions, then we are replicating what had been done to Jenny during the times she was being sexually exploited. For example, in her previous experiences with boys, she thought she was in a relationship, but the relationship was what was in it for the boys and not what was in it for her. In our work, reciprocal relationships between horses and humans are fundamental to the process, with the horses having free choices to leave if they are not enjoying the interaction. If that were to happen (it hasn't happened yet), we as therapists are qualified to work with the family without the equines being present and to use that experience of free choice and self-efficacy to help clients think about reciprocity in relationships. If animals were not given choices and if they were expected to remain in situations where the human needs are paramount, then we would be perpetuating the metaphor of helplessness and force. This ill approach would convey to our clients that one sentient being's feelings, wishes, and needs are more important than another's.

To show respect to the horses, we are careful to keep the barrier activity session of denying horses their treats to 5 minutes only so that the horses don't get frustrated at not getting to the treats. At the end of the session the horses get to eat all the treats, which are then no longer labeled self-esteem. This is an important part of the session as it keeps the animals in mind as sentient beings. All clients love to feed the horses and offer them praise for their participation. This positive interaction helps clients integrate their own self-determination in relationships.

Conclusion

EAFPT can be incredibly effective by enhancing the development of empathy, efficacy, confidence, relationship, and much more. This work is far more complex than individual work, however, and requires considerably more training and skill than many assume. With that said, simple activities in nature with animals who have both voice and choice alongside well-qualified and experienced group therapists have the potential to make significant differences in short periods of time. By being in the moment and working within safe therapeutic space with animals who are free to be themselves, clients discover their own freedom to let down their guard and be themselves as well. Working with families is totally different from working individually and needs a heightened skill set. Therapists in this field need to be:

- skilled and trained in systemic family therapy;
- fluent in equine ethology and behavior;
- skilled in knowing when to use humor as a defuser, and adaptable and able to switch the session plan immediately depending on what the family present, the animals present, and the wider environment presents;
- skilled in splitting attention—if you have found it difficult to split attention between one person and one animal, it's magnified with a group of people and animals; and
- able to work as part of a good human therapy team. There is no room for therapists' egos in EAFPT.

Resources

EAGALA, https://www.eagala.org/
IIAAPT, https://iiaapt.org/
https://www.tourettes-action.org.uk/
http://www.turnaboutpegasus.co.uk/

Discussion Questions

1. What does the human therapist need to be adept in when doing Equine Assisted Family Play Therapy™?
2. What else is important when undertaking group work?
3. In your opinion, would this intervention have been as effective if the horses were not free to choose whether to attend sessions?
4. What else might have helped this family?

References

Almon, J. (2013). *Adventure: The value of risk in children's play.* Alliance for Childhood.

Cattanach, A. (1992). *Play therapy with abused children.* Jessica Kingsley Publishers.

Centers for Disease Control and Prevention. (2022). *Data and statistics on Tourette syndrome.* https://www.cdc.gov/ncbddd/tourette/data.html#:~:text=About%201.4%20million%20people%20in%20the%20U.S.

Equine Assisted Growth and Learning Association. (2018). *EAGALA model.* https://www.eagala.org/model

Faa-Thompson, T. (2022). Horse play and canine capers: The importance of play to facilitate learning and healing. In M. Kirby (Ed.), *Nourished: Horses, animals and nature in counselling and psychotherapy & mental health* (pp. 213–228). Australia Aware Publishing.

Fearn, M. (2014). Working therapeutically in the outdoors. In E. Prendiville & J. Howard (Eds.), *Play therapy today: Contemporary practice with individuals, groups and carers.* Routledge.

Finkelhor, D., Turner, H. A., Shattuck, A., & Hamby, S. L. (2015). Prevalence of childhood exposure to violence, crime, and abuse: Results from the national survey of children's exposure to violence. *JAMA Pediatrics, 169*(8), 746–754. https://doi.org/10.1001/jamapediatrics.2015.0676

Genetic and Rare Diseases Information Center (n.d.). *Tourette syndrome.* https://rarediseases.info.nih.gov/diseases/7783/tourette-syndrome

Gilligan, R. (2001). *Promoting resilience: A resource guide on working with children in the care system.* BAAF.

Howe, D. (2005). *Child abuse and neglect: Attachment, development and intervention.* Palgrave Macmillan.

Jordan, M. (2015). *Nature and therapy: Understanding counselling and psychotherapy in outdoor spaces.* Routledge/Taylor & Francis Group.

Linde-Krieger, L. B., Moon, C. M., & Yates, T. M. (2021). The implications of self-definitions of child sexual abuse for understanding socioemotional adaptation in young adulthood. *Journal of Child Sexual Abuse: Research, Treatment, & Program Innovations for Victims, Survivors, & Offenders, 30*(1), 80–101. https://doi.org/10.1080/10538712.2020.1841352

Martin, H., & Beesley, P. (1977). Behavioural observations of abused children. *Developmental Medicine and Child Neurology, 19*, 373–387.

Tourettes Action. (2023). *Information and resources for health professionals about Tourette syndrome.* https://www.tourettes-action.org.uk/

Treacy, A. C., Taylor, S. S., & Abernathy, T. V. (2018). Sexual health education for individuals with disabilities: A call to action. *American Journal of Sexuality Education, 13*(1), 65–93. https://doi.org/10.1080/15546128.2017.1399492

Trickett, P. (1997). Sexual and physical abuse and the development of social competence. In S. Luthar, J. Burack, D. Ciccetti, & J. Weisz (Eds.), *Developmental pathology: Perspectives on adjustment, risk and disorder* (pp. 67–92). Cambridge University Press.

VanFleet, R., & Faa-Thompson, T. (2017). *Animal assisted play therapy.* Professional Resource Press.

VanFleet, R., & Faa-Thompson. T. (2019). *Animal assisted play therapy techniques manual.* Play Therapy Press.

World Health Organization. (n.d.). *Sexual exploitation and abuse.* www.who.int/docs/default-source/documents/ethics/sexual-exploitation-and-abuse-pamphlet-en.pdf?sfvrsn=409b4d89_2

CHAPTER 17

Eating Disorders
Enhanced Cognitive Behavior Therapy with a Mexican American Adolescent
Sara Cantu

Claudia is a 14-year-old, third-generation Mexican American girl who lives with her mother, father, and younger brother. She enjoys school, plays in the band, and plays on the school tennis team. Her mother works in the office of Claudia's school, and her father manages a branch of a bank. During the COVID-19 pandemic, Claudia had a difficult time adjusting to virtual school, feeling disconnected from friends and not being able to enjoy her activities. Claudia's mother also noticed changes in the way Claudia was eating and was concerned that she was frequently throwing up. Her mother brought her concerns to their family doctor, and the doctor recommended making an appointment with a therapist.

When working with Claudia, it is important to consider:

1. What are the symptoms and diagnostic criteria for bulimia? How do these symptoms apply to Claudia's diagnosis?
2. What is the focus of Enhanced Cognitive Behavior Therapy (CBT-E)? How is a CBT-E treatment plan formulated for Claudia? Given Claudia's specific eating disorder, what are the treatment goals?
3. What ethical and cultural considerations should be made when working with Claudia and her family?

Eating Disorders

Eating disorders are a group of psychological disorders related to eating behaviors that result in a lower quality of life and social functioning (Qian et al., 2022). Eating disorders include anorexia nervosa (AN), characterized by restrictive eating; binge-eating, characterized by overeating to the point of pain; and bulimia nervosa (BN), characterized by attempts to control weight through use of compensatory behaviors (e.g., vomiting, laxatives, extreme exercise, or fasting) (NIH,

235

2021). Eating disorders can cause serious damage to the heart, kidneys, intestines, throat, and teeth.

The median age of onset for BN and AN is 18 years old and for binge eating is 21 years old (NIH, 2021). The prevalence of eating disorders in the United States is 1.2% for binge eating disorder with a lifetime prevalence of 2.8%; .3% for BN with a lifetime prevalence of 1%; and .6% for AN (NIH, 2021). Overall, the lifetime prevalence of an eating disorder diagnosis is .91%, with a 12-month prevalence rate of .43% (Qian et al., 2022). However, US adolescents who develop an eating disorder between the ages of 13 and 18 have a lifetime prevalence of 2.7%, which is 33.7% higher than if the onset were 21 years or older. The frequency of anorexia in Hispanics/Latinos is lower compared to the non-Hispanic White population, whereas the frequency of binge eating disorder and bulimia is comparable to the non-Hispanic White population (Perezet al., 2016).

Enhanced Cognitive Behavioral Therapy

In 1981, C. G. Fairburn developed a manual for Cognitive Behavioral Therapy Bulimia Nervosa (CBT-BN). Since this first edition, the manual has been revised to include a more transdiagnostic approach to treating eating disorders and was renamed Enhanced Cognitive Behavioral Therapy (CBT-E) (Fairburn, 2008). The CBT-E transdiagnostic approach focuses on the similarities found between different eating disorder diagnoses (Fairburn, 2008).

Current research (Atwood & Friedman, 2019; Dalhenburg, Gleaves, & Hutchinson, 2019; Groff, 2015; Linardon, 2018) reflects that CBT-E is more effective in decreasing eating disorder behaviors when compared to other treatment models as well as nontreatment control groups. Atwood and Friedman (2019) found that treatment participants experienced a decrease in eating disorder behaviors more quickly using CBT-E when compared with other treatment models. Dahlenburg et al.'s (2019) systematic review concluded that the benefits of CBT-E are maintained to a significant degree after treatment and that some participants continue to experience increased benefits over time. The decrease in eating disorder behavior was found across the spectrum of eating disorder diagnoses, supporting CBT-E's transdiagnostic perspective (Linardon, 2018).

Although researchers have found reasons to support the use of CBT-E, there are limitations to current research proving the efficacy of CBT-E with specific populations. To date, studies applying CBT-E have not included men, the LGBTQ+ community, diversity of races and ethnicities, and use with younger participants and families. The current body of research is also missing a greater depth of understanding of the impact of CBT-E on specific eating disorder behaviors known to significantly impact recidivism, including subjective bingeing, driven exercise, eating disorder behavior marginally below the diagnostic threshold, and lack of systemic support.

Although studies supporting the use of CBT-E have concluded that participants experienced significantly decreased eating disorder behavior, participant symptoms remained above the threshold needed for diagnosis (Atwood & Friedman, 2019). In addition, a significant portion of current research supporting the use of CBT-E has been conducted in connection with Fairburn, CBT-E's creator, creating concern for the possibility of allegiance effect influencing outcomes (Groff, 2015). It is important for counselors to keep these limitations in mind when considering the implementation of CBT-E. For Claudia, I carefully considered these limitations as well as benefits and decided that CBT-E was the best treatment approach for her, as will be described below.

CBT-E Overview and Stages

CBT-E treatment strategies focus on cognitive distortions that reinforce the eating disorder: overemphasis placed on body shape and weight as well as the control that the person has over body shape and weight. A person diagnosed with an eating disorder might behave in different ways, even changing behavior over time, in response to these cognitive distortions, but the psychopathology that maintains the eating disorder remains the same.

The overall treatment goals for CBT-E are to (a) disrupt the maintaining mechanism composed of cognitive distortions and disordered eating behaviors and (b) develop healthy cognitions about eating and healthy routine eating behaviors. These goals are accomplished in four stages within a typical 20-week CBT-E treatment protocol (Fairburn, 2008). In week one of stage one, the initial assessment takes place. In the following three weeks of stage one, the clinician meets with the client two times per week, sessions 2–7. During the intense first four weeks of stage one, the goal is to align with the client by focusing on treatment and change, create a personalized formulation, provide education, and introduce the importance of in-session weighing and regular eating. In stage two, weeks 5 and 6, sessions 8 and 9, the client and clinician assess progress made, identify challenges or barriers to progress, and adjust the formulation if needed. In stage three, weeks 7 through 14, weekly appointments address the primary maintaining mechanisms of the eating disorder in an individualized way, providing strategies and alternatives to behaviors and thinking. In stage four, sessions 18, 19, and 20 are held every other week, and focus is on maintaining changes made and minimizing risk of relapse. A final appointment is held 20 weeks after the end of stage four to review progress.

CBT-E Stage 1

In the initial assessment, the client will begin to engage in treatment, will be provided information related to their eating disorder, create a formulation with the help of the clinician, discuss expectations of treatment, plan for real-time self-assessment, discuss homework, and confirm the next appointment (Fairburn, 2008). To better understand the client's eating disorder, clinicians gather information related to current disordered eating behavior, current concerns related to the eating disorder, development and history of the eating disorder, coexisting mental health or medical concerns, personal and family history related to health and mental health, a quick personal history, current life circumstances, and the client's attitudes toward treatment. In addition, height and weight are taken at the conclusion of the first session. The initial assessment typically can be conducted in a longer first session, no longer than an hour and a half.

It is important that the clinician consider medical concerns and the possible need for medical oversight during treatment. The clinician should gather medical information in the initial assessment including recent blood work results, recent EKG and bone density results if available, risk of suicide or self-harming behavior, current significant mental health concerns, current substance use, as well as a release to work with other medical providers supporting the client. Potentially, significant medical concerns, suicidality, or substance use could preclude a client from participating in CBT-E before addressing outstanding risks.

During the first session, the clinician collaboratively creates with the client a formulation, a tool to conceptualize the eating disorder with the client used throughout treatment. A formulation is a visual diagram of cognitive distortions that represent overemphasis on body shape, weight, and control over body shape and weight; subsequent behavior; and reactions that perpetuate the cognitive distortion and behavior that keep the client in her eating disorder. The formulation is created using the client's words and focuses on the pattern that maintains the eating disorder. Common maintaining mechanisms include overevaluation of shape and weight, overevaluation of control, dietary restriction, dietary restraint, being underweight, and changes in eating triggered by situations. The client is given a copy of the formulation to review. The formulation will be at the center of treatment planning.

The clinician explains to the client what to expect in treatment, with emphasis placed on the importance of completing each step of treatment such as sessions, self-assessment, homework, and in-session weights. In-session weights are an opportunity for the client to be responsible as well as face reality; this happens through weighing during sessions only, speaking the number out loud, graphing weights showing trends, and addressing concerns with the clinician.

The remaining sessions in stage one, each 50 minutes in length, follow a pattern: weight once a week, review records for quality, discuss attitude and patterns, determine and follow agenda with client, summarize, and discuss homework. The goals of these sessions are to provide education related to eating disorder diagnosis, establish a regular eating pattern, and arrange for family support. A regular eating pattern focuses first on routine rather than changing what a client is eating. The client is asked to eat breakfast, lunch, snack, dinner, snack, and sometimes a snack before lunch. Fairburn (2008) emphasizes, "Implementing the regular eating intervention is a skill that all CBT-E therapists need to acquire. It involves conveying the rationale well, being persuasive, tackling objections and obstacles, and praising all signs of progress" (p. 81). Involvement of family is based on their family's ability to support change and limited by family's contribution to the difficulty of creating change.

CBT-E Stage 2

During stage two, the clinician and client review progress using informal assessment or formal assessment completed outside of session, identify barriers, review formulation to gain a deeper understanding, and design stage three, prioritizing the most pressing maintaining mechanisms. During stage two, it is determined whether a longer version of CBT-E over 40 weeks rather than 20 would be most appropriate, based on the client's needs and health.

CBT-E Stage 3

Stage three includes the same components as stages one and two, as well as targeting maintaining mechanisms in individualized ways. Depending on the client, stage three can include identifying overevaluation; creating greater importance in other domains; addressing shape checking, avoidance, and the idea of feeling fat; historical review; managing mind-set; education on dieting; dietary restriction; mood intolerance; addressing dietary rules; learning problem-solving skills; and functional mood modulatory behavior.

CBT-E Stage 4

Finally, stage four follows the same structure as sessions in stage three. The difference in stage four compared to stage three is that sessions become increasingly more future focused and less focused on the present. It is recommended that treatment concludes once maintaining mechanisms have been disrupted and the client has begun to change patterns. It is not expected that all symptoms or behavior of the eating disorder have completely ceased. A final session is held 20 weeks following the last session of stage four. In the final session, the clinician and client determine whether there is a need for additional treatment based on significance of eating disorder symptoms.

Case Study

Given the evidence-based research, I implemented CBT-E to treat Claudia's eating disorder. I believed CBT-E would help disrupt the maintaining mechanisms of her eating disorder and begin to alleviate her eating disorder symptoms quickly. Her parents and health care providers were willing to be part of her treatment by supporting her change in behavior.

Goals for Claudia's first session included building rapport, gathering information about Claudia's current eating disorder symptoms, providing information related to eating disorders, creating a formulation together, discussing expectations of treatment, planning for real-time self-assessment, discussing homework, and confirming the next appointment. Once I introduced myself, I discussed confidentiality and Claudia's current eating disorder symptoms and provided some basic information to Claudia about eating disorders and the idea of a formulation, I encouraged Claudia to work with me to create a formulation of her eating disorder.

TABLE 17.1. CLAUDIA: TRANSCRIPT/ANALYSIS

Transcript	Analysis
T: "You and I are going to work together to draw a picture of how your eating disorder works. We will call it a formulation. Here is a picture of how some eating disorders work."	Using the diagram of a formulation helps someone to understand the steps that reinforce the behavior of an eating disorder.
C: "What does overevaluation mean?"	Overevaluation and other terms used in a formulation may not be familiar to an adolescent; these words can be personalized by therapist and adolescent.
T: "Overevaluation means giving something a lot of importance. What word would you use to describe this? How would you describe the things you do to try to control your weight or the shape of your body?"	Personalizing the formulation makes the process more meaningful and clearly identifies the steps in the formulation that must be taken to create change in the eating disorder.
C: "I think I would call it highlighting instead of overevaluation. I tell myself I am taking care of my food when I throw up."	Claudia's words will be added to the formulation; the formulation is a working document and will be updated as Claudia and her therapist work together.

After introducing the idea of the formulation and beginning to personalize it using Claudia's input, I gave Claudia a copy of the formulation to take home with her so she could continue to think about it between sessions. During the first session, Claudia and I also talked about the importance of real-time self-assessment, homework, and establishing a regular eating pattern. Real-time self-assessment involved Claudia keeping a detailed record of her eating patterns and eating disorder behavior that were reviewed during each session (see My Monitoring Record work sheet from Credo Oxford, https://www.credo-oxford.com/pdfs/F5.3_Blank_monitoring_record.pdf). At first, I emphasized eating at regular intervals, rather than focusing on what was eaten. I addressed concerns Claudia had about implementing a regular routine for eating. After Claudia and I created a formulation and plan for a regular eating routine, she will share it with her family. In a later session, I encouraged her to share it with both of her parents.

During stage two of treatment, Claudia and I continued talking about her formulation and examined the maintaining mechanism more closely. By creating the formulation with Claudia, we identified that Claudia's maintaining mechanism in her eating disorder was an overevaluation of her appearance. The heightened value she placed on her appearance resulted in Claudia wanting to control her body through eating disorder behaviors. Helping Claudia to see the pattern that she was in, and its consequences, was an important step in changing the behavior. I made this process developmentally appropriate for Claudia by integrating in art activities.

TABLE 17.2. **CLAUDIA: TRANSCRIPT/ANALYSIS**

Transcript	Analysis
T: "I am asking you to begin to eat breakfast, lunch, and dinner, with a snack between breakfast and lunch, and a snack between lunch and dinner."	This routine allows for Claudia to feel both hungry and satisfied at regular intervals throughout the day. She will avoid feeling overly hungry or overly full if she maintains this routine.
C: "I don't have time to eat that many times; no one eats that often. I can't eat dinner on the nights I have tennis."	Claudia could be fearful of the change in routine that could result in a change in herself or a change in the control she feels.
T: "This will take some planning, and I understand that it will be a change for you. A lot of people have this routine; I know you can do it. Let's make a plan together to help you be successful."	I will be patient and empathetic when responding to her concerns. Normalizing a new routine will help Claudia to feel like the change is possible.
C: "I don't usually eat breakfast before school; I am always running late."	It is reasonable that this change will require adjustments that need to be discussed.
T: "Okay, let's think of something that will be easy for you to do in the morning."	Initially, emphasis is placed on the routine and not what Claudia will be eating.

TABLE 17.3. **CLAUDIA: TRANSCRIPT/ANALYSIS**

Transcript	Analysis
T: "Today I would like you to create a picture that shows me the importance you give to different parts of who you are. We are going to use these art supplies to help us. [Provides paper, markers, glue, assorted materials including glitter, construction paper, yarn, pipe cleaners] Let's start by making a large circle."	Providing a variety of materials and flexibility for Claudia to depict her self-evaluation gives her freedom and control to express herself in a developmentally appropriate way.
C: Agreeably drew a large circle using markers.	
T: "Let's name important parts of you together."	This could be difficult for someone with an eating disorder, who places a lot of value on a few domains of themselves, to do without support.
C: "How I look is important, being a friend is important, helping around the house is important . . ."	
T: "Now that you have named valuable parts of who you are, use the circle you drew and any of our materials to show me how much you value each part. Like this one I drew."	I will provide Claudia with an example. I will be careful not to indicate a right or wrong way to complete this activity, giving Claudia the opportunity to create something unique.
C: [Worked silently while I waited. When she was done, she looked up, indicating that she was finished.]	
T: "I notice there are some parts of your circle that are larger and some that are smaller. What do you think it would be like if this small piece were gone? Or this big piece were even bigger?"	Reflecting with Claudia on what it would be like if the representation of herself is changed will help her to see the impact that this thinking has on her and her behavior.

After Claudia and I identified and gained an understanding of how her overevaluation of her appearance impacted her, she and I began to define a plan to create greater importance in other domains of her self-evaluation. Together Claudia and I identified new activities that Claudia was interested in becoming involved in. These new activities provided her with new or strengthened domains from which her evaluation of self was created. Ideas for new activities often come from activities that the client was previously interested in, activities they have been curious about, or interests they saw friends and family involved in. It was important to agree on one to two new activities that Claudia was willing to start. Creating specific goals that were related to activities was important because general goals were difficult to achieve, and setting too large a goal would have prohibited her from reaching the goal. Claudia and I agreed on a way to ensure that she started her new activity of playing 10 minutes with her dog three times a week and agreed that this goal would be reviewed during each session.

In the remaining sessions, Claudia and I continued to examine and adjust her formulation and explored what changes could be made to disrupt the maintaining mechanisms of her eating disorder. Sessions involved reviewing self-assessments and weekly goals to better understand the formulation as well as establishing goals for the following weeks. Claudia was ready to conclude her counseling when her eating disorder's maintaining mechanism had been disrupted, as evident by changes in her behavior related to body and eating behavior.

Ethical and Cultural Considerations

When working with a client who has been diagnosed with an eating disorder, it is very important to be aware of health and safety concerns that could be affecting the client. By regularly communicating with other professionals working with a client, clinicians can ensure that potentially life-threatening health and safety concerns are managed appropriately.

Family involvement is also vital to the treatment process when working with an adolescent diagnosed with an eating disorder. Family members are an important part of supporting change. They are also largely responsible for shopping for and preparing food, which is important to forming a regular eating routine.

Clinicians should be thoughtful of the client's cultural relationship with food and cultural expectations for body image when treating an eating disorder. Treatment is influenced by culturally appropriate food, traditions around food, and cultural differences related to the idea of an ideal body. The degree of assimilation or acculturation that a client experiences also impacts cultural aspects of treatment. For example, the degree to which Claudia identifies as Mexican American, Mexican, or American impacts her body satisfaction. Culture influences body-related values important for body image perception (Çakıcı, Mercan, & Denizci Nazlıgül, 2021). Claudia's maintaining mechanism may have been rooted in the thin ideal portrayed by Western culture and her overevaluation of the importance of her appearance.

Parent Consultations

Parents or other family members are an integral part of treatment when working with adolescents who have been diagnosed with an eating disorder. Family plays an important part in supporting the client to log real-time self-assessments and providing the opportunity for the client to establish regular eating patterns. Family members are often included in sessions to make them aware of the specific nature of the client's eating disorder, the nature of treatment, and how they can play a supportive role.

Conclusion

Through the course of CBT-E, Claudia learned about the maintaining mechanisms of her eating disorder, how her thoughts and behavior were reinforcing the importance of the maintaining mechanisms, and how she can disrupt this pattern and create new healthier patterns for herself. Claudia and her family worked together to create a routine of regular eating supporting Claudia's new outlook. Working with Claudia, I learned the importance of collaborating with Claudia to regularly revise and fine-tune her formulation. These updates ensured that Claudia's sessions were specific to her needs and relevant to her progress each session.

Sample Case Notes

Session 1

Subjective: Client was hesitant to describe eating disorder behavior; she attempted to justify her behavior and focused on decrease in eating disorder behavior after parents become concerned; she expressed lack of motivation when talking about creating a regular eating routine. Client stated, "It's really not a problem anymore."

Objective: Client sat with arms and legs close to body, hands in lap, she made direct eye contact when spoken to. Client spoke clearly and thoughtfully. When working together to create formulation, the client was cooperative and careful to follow directions.

Assessment: Reflected in the client's formulation, she is involved in thinking errors and behavior related to her body and weight that perpetuate the pattern of the eating disorder.

Plan: Counselor will follow prescribed steps in CBT-E manual; the remaining sessions of stage one will emphasize pattern and attitude of self-assessment, and establish a regular eating pattern.

Session 8

Subjective: Client was smiling and cooperative. Client was engaged with craft materials, expressive and thoughtful in the way that she chose to use them. Client adjusted what she created as she thought about different parts of herself, demonstrating reflectiveness.

Objective: Client was relaxed, sitting with relaxed posture, making direct eye contact throughout the session. She was actively engaged in creating a visual representation of herself, adding new ideas and details as she worked.

Assessment: Client demonstrated an overevaluation of her appearance through discussion and visual representation that she created. She can identify other areas of herself that are important and recognize the impact that placing significant emphasis on her appearance has on other areas of her life.

Plan: Client and I will work together to enhance the importance of other domains for self-evaluation by identifying activities that she will become involved in and creating a specific plan for her to begin these activities.

Resources

For Professionals

Eating Disorders: A Guide to Medical Care, https://higherlogicdownload.s3.
    amazonaws.com/AEDWEB/27a3b69a-8aae-45b2-a04c-2a078d02145d/
    UploadedImages/Publications_Slider/2120_AED_Medical_Care_4th_Ed_
    FINAL.pdf

Instructions for Self-Monitoring, https://www.cbte.co/download/t5-1-instructions
    -for-self-monitoring/?wpdmdl=2298&masterkey=5f4cd05c9f8e6

Topics to Cover When Assessing the Eating Problem, https://www.cbte.co/site/
    download/t5-1-topics-to-cover-when-assessing-the-eating-problem/?wpdmdl
    =654&masterkey=5c6fc29ef10b9

For Adolescents

Individuals 10 Actions, https://higherlogicdownload.s3.amazonaws.com/AED
    WEB/27a3b69a-8aae-45b2-a04c-2a078d02145d/UploadedImages/Publica
    tions_Slider/ExE_Individuals_10_Actions.pdf

National Association of Anorexia Nervosa and Associated Disorders, https://
    anad.org/

National Eating Disorders Association, https://www.nationaleatingdisorders.org/

For Parents

*Cognitive Behavior Therapy for Eating Disorders in Young People: A Parent's
    Guide* by Riccardo Dalle Grace and Carine el Khazen (2021).

Nine Truths about Eating Disorders, https://www.aedweb.org/publications/
    nine-truths

Your Child's Weight: Helping without Harming Birth through Adolescence by
    Ellyn Satter (2005).

Discussion Questions

1. What health-related information would you gather to ensure that Claudia is ready for CBT-E?
2. What are the benefits of creating a formulation in collaboration with Claudia?
3. What ethical considerations are important to consider when working with Claudia and her family?
4. When working with Claudia, or another adolescent diagnosed with an eating disorder, what personal beliefs or opinions about food and body would you need to be aware of?

References

Atwood, M. E., & Friedman, A. (2019). A systematic review of enhanced cognitive behavioral therapy (CBT-E) for eating disorders. *International Journal of Eating Disorders, 53*(3), 311–330. https://doi.org/10.1002/eat.23206

Çakıcı, K., Mercan, Z., & Denizci Nazlıgül, M. (2021). A systematic review of body image and related psychological concepts: Does ethnicity matter? *Psikiyatride Güncel Yaklaşımlar, 13*(4), 707–725.

Dahlenburg, S. C., Gleaves, D. H., & Hutchinson, A. D. (2019). Treatment outcome research of enhanced cognitive behaviour therapy for eating disorders: A systematic review with narrative and meta-analytic synthesis. *Eating Disorders, 27*(5), 482–502. https://doi.org/10.1080/10640266.2018.1560240

Fairburn, C. G. (1981). A cognitive behavioural approach to the treatment of bulimia. *Psychological Medicine, 11*(4), 707–711. https://doi.org/10.1017/S0033291700041209

Fairburn, C. G. (2008). *Cognitive behavior therapy and eating disorders.* Guilford Press.

Groff, S. E. (2015). Is enhanced cognitive behavioral therapy an effective intervention in eating disorders? A review. *Journal of Evidence-Informed Social Work, 12*(3), 272–288. https://doi.org/10.1080/15433714.2013.835756

Linardon, J. (2018). Meta-analysis of the effects of cognitive-behavioral therapy on the core eating disorder maintaining mechanisms: Implications for mechanisms of therapeutic change. *Cognitive Behaviour Therapy, 47*(2), 107–125. https://doi.org/10.1080/16506073.2018.1427785

National Institutes of Health. (2021). *Eating disorders.* https://medlineplus.gov/eatingdisorders.html

Perez, M., Ohrt, T. K., & Hoek, H. W. (2016). Prevalence and treatment of eating disorders among Hispanics/Latino Americans in the United States. *Current Opinion in Psychiatry, 29*(6), 378–382. https://doi.org/10.1097/YCO.0000000000000277

Qian, J., Wu, Y., Liu, F., Zhu, Y., Jin, H., Zhang, H., Wan, Y., Li, C., & Yu, D. (2022). An update on the prevalence of eating disorders in the general population: A systematic review and meta-analysis. *Eating and Weight Disorders—Studies on Anorexia, Bulimia and Obesity, 27*(2), 415–428. https://doi .org/10.1007/s40519-021-01162-z

TABLE 17.4.   **MY MONITORING RECORD**

Day_____   Date_____

Time	Foods and drink consumed	Place	V/L/E*	Context and comments

*V = vomiting, L = laxative misuse, E = exercise

Note: From "F5.3—Blank monitoring record," Online Training Program in CBT-E, CREDO, Oxford, 2017. https://www .cbte.co/for-professionals/cbt-e-resources-and-handouts/

CHAPTER 18

Substance Use Disorder
Motivational Interviewing and Creative Approaches with an African American Adolescent
Allison Crowe and Jason O. Perry

Robby is a 17-year-old African American high school cisgender male who lives with his grandparents in a small town in North Carolina. His mother intermittently stayed with them for extended periods but would leave due to her struggles with illicit substances. Robby's father left his mother and him when he was 8 years old, and the father later remarried. Throughout his school years, Robby had managed to stay out of any sort of legal trouble. However, recently he was arrested for breaking and entering into a store and stealing a vaping device and a small package of synthetic THC. As part of his sentence, Robby was court ordered to receive a mental health assessment and treatment. He was diagnosed with depression and substance use disorder.

For the case of Robby, please consider the following:

1. For teenagers such as Robby, what are common considerations for counselors when working with mental health and substance use disorders?
2. How can Motivational Interviewing be especially impactful for this age group, and why is it a useful theory to draw from?
3. How can creative techniques enhance more traditional frameworks when working with teenage clients? What benefits and challenges should counselors consider with creative approaches?

Depression

The Substance Abuse and Mental Health Services Administration (SAMHSA, 2020) estimates that 21 million adults (8.4%) in the United States had at least one major depressive episode in 2020. This was highest among individuals ages 18–25 (17.0%). Among adolescents (ages 12–17), it is estimated that 4.1 million adolescents (17%) in the United States had at least one major depressive episode in 2020. In 2020, an estimated 41.6% of US adolescents with a major depressive episode received treatment. Depression in adolescents can look like the following—feelings of sadness, anxiousness, worthlessness, or emptiness. Also, the teen might lose interest in activities he used to enjoy. Feelings of irritability, frustration, or anger are frequently experienced. In addition, there might be withdrawal from family and friends, a drop in grades, changes in eating and sleeping habits. Fatigue or memory loss, as well as harming oneself or thoughts of suicide, are other symptoms of depression (National Institute of Mental Health, NIMH, 2022).

Substance Use Disorders

It is well known that substance use disorders (SUDs) often co-occur with mental health concerns and vice versa. Although they commonly co-occur, they don't "cause" each other. Three possibilities have been established as to why they are seen together (NIMH, 2021). First, the same risk factors can contribute to both mental health struggles and substance use disorders. Environmental factors such as trauma, experiences of discrimination and racism, or poverty impact both. When experiencing a mental health concern such as depression or anxiety, a person self-medicates or seeks a way to cope with the symptoms through substances, which can lead to a substance use disorder. Finally, substances or a substance use disorder can contribute to the development of other mental health concerns due to changes in the brain (NIMH, 2021).

Among adolescents in the United States, substance usage is a public health concern, with at least one in eight teenagers abusing an illicit substance in the past year (National Center for Drug Abuse Statistics, 2023). Specifically, substance use increased by 61% among eighth graders between 2016 and 2020. Sixty-two percent of twelfth graders have abused alcohol, and 50% of teenagers have misused a substance at least once.

Motivational Interviewing

For the case of Robby, we draw from the major tenets of Motivational Interviewing (MI). MI is a counseling approach for eliciting change with a particular emphasis on helping clients explore and resolve ambivalence, defined as a struggle to articulate conflicting values that work against positive change (Miller, 1995; Miller & Rollnick, 2002, 2004, 2009). This emphasis on resolving ambivalence is essential because ambivalence often creates stumbling blocks along a client's road to living a healthier, more fulfilling lifestyle (Miller & Rollnick, 2002; Rollnick & Miller, 1995). MI is a client-centered approach in which the counselor accepts people as they are by viewing clients' own values, motivations, abilities, and resources as important and valuable. MI is based on the Rogerian fundamental principle of empathic understanding (Rogers, 1951), although MI differs from traditional Person-Centered theory, as it is more focused and goal-directed toward resolving client ambivalence (Miller & Rollnick, 2002, 2009). It is a collaborative approach, supported by the belief that every person has the motivation and resourcefulness to change. Clients who are ambivalent may not have had the opportunity to feel understood (Miller & Rollnick, 2002).

MI encourages counselors to assist the client with examining and resolving ambivalence, because ambivalence is understood as the main obstacle to overcome when attempting to change. As the counselor, we must remember that motivation must originate from the client. The counselor relies on the client's intrinsic goals and values to create change. The counselor works with the client to express all feelings related to changing a behavior to resolve ambivalence. Readiness for change is understood as a product of interpersonal communication, and the counselor should remain open and responsive to a client's motivational signals. For example, resistance from the client could mean that treatment is moving too fast. A counselor can notice this and adjust his or her motivational strategies to remain flexible with the client. Finally, the counseling process is supported by a collaborative relationship.

Four MI Principles

Miller and Rollnick (2002) share four key principles that are central to MI. The first, *expressing empathy*, focuses on the importance of seeing the world through the eyes of the client. This is critical, because when a client feels understood, an open expression of thoughts and feelings is possible. Reflective listening is an important part of expressing empathy, as well as normalizing ambivalence about change (Miller & Rollnick, 2002). This reflection and normalization of ambivalence not only helps the client to feel understood, but also helps to reduce defensiveness and resistance.

The second principle, *developing discrepancy*, describes how exploring discrepancies can facilitate change. When the client can see that there is a difference (or discrepancy) between behavior and goals, or values and goals, they may be more likely to make changes. *Rolling with resistance* refers to avoiding arguments for change. When a counselor notices opposition from the client, they should not oppose it directly. Instead, resistance is the client signaling for the counselor to adjust their approach. By inviting new perspectives without imposing, the counselor maintains a supportive stance, affirming clients' autonomy and ability to solve problems with their own insight (Miller & Rollnick, 2002).

The final principle, *supporting self-efficacy*, describes a self-fulfilling prophecy that occurs from a counselor's belief in the client's capacity to lead their own change. Operating under this principle, a counselor acknowledges that his or her own expectations have a profound impact on client outcomes. By understanding that the power to choose is inherent within the client, not the counselor, a counselor can advocate for change through expressing belief in the client's abilities, personal responsibility, and by offering to help, but not create, the process of change.

Since the original approach, authors have applied MI to different types of clients and presenting concerns. We encourage readers to consult literature on MI and adolescents (e.g., Naar & Suarez, 2021) to ensure that it is tailored to developmental needs of the age group. In the following case study, we offer the case of Robby through the eyes of Motivational Interviewing principles. In addition, we apply a creative approach taken from an earlier article on creative approaches to Motivational Interviewing (Crowe & Parmenter, 2012). This is just one activity from the article, and readers are encouraged to consult the full article to see more creative approaches that align with each of the MI principles.

Case Study Application

Seventeen-year-old Robby Denton spent most of his childhood living in the home of his maternal grandparents, in a small rural town in northeastern North Carolina. By all outside appearances, Robby had a good life, as his grandparents were held in high regard by members of the community. Though their home was modest, he lived in a desirable neighborhood and had a few friends close to his age. His mother sometimes stayed at the home for extended periods of time, but she seemed to slip in and out of her son's life, and her level of involvement in Robby's development proved to be inconsistent at best. This was mainly due to her struggles with illicit substances and unemployment. Robby's father had moved out of the state for employment purposes when Robby was in elementary school and remarried soon after, when Robby was about 8 years old. His father's and stepmother's relationship resulted in producing two siblings, both boys, now ages 6 and 7, respectively. He heard from his dad and stepmom from time to time, but his grandparents were the most constant "family" to Robby. He struggled with adjusting to his parents' lack of involvement in his life. Although his grandparents were aware that the familial situation caused him to become irritable and angry, they avoided seeking counseling services for Robby and did not talk about the problems at home.

When two law enforcement officers knocked on the front door asking to speak to Robby one afternoon, his grandparents were in shock. This was the first time Robby had ever been in any sort of potential trouble. The officers explained that Robby was a suspect in a recent breaking and entering and robbery at a local tobacco store. When the officers searched his room, Robby was found to have a vaping device and a small package of synthetic THC in his backpack matching the description of the items stolen from the store. He was arrested and was released to his grandfather, who paid the $300 cash bail, and a court date was set to take place in four weeks. The attorney, who was appointed by the court, strongly advocated on Robby's behalf and asked the judge to take into account his client's age and the fact that he had no prior record. The judge, who was known for being creative and progressive, ordered Robby to comply with supervised probation for a period of one year and entered a deferred prosecution judgment, which meant that the case would be dismissed once all conditions were met. As special conditions of Robby's probation, the judge ordered him to obtain an assessment from a clinical mental health provider and follow any recommended treatment. The judge also ordered Robby to pay restitution, in the amount of $350, to replace the window he broke when he entered the tobacco store, and to participate in victim-offender conferencing, a practice consistent with the principles of Restorative Justice (Karp, 2019).

Although Robby was happy to not be in jail, he was angry that he got caught and was resistant to change. He was not one to talk about and share his feelings and was upset about having to meet with a mental health counselor. From Robby's perspective, he was managing his life well enough and wished he could cancel the appointment with the counselor, avoiding it. Although Robby recognized that he had been unhappy for quite some time, he was not interested in seeking help or making changes in his life.

Treatment Goals and Objectives

The treatment aim was to work according to MI principles, particularly expressing empathy, rolling with any resistance, and developing a discrepancy with Robby. The objective was to allow Robby to be the one to decide that something needs to change and be the driver of this change.

First Sessions

Prior to the first appointment, at the urging of his grandmother, Robby reviewed my (second author's) counseling website. The website mentioned that I was skilled in using the method of Motivational Interviewing. Robby was slightly interested in knowing more about what to expect, especially because this would be his first visit with a mental health counselor. He was less than excited when he entered my counseling office for his first appointment, but by the end of the session Robby was surprised that he had talked more than he thought he would. In fact, he noticed that he felt like a big weight had been lifted after that initial visit. As his counselor, I did not judge him, even when he admitted that when he felt down, he used his vape to smoke THC to take his mind off things. And when he told the story of why he'd broken into the convenience store, Robby was relieved that he did not feel judged.

When Robby realized that he was about to enter his third session, he was surprised to find himself not experiencing feelings of dread. As the alliance between Robby and me continued to develop, grow, and strengthen, he felt more comfortable sharing his thoughts and feelings related to his life. As he could safely talk about and share how he was feeling, details about his parents and the deep depression that used to remain beneath the surface began to bubble up to the top. Robby spoke of feeling confused, especially when he was little, why his mom would come back and then leave again, and why his grandparents never wanted to talk about it.

Keeping true to the spirit of MI (Rollnick & Miller, 1995), I worked to build a partnership, working together in a collaborative way, and I avoided the role of the expert. Robby noticed feelings of being valued and accepted as I demonstrated respect for his ability to make decisions for himself and be autonomous. Robby also sensed that I was compassionate and caring, most especially because, on several occasions, I discussed the importance of us working to understand what was in his best interest. Lastly, the concept of evocation was quite evident, as I encouraged Robby to generate ideas during our sessions.

River of Life Activity

In the third session I introduced the River of Life activity (Crowe & Parmenter, 2012), which involved having Robby draw a large river, and then map out major life events, people, places, and things that have influenced him along the way. The principle that we consider most in this session is *expressing empathy*. Robby needed to feel that I had empathy for him and his experiences in his river of life. According to MI and the stages of change, when the client can sense this from the counselor, the likelihood is greater that the client feels understood, and the therapeutic relationship can strengthen. The goal of the session was for me to accept Robby "as is" and to convey this back to Robby. By using visual art, I worked with Robby to draw his river so that I could see the world through his eyes. This principle is critical, because when a client feels as though he or she is understood, an open expression of thoughts and feelings is possible. If we accept the client as is and communicate this to the client, the possibility for change increases. Below we list materials, instructions, and a part of the transcript between Robby and me as the counselor.

Materials: Large piece of paper, such as butcher-block paper. Smaller pieces of paper can also be used if the counselor does not have butcher block paper.

Instructions:

1. Instruct client to create their "river of life" by drawing an image of a river that represents events, activities, and important milestones that the client has faced before coming to counseling. This gives the counselor an opportunity to learn more about the client and their river of life or personal story.
2. After drawing their river image and sharing this with the counselor, the counselor and client together discuss the themes, events, and other important information.
3. The counselor is to focus on acceptance of the client as they are and conveying this to the client. This is done using person-centered skills such as unconditional positive regard and communication of empathy using reflection of content, feeling, and meaning.

Later in the session, Robby shared about the first time he tried vaping with THC with a friend from school. It helped him forget about some of the pain and anger that he had with his parents, and it felt good to "numb out" the loneliness he felt when he looked back on his dad's leaving and his mom's inconsistent relationship. It also helped him forget his resentment toward his grandparents for never talking to him about his parents or letting him ask questions. He also admitted to me that a big part of him did not want to stop vaping. Why should

TABLE 18.1. **ROBBY: SESSION 3**

Transcript	Analysis
C: "Robby, you will notice this large piece of paper I have today. I would like you to draw what I call your river of life that has major events, activities, and milestones that you have been through before coming into counseling."	By understanding more about Robby, the counselor can express empathy for Robby.
R: "Umm, okay, I guess I can do that. Isn't this drawing stuff for little kids though?"	Adolescents often feel awkward in general and are sometimes surprised by expressive arts.
C: "The arts can be for everyone, regardless of age. You do not have to be good at drawing to do this. Would you be willing to try it? I know you have done a lot of new things with me so far, so I wonder if you would do the same today."	The counselor develops a small discrepancy by pointing out that Robby has been willing to try a few new things just by coming into counseling as a willing participant.
R: "Sure. I guess my first rock in the river was when my dad left. I did not understand what was going on and why he and my mom were not happy. He left North Carolina without any explanation."	Robby had talked about his dad's leaving and what it meant to him, but this was the first time he had really considered it as a major upsetting event, or "rock" in his river. This creative activity helped Robby more fully understand the significant impact this had on him at an early age.
C: "I can imagine how confusing that must have been for you."	More expression of empathy.
R: "Yes, it was. And my mom—she was not much better. She would live with us for a while and things would be great. I would be happy again. But then something would happen, and the next morning, she would be gone. My grandparents would just tell me it was 'for the best' and that I would understand when I was older."	Robby shares further pain and confusion with greater depth than he had before.
C: "So, how about we draw this as your next rock . . . when your mom first moved out."	The counselor continues to draw out the events of Robby's River of Life and express empathy.
R: "I would be so upset and confused when she left, but then feel excited when she would call, saying that she was coming back."	Robby is gaining insight into his own patterns of up-and-down feelings.
C: "So, on one hand it was hurtful that she would leave with no warning, but at the same time when she had come back it felt good."	The counselor begins to implement the technique of developing a discrepancy.

he? It does not impact his grades at school or anything else. What was the big deal? I heard this ambivalence and planned to highlight this in a future session, instead still focusing on expressing empathy to continue to build the therapeutic alliance. In a future session, I began to plant the seed that there might be ways for Robby to cope with his feelings other than using substances, and that Robby's legal trouble might indicate that something needs to change.

Case Discussion

The River of Life activity was a creative exercise coupled with Motivational Interviewing techniques that helped Robby see more deeply the impact of his parents' leaving when he was young. Although he had some knowledge of this impact, the visual arts allowed him to conceptualize this as a rock in his river. As the counselor, I drew out pain and unhappiness from Robby's childhood based on these events and his grandparents' tendencies to bottle up their own thoughts and feelings related to this. In addition, I continued to work with Robby to see the connection between the THC vaping and how this was a negative coping behavior for the pain he felt. As sessions continued, I used additional creative techniques and MI principles to change Robby's behavior so that he replaced his substance use with other, more positive, healthy coping strategies.

Ethical and Cultural Considerations

According to Sullivan et al. (2017), nearly 17% of Americans live in rural areas, including some of the poorest and most underserved areas of the nation (Sullivan et al., 2017). In addition, African Americans are like other rural residents in that they hold rural values (i.e., close relationships with family, strong ties to religion, independence, and stoicism) but have endured decades of discrimination and poverty and have legitimate reasons to mistrust the health-care system (Sullivan et al., 2017). Although African Americans experience mental disorders (such as depression and anxiety) at rates similar to Whites, they are significantly less likely to receive treatment (Sullivan et al., 2017). Individuals who delay entering treatment may sometimes wait until a higher level of care is needed, such as in-patient hospitalization. Consequently, avoiding treatment can result in marked functional impairment (Sullivan et al., 2017).

MI can be used with culturally diverse clients such as Robby. Lee and colleagues (2013) suggest that counselors expand their scope beyond the individual to the family and community and acknowledge discrimination and racism as causes of distress rather than factors that impact levels of distress. Counselors using MI with diverse clients must also be aware of their own implicit cultural bias to avoid microaggressions that will do more damage to the client. In addition, to deliver culturally competent MI, the counselor should bring up culture, cultural norms, and cultural communities to gain a full understanding of the client.

Parent and Teacher Consultations

Because Robby's grandparents were his legal guardians, I provided biweekly feedback to whichever grandparent drove him to the counseling appointment. To maintain trust with Robby, I always asked him if I could tell his grandparent something general about our session, without disclosing anything private, by inviting his grandparent to the last five minutes of the session. I informed Robby that usually adults will "stay off your back" if they know you are making progress. Robby was agreeable to this and would decide which sessions he wanted to invite in his grandparent. I would tell the grandparent something general, such as,

Today, we discussed difficult events in Robby's life, that I will keep private, and I provided empathy without judgment by statements such as "You felt confused and hurt." I believe doing this without giving advice is helping Robby develop his own motivation to move toward his goals of living a better life. Grandpa, one thing that might be helpful for you to try is to ask Robby during dinner to share one positive and one negative about his day, without giving advice. Then, you share one positive and one negative about your own day.

I also invited his grandparents and mother to feel free to schedule a consultation session with me. I made it clear that I would keep Robby's privacy but would help them understand MI principles and interactions with Robby that may be helpful. If Robby had difficulties with teachers at school, I would ask Robby's permission to send his teachers and school counselors an email with brief suggestions on how to help him (i.e., say "I know you want to do well in this class. You seem down today. What's going on? How can I help?").

Conclusion

Robby made considerable progress through MI. The immediate empathy he experienced substantially decreased his resistance to counseling to the point of not just seeing it as a meaningless obligation forced on him by the judge but, rather, seeing it as a valuable experience to help him achieve his own goals. Robby was able to explore the discrepancies between his substance use and his desire to one day be a respectable father. He developed a new perspective of self-efficacy in taking steps toward managing his depression now and in the future; using healthy coping strategies; setting realistic expectations and boundaries with his parents; and building reputable relationships so that he could become an engaged and respectable father one day.

Seeing Robby's progress confirmed our belief that creative techniques coupled with MI principles can add dimension, especially when working with young people experiencing depression and substance use.

Sample Case Notes

Session 1

Subjective: Client entered session due to court mandate and appeared reluctant to share.

Objective: Mandated counseling due to legal issues, THC use, and recent behavior changes at home. Lives with grandparents and charged with breaking and entering.

Assessment: Client will benefit from counseling using Motivational Interviewing with a focus on empowering himself to be the motivator of change. Will focus on expressing empathy to build alliance.

Plan: Use MI principles to begin to build the therapeutic relationship, roll with resistance to change, develop discrepancies. Consider creative techniques to illustrate life events and take pressure off talk therapy alone.

Session 3

Subjective: Client appeared more comfortable and willing to share with this counselor. Started processing feelings related to parents' departures, grandparents' unwillingness to communicate, and the role THC played in coping with this.

Objective: Engaged in River of Life activity that encouraged client to use visual art to create his own river that depicted major life events that impact him today. Used MI techniques to continue the relationship and begin to develop discrepancies and roll with resistance.

Assessment: Client understood impact of parents' departures and grandparents' lack of communication in a deeper sense. Began to understand and explore THC and its relationship to coping.

Plan: Will continue to use creative applications of MI with client to reinforce change.

Resources

For Professionals

Crowe, A., & Parmenter, A. (2012). Creative approaches to Motivational Interviewing: Addressing the principles. *Journal of Creativity in Mental Health, 7,* 124–140, doi: 10.1080/15401383.2012.684662

Holt, E., & Kaiser, D. H. (2009). The first step series: Art therapy for early substance abuse treatment. *Arts in Psychotherapy, 36,* 245–250. doi: 10.1016/j.aip.2009.05.004

Horay, B. J. (2006). Moving towards gray: Art therapy and ambivalence in substance abuse treatment. *Art Therapy: Journal of the American Art Therapy Association, 23*(1), 14–22. doi: 10.1080/07421656.2006.10129528

Miller, W. R. (1995). *Motivational enhancement therapy with drug abusers.* University of New Mexico. http://motivationalinterview.org/Documents/MET DrugAbuse.PDF

Naar, S., & Suarez, M. (2021). *Motivational interviewing with adolescents and young adults* (2nd ed.). Guilford Press.

For Adolescents

Wood, A. (2020). *The motivational interviewing workbook: Exercises to decide what you want and how to get there.* Rockridge Press.

Discussion Questions

1. Based on the case study of Robby as presented in this chapter, what would you do next in session if you were the counselor working with Robby?
2. As the counselor working with Robby, you pick up on some defensiveness and resistance from Robby in session 6. Use MI language to describe how you would conceptualize this and outline your "next steps" for treatment.
3. What other creative techniques could you imagine using with Robby? How would you use these in combination with MI?

References

Carroll, K., Ball, S., Nich, C., Martino, S., Frankforter, T., Farentinos, C., Woody, & G., Kunkle, L. E. (2006). Motivational interviewing to improve treatment engagement and outcome in individuals seeking treatment for substance abuse: A multisite effectiveness study. *Drug and Alcohol Dependence, 81*(3), 301–312.

Crowe, A., & Parmenter, A. (2012). Creative approaches to Motivational Interviewing: Addressing the principles. *Journal of Creativity in Mental Health, 7*, 124–140. doi: 10.1080/15401383.2012.684662

Karp, D. R. (2019). *The little book of restorative justice for colleges and universities: Repairing harm and rebuilding trust in response to student misconduct.* Good Books.

Lee, C. S., López, S. R., Colby, S. M., Rohsenow, D., Hernández, L., Borrelli, B., & Caetano, R. Culturally adapted motivational interviewing for Latino heavy drinkers: Results from a randomized clinical trial. *Journal of Ethnic Substance Abuse, 12* (4): 356–373. doi: 10.1080/15332640.2013.836730

Miller, W. R. (1995). *Motivational enhancement therapy with drug abusers.* University of New Mexico. http://motivationalinterview.org/Documents/MET DrugAbuse.PDF

Miller, W. R., & Rollnick, S. (2002). *Motivational interviewing: Preparing people for change* (2nd ed.). Guilford Press.

Miller, W. R., & Rollnick, S. (2004). Talking oneself into change: Motivational interviewing, stages of change, and therapeutic process. *Journal of Cognitive Psychotherapy: An International Quarterly, 18*(4), 299–308. doi: 110.1891/088983904780944306

Miller, W. R., & Rollnick, S. (2009). Ten things that motivational interviewing is not. *Behavioural and Cognitive Psychotherapy, 37*, 129–140. doi: 10.1017/S1352465809005128

Naar, S., & Suarez, M. (2021). *Motivational interviewing with adolescents and young adults* (2nd ed.). Guilford Press.

National Center for Drug Abuse Statistics. (2023). *Illicit drug use.* from https://www.cdc.gov/nchs/fastats/drug-use-illicit.htm

National Institute of Mental Health. (2021). *Depression.* https://www.nimh.nih
.gov/health/topics/depression

NIMH. (2022). *Substance use and co-occurring mental disorders.* Retrieved April
3, 2023, from https://www.nimh.nih.gov/health/topics/substance-use-and
-mental-health

Papp, J., Campbell, C., Onifade, E., Anderson, V., Davidson, W., & Foster, D.
(2016). Youth drug offenders: An examination of criminogenic risk and juve-
nile recidivism. *Corrections: Policy, Practice and Research, 1*(4), 229–245.
doi: 10.1080/23774657.2016.1218804

Rogers, C. (1951). *Client-centered therapy: Its current practice, implications and
theory.* Constable.

Rollnick, S., & Miller, W. (1995). What is motivational interviewing?
Behavioural and Cognitive Psychotherapy, 23(4), 325–334. doi: 10.1017/
S135246580001643X

Substance Abuse and Mental Health Services Administration. (2020). *Key substance use and mental health indicators in the United States: Results from
the 2020 national survey on drug use and health.* https://www.samhsa
.gov/data/sites/default/files/reports/rpt35325/NSDUHFFRPDFWHTML-
Files2020/2020NSDUHFFR102121.htm

Sullivan, G., Cheney, A., Olson, M., Haynes, T., Bryant, K., Cottoms, N., & Cur-
ran, G. (2017). Rural African Americans' perspectives on mental health: Com-
paring focus groups and deliberative democracy forums. *Journal of Health
Care for the Poor and Underserved, 28*(1), 548–565. doi: 10.1353/hpu.2017
.0039

Timko, C., Booth, B. M., Han, X., Schultz, N. R., Blonigen, D. M., Wong, J. J.,
& Cucciare, M. A. (2017). Criminogenic needs, substance use, and offend-
ing among rural stimulant users. *Rural Mental Health, 41*(2), 110–122. doi:
10.1037/rmh0000065

CHAPTER 19

LGBTQ
Gestalt Therapy and Liberatory Approaches with a Dominican American Adolescent
Ana Guadalupe Reyes

Jose Luis identifies as a 16-year-old queer nonbinary person of Dominican descent. They live with their parents, two younger siblings, and paternal grandparents in a three-bedroom house. Their parents and grandparents are devout Catholics who attend mass every Sunday. Jose Luis recently came out as queer and nonbinary to some of their best friends and swore them to secrecy because they are afraid of how their parents will respond. Jose Luis was referred to counseling by their school counselor due to their experience of anxiety, increased bullying at school, and exploration of their gender identity and sexuality. Jose Luis's parents were reluctant to seek counseling until the school counselor provided additional information regarding the counseling process. Their parents, Rosie and Carlos, accompanied Jose Luis to the intake session. Jose Luis's parents reported concerns about the client's grades, lack of communication with family, anxiety, isolation, clothing style, and bullying at school. Josie Luis appeared quiet and anxious as their parents shared their concerns.

For this case study, consider the following:

1. What are some of the most common concerns queer adolescents may experience during the coming-out process?
2. What may be underneath the parents' reluctance to seek counseling?
3. How can we build trust and rapport with the parents and client? How can we work collaboratively with the parents to support Jose Luis?
4. What are some cultural considerations we need to be aware of?

LGBTQ People

According to the National Alliance on Mental Illness (NAMI, 2023), lesbian, gay, bisexual, transgender, and queer (LGBTQ) people are at greater risk for poor mental health across all developmental stages, highlighting the importance of culturally responsive mental health services across the life span. Some of the issues most commonly reported among LGBTQ youth are depression, anxiety, substance abuse, suicidality, self-harm, internalized homophobia, biphobia, or transphobia, and comorbid mental health disorders (Batejan, Jarvi, & Swenson, 2015; Hunt, Vennatt, & Waters, 2018; Mustanski, Newcomb, & Garofalo, 2011; Trevor Project, 2022). In addition, LGBTQ youth often report feelings of isolation, shame, guilt, and internalized oppression; history of traumatic events such as physical, emotional, or sexual abuse; and familial rejection and lack of social support (Hunt et al., 2018). Based on what we know about Jose Luis thus far, it is essential to remember that they may be experiencing feelings of shame, isolation, and fear as they continue coming out and exploring their gender identity. As I work with Jose Luis, I will continuously assess how they've internalized oppression and work with them to heal from internalized oppression. Further, I will work with Jose Luis's parents through parent consultation and potentially refer them to an LGBTQ Latin parent support group.

Multiple researchers have found correlations between experiences of discrimination and increased levels of depression, anxiety, and internalized negativity about one's sexual identity (Meyer, 2003; Mustanski et al., 2011). One of the factors contributing to increased mental health concerns experienced by LGBTQ youth is minority stress (Meyer, 2003). Minority stress is the compounding effect of the intersecting stressors LGBTQ youth experience from ongoing institutional, systemic, and individual discrimination, stigmatization, and harassment, such as racism, homophobia, biphobia, transphobia, cisgenderism, sexism, and heterosexism due to their race/ethnicity, sexual identity, gender identity, and/or gender expression (Hunt et al., 2018; Meyer, 2003). Further, LGBTQ youth experience disproportionate physical and mental health disparities in the United States (Hafeez, Zeshan, Tahir, Jahan, & Naveed, 2017; Hunt et al., 2018). Jose Luis may experience various forms of discrimination as a queer nonbinary person of Dominican descent. Thus, it is crucial to explore Jose Luis's social and cultural identities, what their identities mean to them, and assess their experiences of oppression.

Mental health professionals must understand the experiences of LGBTQ youth as multidimensional and interdependent with other salient personal, racial/ethnic, cultural, and social identities (Paradies et al., 2015). From an intersectional lens, it is essential to acknowledge that LGBTQ youth may experience discrimination, oppression, and victimization based on the intersections of systemic and structural oppression that target people based on their racial/ethnic identity (e.g., racism), gender identity (e.g., cisgenderism, transphobia), gender expression (e.g., heterosexism, cisgenderism, transphobia), sexual identity (e.g., heterosexism, homophobia, biphobia), socioeconomic status (e.g., classism), religion, spirituality, country of origin (e.g., nationalism), documentation status, and ability status (Paradies et al., 2015), creating a unique experience of power, privilege, and oppression based on their social locations. For example, as a queer nonbinary Latine adolescent, Jose Luis may experience racism, heterosexism, cisgenderism, homophobia, transphobia, and xenophobia in various forms daily.

The intersection of various target identities has been linked directly to increased susceptibility to discrimination, oppression, and victimization (Collins & Blige, 2016; Crenshaw, 1989), compounding the psychological and physiological effects of discrimination. For example, transgender adolescents of color are vulnerable to increased violence, harassment, and discrimination resulting from the intersection of heterosexism, cisgenderism, homophobia, and transphobia. In 2017, the National Coalition of Anti-Violence Programs (NCAVP; 2018) gathered data on 52 anti-LGBTQ homicides in the United States and found that LGBTQ people of color (POC) accounted for 71% of the reported anti-LGBTQ homicides (n = 31). Twenty-four out of the 31 LGBTQ POC killed in anti-queer violence were transgender womxn of color (NCAVP, 2018). The introduction of anti-LGTBQ legislation across the United States significantly impacts the mental health of LGBTQ people, including youth. For example, "93% of transgender and nonbinary youth said that they have worried about transgender people being denied access to gender-affirming medical care due to state or local laws" (Trevor Project, 2022, p. 14). Thus, I will explore Jose Luis's experiences of anti-LGBTQ legislation and how current legislation may directly or indirectly affect them. Jose Luis may be hypervigilant and afraid of how their life could be impacted by anti-trans legislation. In addition, I will explore their interest in gender-affirming medical care and connect them to resources as needed.

Guiding Theory and Frameworks

I will tailor my approach to meet Jose Luis's needs as they arise. Thus, I will be using Gestalt therapy as my guiding theory and intersectionality theory as a framework to honor Jose Luis's cultural wisdom and to guide my clinical work with Jose Luis and their family. I will also integrate expressive arts to assist Jose Luis in exploring their identity as a queer nonbinary Latine adolescent, including their experience of anxiety, bullying, and gender and sexuality.

Gestalt Therapy

Gestalt theory is a holistic, phenomenological, experiential, process-oriented, and relational approach to counseling (Perls, Hefferline, & Goodman, 1951; Yontef, 1993). Gestalt therapy focuses on the totality of living organisms (i.e., emotions, senses, bodily sensations, and thoughts) to increase clients' moment-to-moment awareness, thus increasing their ability to live fully, make choices, and accept responsibility (Perls et al., 1951; Yontef, 1993). The therapeutic relationship is considered an opportunity for authentic encounters between the client and counselor, with moment-to-moment experiments co-created by the client and counselor. Experiments provide opportunities for the client to fully engage in exploration, growth, and self-acceptance while being in a relationship with the counselor and experiencing the relationship, and exploring their intrapersonal process (i.e., physical sensations, emotions, thoughts) in the here and now (Perls et al., 1951; Yontef, 1993).

Gestalt therapy will benefit Jose Luis because our initial focus will be building a therapeutic relationship where Jose Luis can authentically experience themselves and me. Being in a caring and authentic relationship with a counselor who shares some social and cultural identities (i.e., queer, nonbinary, Latine) may also support Jose Luis in exploring and accepting their intrapersonal experience. The experiential nature of Gestalt therapy will also provide opportunities for Jose Luis and me to co-create different experiments to help them further explore different ways of being and to experience themselves differently.

Intersectionality Theory

Intersectionality theory aims to explore and understand people's social locations, power relations, and the impact of systemic and structural oppression on those with marginalized identities (Collins & Blige, 2016; Crenshaw, 1989). Consequently, intersectionality theory demands the understanding and interrogation of our historical and current social, political, and ideological context "to bring the often-hidden dynamics forward in order to transform them" (Carbado, Crenshaw, Mays, & Tomlinson, 2013, p. 312) through reflexivity, practice, scholarship, research, and activism (Collins & Blige, 2016). In counseling, intersectionality theory can be used as a lens or framework to explore clients' social and cultural identities, the impact of systemic and structural oppression on their overall well-being and create comprehensive treatment plans that include advocacy inside and outside of the counseling room.

Using intersectionality theory as a framework with Jose Luis will help me explore their social and cultural identities, such as their race, ethnicity, sexuality, gender identity, language(s) spoken, ability status, and religion/spirituality during the initial phases of our work together, so that I can engage in ongoing reflection and exploration of their experiences of oppression outside of sessions and in sessions with Jose Luis. Further, I will engage in reflection and exploration of ways to dismantle the power structures present in our work (i.e., moving from power over the client to practicing power sharing with the client) and the power structures present in the client's life (i.e., at school, at home, and within their community).

Expressive Arts

Expressive arts, also called "creative interventions," are creative, nonverbal therapeutic modalities used to facilitate clients' connections to implicit experiences and deeper feelings that may otherwise be absent from conscious awareness (Purswell & Stulmaker, 2015). Expressive arts in counseling offer opportunities for creative expression, catharsis, and the development of insight and awareness. Examples of expressive arts techniques include bibliotherapy, poetry, film, music, music videos, drawing, painting, puppet shows, clay, role-play, and sand tray (Purswell & Stulmaker, 2015; Riley, 1997). Integrating expressive arts into clinical work with adolescents is a developmentally appropriate intervention as it allows adolescents to explore potentially distressing material in nonthreatening and abstract ways to help them explore what may be forbidden for them to verbalize (Riley, 1997). In addition, expressive arts may teach adolescents different ways to express their inner experiences inside and outside counseling (Riley, 1997).

Integrating sand tray and other creative interventions that resonate with Jose Luis may provide another way for them to explore their inner world and express their experiences in session, especially during the initial stages of our work together. Depending on Jose Luis and their parents' receptivity, I may integrate creative interventions into family sessions to support them in communicating with each other.

Case Study Application

As a Gestalt therapist, I conceptualize Jose Luis as a courageous, creative, and dynamic adolescent doing their best to explore who they are and how they can honor who they are in the face of ongoing oppression and discrimination. Jose Luis's experience of anxiety is a typical response to discrimination, bullying, and oppression. Their school climate is a microcosm of the larger sociopolitical climate in the United States, directly impacting Jose Luis's experience of safety, acceptance, and belonging. Thus, Jose Luis is experiencing inner conflict as they explore their safety, who they are, and who they want to be. To cope with the increase of bullying and anti-LGBTQ legislation, Jose Luis engages in deflection (i.e., shifting their attention away from distressing aspects of their experience) and introject (i.e., internalizing beliefs, values, attitudes, and cultural norms without examination).

Jose Luis withdraws from their family and others because they are terrified of rejection. To protect themselves, they've learned to disconnect from others (e.g., isolating from friends and family, sharing minimal information with family, being selective regarding who they come out to as queer and/or nonbinary) and, at times, to disconnect from parts of themselves (e.g., queer identity, nonbinary identity, desire to dress more "feminine").

I believe their parents are also courageous, creative, and dynamic people trying to meet their needs as they arise while meeting Jose Luis's needs. Although Jose Luis's parents are not my clients, I need to partner with them as I work with Jose Luis because they are from a collectivist culture and are skeptical about the counseling process. Building a collaborative and compassionate relationship with Jose Luis's parents helps me to build trust, increase their willingness to continue seeking mental health services, and ultimately explore ways we can support Jose Luis. Familial and parental acceptance and support are protective factors for LGBTQ youth mental health (Trevor Project, 2022); thus, I must provide ongoing support to Jose Luis's parents as they process and accept their child's sexuality and gender identity.

As I approached my work with Jose Luis and their parents, I kept in mind that LGBTQ youth, particularly youth of color, experience significant disparities in mental and physical health concerns due to ideological, institutional, interpersonal, and internalized oppression. Yet, a deficit-based view of LGTBQ youth of color is limiting and can promote harmful narratives. Thus, I explored ways to honor the strengths, resilience, and resistance of Jose Luis. During my initial sessions with Jose Luis and in parent consultations, I explored Jose Luis's Community Cultural Wealth (CCW; Yosso, 2005) to help inform Jose Luis's treatment plan, including the clinical interventions implemented. The CCW model helped me recognize and honor the different forms of capital (i.e., aspirational capital, linguistic capital, familial capital, social capital, navigational capital, and resistant capital) that helped Jose Luis "survive and resist racism," cisgenderism, heterosexism, and linguicism (Yosso, 2005, p. 154). I encourage you to learn more about Yosso's (2005) CCW model. Unfortunately, an in-depth overview of the CCW model is outside this chapter's scope.

Intake Session

My goals for the intake session were to develop rapport with Jose Luis and their parents, obtain informed consent from the parents, and informed assent from Jose Luis. Further, I aim to complete an initial assessment of family dynamics and explore Jose Luis's presenting concerns from their and their parents' perspectives.

Session 1

My goals for the first session were to develop rapport, assess Jose Luis's CCW, start exploring their social and cultural identities, and delve into what brought them to counseling from their perspective. After reintroducing myself, I invited Jose Luis to ask me any questions they had for me to shift the power dynamic between us and start building a collaborative therapeutic relationship.

At the end of the first session, I thanked Jose Luis for trusting me enough to share their sexuality and gender identity and experiences coming out to friends. I reminded them that we will start exploring their treatment goals during our next session. See Sample Case Note for a summary.

TABLE 19.1. **JOSE LUIS: SESSION 1**

Transcript	Analysis
Jose Luis: "I remember you saying that you speak Spanish and English. Can we use Spanish in our session?"	Jose Luis was trying to understand what language(s) were acceptable during their sessions. As a student, they are used to being in English-dominant spaces unless they are home with their family. Their first language is Spanish, yet due to linguicism, they've internalized the message that English is the preferred language. Thus, they are exploring what parts of themselves they can share with me and how receptive I will be.
Ana: "Of course, we can speak en español y también podemos mezclarlo un poco y agregar algo de Spanglish [translation: in Spanish and we can also remix it a bit and throw in some Spanglish.] Whatever you are most comfortable with. How does that sound?"	Communicating acceptance and sharing that in this space we speak multiple languages
Jose Luis: "I guess that is cool. I didn't know we could do that . . ."	Jose Luis was trying to make sense of my response.
Ana: "This is your space. Sometimes we will do things that may seem a bit weird at first to help you explore how you feel and what is going on for you. However, you get to decide what you want to share and do in here. Our time together is for you to explore what is going on for you in ways that help you."	I took the opportunity to provide some psychoeducation regarding our sessions to remind Jose Luis that they have the autonomy to decide what and how they share.
Jose Luis: "Okay . . . I've been telling my parents that I need help for a few months. Pero no entienden por qué no saben que me identifico como una persona queer y no binaria. [translation: But they don't understand because they don't know that I identify as queer and nonbinary.] They just think I am a little weird because most of my friends are also queer, but my parents don't know that. They just think we dress and act weird."	Josè Luis starts opening up and exploring what brings them to counseling.

Session 2

My goal for the second session was to continue facilitating Jose Luis's expression of their feelings, thoughts, and experiences and identify their treatment goals. After exploring Jose Luis's feelings and thoughts, I invited them to write down three things they wanted to accomplish during our sessions. We agreed to work on the following:

Treatment Goal #1: Increase self-awareness and integration of various aspects of self as evidenced by Jose Luis's self-report.

Objectives:

1. Engage in self-reflection exercises such as journaling or guided reflection prompts to help them explore thoughts, emotions, and experiences.
2. Identify and explore core beliefs and values.
3. Foster self-acceptance and self-compassion.
4. Practice mindfulness and present-moment awareness.
5. Encourage exploration of different aspects of self.

Treatment Goal #2: Increase Jose Luis's acceptance of emotions as they arise, as evidenced by Jose Luis's ability to label, express, and experience their emotions.
Objectives:
1. Develop emotional awareness by encouraging them to identify and label different emotions as they arise and explore their physical sensations and accompanying thoughts.
2. Normalize the experience of emotions.
3. Identify triggers and patterns.
4. Explore the functions of their emotions.

Treatment Goal #3: Increase ability to communicate needs as they arise to others as evidenced by Jose Luis's ability to verbalize their needs in the counseling sessions, their parents' report, and Jose Luis's self-report.
Objectives:
1. Identify and clarify personal needs.
2. Explore barriers to communication.
3. Develop communication skills.
4. Practice expressing needs in counseling sessions.
5. Collaborate with Jose Luis's parents/family to support and reinforce their progress in communicating needs.

Jose Luis and I agreed to periodically assess their progress and revise their treatment goals.

Later Sessions

As we enter the working phase of our time together, I aim to explore Jose Luis's contact boundary disturbances (i.e., how they make and break contact with themselves, me, and others) in session to co-create experiments with them that help them achieve their treatment goals. For example, we will practice mindfulness and present-moment awareness in sessions to help Jose Luis connect with their inner experience. In later sessions, we will continue shifting the treatment plan and approach to meet the emerging needs of Jose Luis (e.g., referrals to support groups and gender-affirming medical care). Further, Jose Luis and I will continue exploring ways to integrate their parents and family members into their counseling sessions, as needed, especially as they continue exploring their desire to come out to their parents.

Session 4

Now that we've developed more trust and established a sense of safety in our therapeutic relationship, I aimed to support Jose Luis in exploring their somatic experience of anxiety through an expressive art intervention in the fourth session. On the following page is a short transcript of our session.

TABLE 19.2. JOSE LUIS: SESSION 4

Transcript	Analysis
Ana: "Gently close your eyes and simply become aware of your breath. There is no need to change it—simply notice the natural rhythm of your breath [pause]. Allow your body to move with each inhale and exhale [pause]. Now, gently shift your awareness to any part of your body where you feel anxiety and notice what you feel or sense [pause]. Now, gently shift your awareness back to your breath and notice your breathing—again, there is no need to change anything. Just become aware of your breathing [pause]. Now slowly start wiggling your toes and moving your arms. When you are ready, open your eyes." [Jose Luis opens their eyes.] "Now, I want you to draw how you experience your anxiety."	I facilitated a grounding practice to help Jose Luis connect to their somatic experience in preparation for the expressive arts intervention.
Jose Luis: "Okay, this should be interesting [smiles]."	Jose Luis appeared both excited and nervous about the expressive arts. Yet, they were willing to draw their experience of anxiety.
Ana: "First, you are going to draw the outline of your body—think of it as drawing a gingerbread person (Drewes, 2001). Then you are going to draw/write how you experience your anxiety inside your body (the gingerbread person) or anywhere on the page. You can use any of the materials here."	I described the expressive arts activity and allowed space for Jose Luis to ask any clarifying questions.
Jose Luis: "Can I play some music as I draw?"	Jose Luis expressed a desire to play music and is still asking for permission to bring themselves into our clinical work.
Ana: "Of course, you will have about 15 minutes to draw; if you need more time we can adjust as needed. How does that sound?"	There are several pros and cons regarding whether we play music during an expressive arts activity because music is evocative. However, it seems important for Jose Luis to play music, and the music they choose to play is something we can explore at the end of the expressive arts intervention while we process their drawing.
Jose Luis: "Sounds good. But I don't think it will take me that long at all." [starts playing music]	
Ana: "It sounds like you have a sense of what you are going to draw. Jose Luis: "Yup." Ana: You have fifteen minutes starting now."	
Ana: "You have five minutes left."	
Ana: "You have about one minute left."	
Jose Luis: "Ya casi [translation: Almost ready]."	
Jose Luis: "Ya termine [translation: I am done]." [showing Ana their drawing]	See Figure 19.1 for sample artwork.
Ana: "Estabas enfocade mientras dibujabas [translation: You were focused while you drew]."	
Jose Luis: "No pensé que me iba a conectar de esa manera. Pero cuando comencé a dibujar puedo conectar más [translation: I didn't think I was going to connect that way. But when I started drawing, I was able to connect more] with my anxiety and how it feels like in my body . . . you know. I am surprised by what I drew."	Jose Luis found this expressive arts intervention helpful, allowing them to connect with their experience in ways they hadn't before.

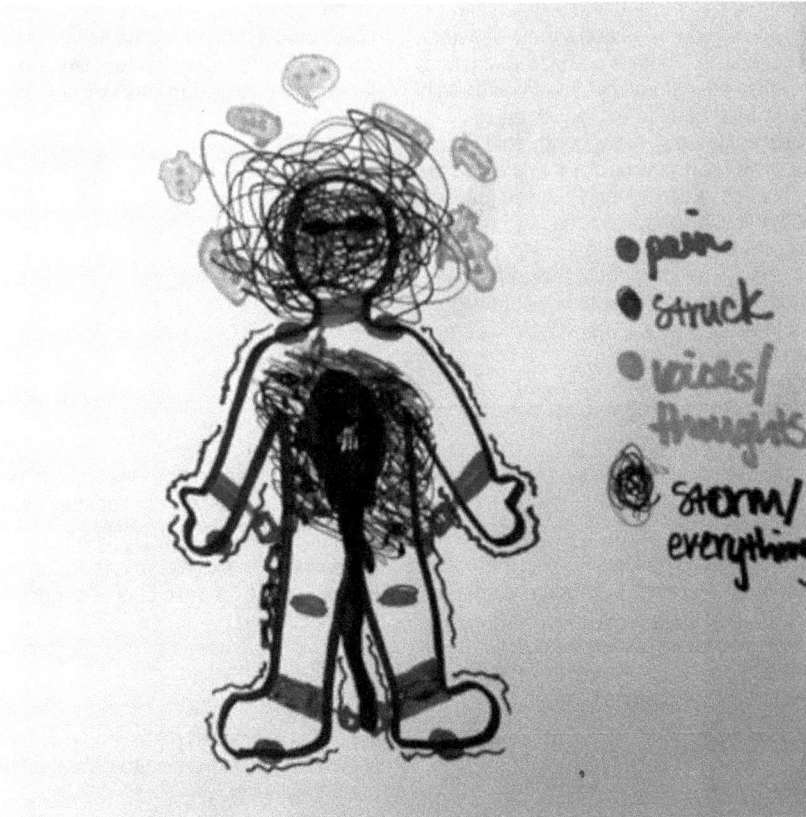

Figure 19.1. *La Tormenta Adentro* [translation: The Storm Within]
Figure courtesy of Ana Guadalupe Reyes, based on client(s)' representations.

For the remainder of the session, we processed Jose Luis's experience of the expressive arts intervention, what the drawing presents to them, and their experience of anxiety. Jose Luis was able to vocalize how their experience of anxiety feels like a storm within that leaves them feeling trapped and stuck.

In the following sessions, Jose Luis's ability to experience and express their emotions increased as they explored and integrated previously disowned parts of themselves. In addition, Jose Luis started identifying environmental triggers such as experiences of discrimination, bullying, and tension within their family system, which increased their anxiety.

Ethical and Cultural Considerations

No relevant ethical considerations, beyond the standard informed consent, came up during my work with Jose Luis. However, many cultural considerations were crucial in providing trans and queer affirming and linguistically and culturally responsive services when working with Jose Luis and their parents. My awareness of the Multicultural and Social Justice Competencies (Ratts, Singh, Nassar-McMillan, Butler, & McCullough, 2016) helped me explore counseling and advocacy interventions that benefited Jose Luis. For example, during parent consultations, I provided psychoeducation regarding adolescents and mental health. I also consulted with the school counselor and principal regarding school policies that were negatively impacting the client and engaged in advocacy against anti-LGBTQ legislation. I also reviewed the Competencies for Counseling with Transgender Clients (ACA, 2009) to support my work with Jose Luis.

Parent Consultations

The language I spoke when I provided mental health services was an ongoing cultural consideration because Jose Luis's parents are monolingual Spanish speakers. Thus, during the intake session, I spoke primarily in Spanish, especially when speaking to the parents, and at times talked to Jose Luis in English and would translate what Jose Luis or I said into Spanish to ensure that the parents understood what was being said. Another important cultural aspect was ensuring that the parents felt a sense of *respeto* and *personalismo* during the first few sessions. Therefore, I met with them often for parent consultations and offered brief parent consultations over the phone as needed. During parent consultations, I only spoke Spanish and ensured that all resources and referrals provided offered culturally and linguistically responsive services.

Conclusion

Throughout our work together, Jose Luis met all the treatment goals they established, and they came out to their parents, who at first struggled with supporting the client as they explored what this meant for them as parents. Jose Luis's parents attended a local group for parents of LGBTQ youth, learned ways to support Jose Luis, and started using nonbinary and inclusive language in Spanish. With their increased self-awareness and self-acceptance, Jose Luis started exploring their experiences of internalized oppression and became playful with their gender expression.

As a therapist, I remembered the power of self-acceptance and family of origin and creation. As Jose Luis grew in their self-awareness and self-acceptance, they became more creative and playful in session and outside of session, which served as a reminder of the importance of healing from internalized oppression to experience a sense of liberation and empowerment.

Sample Case Note

TABLE 19.3. **CASE NOTE: DATA/ASSESSMENT**

Client Name: Jose Luis Del Carmen	**Case Number:** 20230517
Session #: 1	**Session Date:** 5/20/2023

Data: The client explored their experiences as a queer nonbinary person within their family system. The client explored their experiences coming out to their friends. The client reported that most of their friends have been supportive except for a couple who seemed to be uncomfortable after the client shared identifying as nonbinary. The client and counselor explore the client's desire to come out to their family. The client expressed fear that their parents would "disown" them due to their religious and cultural values. The client reported feeling "trapped" and "isolated."

Assessment: The client appears self-aware, as evidenced by their ability to recognize their need for additional support and willingness to advocate for themselves. The client appears highly motivated and engaged in counseling, as evidenced by their participation and open responses. The client seemed anxious as they discussed their coming-out process, especially as they explored their desire to come out to their parents. The client fidgeted with their hands and fidget toy throughout the session. The client's fidgeting increased when they discussed their coming-out process. The client maintained eye contact and seemed to maintain psychological contact with the counselor throughout the session.

Plan: The counselor and client will start developing the client's treatment plan. The client will continue attending weekly individual counseling sessions with this counselor.

Counselor Signature: _____ Date: _____

Next Appointment: _____

Resources

For Professionals

Gay, Lesbian and Straight Supporters Network (for teachers and students), https://www.glsen.org/about-us

Erasure and Resilience: The Experiences of LGBTQ Students of Color Report, https://www.glsen.org/research/latinx-lgbtq-students

National LGBTQIA+ Health Education Center, https://www.lgbtqiahealtheducation.org/

For Clients

National Queer Trans Therapists of Color Network (NQTTCN)—Mental Health Fund, https://nqttcn.com/en/mental-health-fund/

- The NQTTCN Mental Health Fund provides financial support of up to $100 per session for up to eight sessions with a mental health professional.

GLBT National Youth Talkline: (800) 246-7743

National Coalition of Anti-Violence Programs: (212) 714-1141 (English and Spanish)

Trevor Project:

- Webchat: https://www.thetrevorproject.org/get-help/
- Crisis Line: (866) 488-7386
- Text: Texting "START" to 678-678

For Parents

Somos Familia—resources for families who have a child who identifies with the LGBTQ+ community, in English and Spanish, https://www.somosfamiliabay .org/resources/
Family Acceptance Project, https://lgbtqfamilyacceptance.org/

Discussion Questions

1. How may your social location impact your work with Jose Luis and their parents?
2. How would you work to dismantle the power structures present in our work with Jose Luis and their parents?
3. How would you engage in advocacy to dismantle the power structures present in Jose Luis's life?
4. How would you approach your work with Jose Luis after reading this chapter?
5. Moving forward, how can you approach your work with queer adolescents in ways that are affirming and liberating?

References

American Counseling Association. (2009). *Competencies for counseling with transgender clients*.

Batejan, K. L., Jarvi, S. M., & Swenson, L. P. (2015). Sexual orientation and non-suicidal self-injury: A meta-analytic review. *Archives of Suicide Research, 19*, 131–150. doi: 10.1080/13811118.2014.957450

Carbado, D. W., Crenshaw, K. W., Mays, V. M., & Tomlinson, B. (2013). Intersectionality: Mapping the movements of a theory. *Du Bois Review, 10*, 303–312. doi: 10.1017/S1742058X13000349

Collins, P. H., & Bilge, S. (2016). *Intersectionality*. Polity Press.

Crenshaw, K. W. (1989). Demarginalizing the intersection of race and sex: A Black feminist critique of antidiscrimination doctrine, feminist theory, and antiracist politics. *University of Chicago Legal Forum*, 139–167.

Drewes, A. A. (2001). The gingerbread person feelings map. In C. E. Schaefer & H. Kaduson (Eds.), *101 more play therapy techniques* (pp. 92–97). Aronson.

Hafeez, H., Zeshan, M., Tahir, M. A., Jahan, N., & Naveed, S. (2017). Health care disparities among lesbian, gay, bisexual, and transgender youth: A literature review. *Cureus, 9*(4), 2–7. doi: 10.7759/cureus.1184

Hunt, L., Vennatt, M., & Waters, J. H. (2018). Health and wellness for LGBTQ. *Advances in Pediatrics, 65*(1). https://doi.org/10.1016/j.yapd.2018.04.002

Meyer, I. H. (2003). Prejudice, social stress, and mental health in lesbian, gay, bisexual, populations: Conceptual issues and research evidence. *Psychological Bulletin, 129*, 674–697. doi: 10.1037/0033-2909.129.5.674

Mustanski, B., Newcomb, M., & Garofalo, R. (2011). Mental health of lesbian, gay, and bisexual youth: A developmental resiliency respective. *Journal of Gay and Lesbian Social Services, 23*, 204–225. doi: 10.1080/10538720.2011.561474

National Alliance on Mental Illness (NAMI). (2023). *LGBTQI.* https://www.nami.org/Your-Journey/Identity-and-Cultural-Dimensions/LGBTQI

Paradies, Y., Ben, J., Denson, N., Elias, A., Priest, N., Pieterse, A., Gupta, A., Kelaher, M., & Gee, G. (2015). Racism as a determinant of health: A systematic review and meta-analysis. *PLoS One, 10*(9). doi: 10.1371/journal.pone.0138511

Perls, F., Hefferline, E. R., & Goodman, P. (1951). *Gestalt therapy: Excitement and growth in the human personality.* Gestalt Journal Press.

Purswell, K. E., & Stulmaker, H. L. (2015). Expressive arts in supervision: Choosing developmentally appropriate interventions. *International Journal of Play Therapy, 24*(2), 103–117. doi: 10.1037/a0039134

Ratts, M. J., Singh, A. A., Nassar-McMillan, S., Butler, S. K., & McCullough, J. R. (2016). Multicultural and social justice counseling competencies: Guidelines for the counseling profession. *Journal of Multicultural Counseling and Development, 44*, (1), 28–48.

Riley, S. (1997). *Contemporary art therapy with adolescents.* Jessica Kingsley Publishers.

Trevor Project. (2022). *2022 National Survey on LGBTQ Youth Mental Health.* https://www.thetrevorproject.org/survey-2022/

Yontef, G. (1993). *Awareness, dialogue and process: Essays on Gestalt therapy.* Gestalt Journal Press.

Yosso, J. T. (2005). Whose culture has capital? A critical race theory discussion of community cultural wealth. *Race Ethnicity and Education, 8*(1), 69–91.

CHAPTER 20

Gender
Narrative Therapy with Parents of a Nonbinary Transgender Korean American Adolescent
Brooks Bull

Lisa, a White, 50-year-old mother, called me for help with her 12-year-old child, Alex. According to Lisa, Alex had recently come out as a nonbinary transgender person (they/them pronouns), and the family needed help "figuring out what to do." The family consisted of Lisa, Charlie (Lisa's partner of 10 years); and Alex, who Lisa adopted at age 8 months from Korea. Alex, who was assigned female at birth, had typical development until age 9 when "things started to go off course socially." Lisa explained that Alex has always been extremely socially isolated, has a hard time making friends, and is overall quite depressed and lonely. Lisa's hope was that therapy could provide the emotional support for Alex to "figure out the gender stuff and get back on track." She explained that Alex's disclosure had created a lot of new tension and conflict between Charlie and her, a new dynamic in their relationship.

This case illustrates how work with transgender adolescents and their parents must address both the cultural and familial level of meaning making. On the societal level, oppressive, pathologizing discourses are everywhere (on the internet, around the watercooler, and on the playground). On the family level, individuals are trying to make sense of gender and the emergent unfolding of identity development and creating their own idiosyncratic meanings and stories. Caregivers play a vital role in providing a safer space where the transgender child can be themselves and go through the evolving process of adolescent identity development. In this way, both cultural and familial context are a major part of the diagnostic and treatment planning picture.

For this case study, consider:

1. How does the cultural context of anti-transgender discourse impact the case conceptualization?
2. What is the rationale for a narrative approach with clients such as this?
3. What historical, political, and social knowledge do practitioners need to have to treat transgender families ethically?

Transgender Environmental Context

We are living through a particularly virulent moment of anti-transgender public discourse in the United States, and the impact can be felt in all corners of transgender communities. At this time, more than 30 states have proposed legislation banning gender-affirming care for minors, some states going so far as to define supporting children to socially and/or hormonally transition as child abuse. There is no underestimating the pervasive and oppressive force this type of political discourse exerts on families with transgender members. As this review of the literature shows, minority stress powerfully impacts the well-being of transgender and nonbinary youth. On the other hand, parental support is also shown to be a very real and powerful protective factor.

Johns and colleagues (2019) found that "compared with cisgender males and females, transgender students were more likely to report violence victimization, substance use, and suicide risk" (p. 67). In addition, nonbinary and genderqueer individuals are at even greater risk. Lefevor, Boyd-Rogers, Sprague, and Janis (2019) showed that these individuals experience significantly more adverse health outcomes compared to both their cisgender and binary transgender counterparts. This highlights just how powerful the cultural value on gender conformity is. Transgender people who do not express their gender identity in strictly masculine or feminine ways are targets of discrimination, leaving them vulnerable to violence and mental health problems including suicidality.

Family acceptance is the most potent balm we have against cultural oppression. Indeed, having even one supportive caregiver can make an enormous positive impact on the well-being of transgender and nonbinary children (Andrzejewski, Pampati, Steiner, Boyce, & Johns, 2021; Ryan, Russell, Huebner, Diaz, & Sanchez, 2010). The strong relationship between familial support and child well-being was confirmed by Kuvalanka, Weiner, Munroe, Goldberg, and Gardner (2017). Olson, Durwood, DeMeules, and McLaughlin (2016) found that transgender children who were supported in their identities showed comparable low levels of depression and anxiety compared to control groups. Both Olson and colleagues (2016) and Kuvalanka and colleagues (2017) provide evidence that when children are supported in their gender identities early in life, they show lower levels of depression and anxiety, and report higher levels of satisfaction overall. The clear evidence of both increased risk for transgender and nonbinary youth coupled with the powerful role parental acceptance plays in improving outcomes makes a strong case for direct therapeutic work with parents whenever possible.

Narrative Therapy

Narrative therapy is one of the few family therapy theories that overtly addresses societal and cultural discourses in its view of problem formation and resolution. White and Epston (1990) revolutionized therapy by highlighting the need to separate people from problems, or as Winslade and Monk (2008) later put it, "the problem is the problem. The person is not the problem" (p. 2). Nowhere is this simple intervention, *externalizing*, more obviously important than in therapy with families with transgender and nonbinary children. By separating the child's gender identity from "the problem," the therapist opens up space to identify the actual sources of distress—dominant cultural discourses that oppress members of the family, and the intrapsychic and interpersonal meanings that support those oppressive discourses.

Re-Storying as an Overall Goal

Narrative therapists are keen to identify the problem-saturated stories and work with clients to reshape those stories into ones in which the problem itself plays the main role while the client is secondary, or even a victim of the problem's nefarious influence. For example, rather than endorsing a client's story that they are depressed, a narrative therapist would ask questions to externalize depression from the client and then facilitate conversation to describe how depression as its own entity impacts the client and their family. From this framework, the narrative therapist collaboratively maps the origins, effects, and prognosis of the problem with the client's help. These questions create more and more daylight between the client as a person and the problem, and oftentimes clients will soon begin to talk about "it," the problem, rather than themselves as a flawed person.

Dominant versus Alternative and Local Discourses

Narrative therapists do not hesitate to name the oppressive role of cultural discourses in a client's presenting problem. As a reminder, dominant discourses are simply the bundle of meanings people from a dominant group culturally ascribe to how a person should be, live, relate, and behave. In terms of gender, the dominant discourse is that there are only two "real" genders, and that they hew closely to biological sex. For anyone whose lived experience does not fit this binary construction, the result is to feel othered, wrong, incomplete, or somehow less than. Local and alternative discourses are real-life people and families whose stories do not fit the mold that the dominant discourses would like to pretend is singular. For example, the fact that there have always been people who do not live within the gender binary, in all cultures and in all eras, is a major challenge to the dominant discourse. However, proponents of the "there are only two real genders" position skillfully deploy a strategy of ahistorical discourse to combat the rich, multitudinous history of gender diversity throughout time. Narrative therapists bring this historical and discursive challenge into the room by naming the powerful oppressive force of cisgender privilege, binary thinking, and the strategic erasure of transgender history. They then provide alternative, local discourses about actual transgender people and families currently living in our communities as well as historical figures from near and distant past as an antidote to the silencing, oppressive dominant discourse our culture offers to transgender children.

Remembering

In narrative practice, therapists ask questions to populate a client's narrative with allies and witnesses, and if possible, bring other supportive people into the conversations (White & Epston, 1990). Connecting parents and transgender children with other families like theirs is of paramount importance. The therapy conversation must extend outside the confines of the session room to adequately address the role of oppression. In fact, therapy with transgender families that exists solely within the therapeutic system further reifies the notion that to have a transgender child is a private problem only to be addressed within a mental health setting. Part of a narrative therapist's job is to puncture the pathologizing conception that produces this insular system and connect transgender children and their parents with the mirroring and growth that only come from and within community.

Parallel to connecting client families to other trans families, another form of remembering can come in the form of filling in history. Dominant discourse would have us pretend transgenderism is a new thing, something that has caught on due to the internet or some other venue of social contagion. In contrast, learning about transgender history provides a tapestry of human experience into which the clients can weave themselves. Giving clients books to read and films to watch that provide allies, elders, and ancestors where previously there was a void can be a powerful intervention. No longer is having a transgender child just a modern thing, or a fad, but just another example of a long history of human diversity that has always been present in all cultures including our own.

Case Study Application

Alex is a nonbinary transgender 12-year-old in need of a supportive family environment in which to continue their exploration and development of identity. Lisa and Charlie are engaged, caring parents in need of support and education to show up for Alex in this process. The family is living many stories at once—the cultural story that transgenderism is a fad, an idea spread through social networks and the media that has swooped in to invalidate Alex's disclosure. Alongside that dominant story, the family is also living out their stated values of "everyone being who they are." Lisa and Charlie have both articulated a desire to allow Alex to choose whatever path in life they feel is right for them; however, the fear and panic they feel around gender identity is getting in the way of fully living that value. Therapy for Lisa and Charlie can be a space to flesh out more of the stories that live alongside the dominant discourse that questions the validity of nonbinary transgender identities and pathologizes supportive parents. For Alex, this therapy can be a space of relative safety to continue their articulation of who they are and learn new skills for self-advocacy. All members of this family will benefit from being connected to more community of families with transgender members.

Regarding the role of clinician, assessment of Alex's gender identity is not the primary task of the clinician (Chang, Singh, & Dickey, 2018). On the contrary, helping parents understand how to support their child on a journey of identity exploration is the therapist's primary job. An awareness of oppressive discourses including adultism (the idea that children cannot know themselves due to their age) as well as binarism (the idea that there are only two valid gender identities and that they correspond strictly to biological sex) are key guiding principles.

The overall treatment goal is to increase parental support for Alex's nonbinary transgender identity. The objectives are as follows:

1. Develop a strong working relationship with parents and child.
    a. Meet parents and child apart from the problem.
    b. Engage family with hope and optimism about having a transgender family member.
    c. Clearly articulate therapist's position and beliefs on gender identity.
2. Assess both family-level and societal dynamics.
    a. Identify dominant discourses impacting parents' current understanding of Alex's gender identity.
    b. Externalize this oppressive cultural force as The Problem.
    c. Map the effects of The Problem for each member.
3. Replace problem-saturated narrative with alternative and local narratives that support Alex.
    a. Identify unique outcomes and exceptions (times when Lisa and Charlie are not swayed by oppressive binary discourses).
    b. Thicken alternative narratives with new language, experiences both from within the family and from new allies (remembering).
4. Connect Alex and parents with community of other transgender families.

Treatment Process

Most of the work with this family happened with just Lisa and Charlie. Alex was more of a visitor to this therapy who could redirect and deepen the parents' work. The first session was devoted to letting Lisa talk about how she had previously understood Alex's struggles before they came out as nonbinary. After that, I shifted my attention to helping Lisa and Charlie externalize the problem and find a way to describe the feelings that were getting in the way of them really being there for Alex.

TABLE 20.1. LISA: SESSION 1

Transcript	Analysis
T: "How have you understood Alex's loneliness and isolation in the past? What stories has your family told about why Alex's life is the way it is?"	Clients need space to tell the story as it exists currently before entering into a revising and re-storying.
L: "I always put it in the framework of adoption—that Alex struggled because they were (almost always) the only adopted, only Korean American person in the room. I always thought about it in those terms first."	Lisa was quick to identify the meta-frameworks impacting her understanding, and names "being adopted" as the lens through which she saw Alex's distress.
T: "And now things are starting to shift in your understanding?"	Tentative question from therapist invites the client to language more of the insight.
L: "Right. Gender was not on my radar in any way until recently, even though as I think back on it now, there were lots of gender-related moments of distress throughout the years."	
T: "It makes sense to me that the very real importance you saw in Alex's status as an adopted kid got in the way of you seeing other aspects of their identity. I think that's part of what's so powerful about dominant discourses—the stories we as a culture tell to make sense of experience—they shine a big light on some things and leave so much else in total darkness. So, you're starting to turn your flashlight to other areas, yes?"	The therapist looks for opportunities to frame the work as a process of discovery, a quest the parent is embarking on. This provides the foundation for the new narratives (alternative and local discourses) to be created.

After an initial meeting with Lisa alone, I asked that she come to the next session with Charlie as well. Early on, the main task is to externalize and shift the problem language away from the child's gender identity and locate the problem in whatever is getting in the way of the parents being supportive. This is best done without the transgender person, who does not need to be subjected to the microaggressions of their parents; therapists can be the buffer between the child and their parents' early journey out of the stranglehold of anti-trans discourse.

Charlie and Lisa were very open to shifting the focus to becoming a stronger team again and "getting their car back on the road." This was the first part of externalizing the problem and shifting the problem focus away from Alex's gender itself. In this case, what was getting in the way most for Lisa and Charlie was a feeling of fear and pressure—fear that Alex was more in harm's way as a result of being a nonbinary trans person, and pressure to stop Alex "from making a huge mistake." As part of this therapeutic approach, I always directly address and challenge anti-trans rhetoric as it comes up for clients, and ultimately give the child strategies for self-advocating in different contexts, including with their parents. I explain and demonstrate this therapist posture and intervention in session 3 with Alex's stepfather, Charlie, who brought up a term he learned from a quick internet search called Rapid-Onset Gender Dysphoria.

TABLE 20.2. LISA AND CHARLIE: SESSION 2

Transcript	Analysis
T: "I see you two as very caring, engaged parents. I wonder what it's like for you to be in a situation where you are at odds with Alex and unable to connect. That must be a terrible feeling, and certainly a problem we can work on together. Can we find words to describe this problem? Take it out of Alex, away from gender completely, and give it a name?"	These questions help clients externalize the problem and shift problem talk away from the child's gender identity itself.
C: "I'm not sure I follow you."	Clients can be confused early on and need guidance to shift an entrenched problem away from a family member.
T: "Understandable! I am asking you to think and talk about this in a very different way. Here's what I mean. From everything I've heard thus far, it seems like you two are a great team and can handle just about anything in terms of family and parenting life. [Both parents nod] So, it strikes me as a big problem that you are not able to join together and support your kid through this new development. It has shaken up your family and put you all at odds. That seems like a problem to me."	The therapist uses a strengths-based approach to join the client system and create a collaborative atmosphere.
C: "Ah, I get it now. Like we have to get the car started again before we figure out where to go."	Charlie offers a metaphor that will be used throughout therapy.
T: "Exactly! Your car is limping along on the shoulder of the road right now."	The therapist looks for opportunities to use client language and images and increase the field of possibilities in terms of how the clients story their experience.
L: "It might actually be in the ditch at this point" [both parents chuckle ruefully].	
T: "You need some help getting back on the road, and we can definitely do that together."	Therapist occupies a hopeful position that emphasizes a future with possibilities not yet articulated. Importantly, therapist does not create conversations that guarantee a specific outcome in terms of the child's gender identity but, rather, emphasizes the journey the family is on to be as present and engaged with one another as possible.

TABLE 20.3. LISA AND CHARLIE: SESSION 3

Transcript	Analysis
C: "I found something online that I think is really important. It explains how this stuff comes up so quick, out of nowhere. [Charlie looks to me.] Have you heard of Rapid-Onset Gender Dysphoria (ROGD)? Apparently, it's spreading like crazy."	Anti-trans discourse makes its way into the therapeutic conversation. This is an important moment to intervene upon both to deepen the alliance with Charlie as well as open up alternative, more local discourses.
T: "I've heard those words before, social contagion and ROGD, they keep coming up in conversations like this one and on my computer screen, and it seems like they mean so many different things depending on who is speaking. Charlie, I am wondering what those words mean for you, what they bring up?"	These questions locate the term ROGD firmly in the sphere of cultural/public discourse and then ask the client to find more personal, local meanings. There is more possibility and room for new meanings in the personal, and so the therapist deepens this as much as possible.
C: "I saw it online, in a forum for parents of kids who suddenly come out as trans, just like Alex. It explains a lot for me. [Lisa tries to speak, but Charlie talks over her.] I thought, *OK, there's a name for this thing, and a reason so many kids are coming out nowadays*. I mean, this wasn't happening in my high school!"	The therapist observes the dynamic between Charlie and Lisa at this moment, noting Charlie's need to keep speaking and not allow Lisa's voice to interject. The power of the dominant discourse is directly affecting how the partners interact, changing what is usually a reciprocal give-and-take into a monological speech.
T: "I'm glad you brought this up, Charlie. It's so important to address these messages head-on. It makes sense to me that a part of you would welcome this type of explanation because it makes it feel like this gender thing might go away if you challenge it correctly. Is that right?"	Therapist validates importance of content and potential emotional reasoning behind it before challenging.
C: "Yeah. This all just feels so sudden. I just want to make sure Alex isn't doing something to be cool, or get attention or something, in a way that will later feel like a huge mistake."	Charlie is able to share the fear behind their interest in ROGD and opens the door to talking more about his anxieties about the future.
T: "I hear you. You really want Alex to be safe and feel good. I have some resources to share with you that will help put ROGD into context [see resource list for Serano]. The truth is that term is being deployed in a really sneaky way to invalidate young people's experience. The rapid part is really insidious because it makes it sound like a kid disclosing their identity is the same thing as a kid having an identity. Let's pause there. Can you look back and tell me about how Alex's gender has made itself known to you over the years?"	The therapist validates the emotion and fear behind the parents' content, and then directly challenges the anti-trans discourse by providing context and psychoeducation. Then the therapist asks the client to tell a more personal, local story about how they have seen and understood their child's gender identity over time.
L: "I'd like to jump in here. I've been thinking about this a lot, actually, about how the words Alex is using are so jarring and alarming to us, while at the same time not much has changed. Charlie, you might not agree with me, but I don't think Alex's presentation has changed much at all. Still our little tomboy in most ways. So, I think for me it's about what this means for the future, what being transgender means for Alex in three or five or even ten years. That part really scares me. That is the feeling I really want to shake, it's like a monster comes over me—us?—and all I can think of is the future, and I feel so much worry."	Lisa enters the conversation speaking from more of a personal, local location as opposed to Charlie's talk, which is heavily influenced at the moment by public discourse. The therapist must attend to both levels of talk and always try to create more space for alternative stories to grow. Lisa also offers powerful language that the therapist uses to externalize the problem. The Monster Feeling becomes shared language for when the parents are snagged by fear and start to feel drawn to anti-trans discourses that invite parents to adjudicate their children's identities.

Ethical and Cultural Considerations

Working with families with transgender or nonbinary adolescents will mean starkly different things depending on what state you are practicing in. As I write this, news is coming across my screens about state legislatures moving bills along that would limit or outright ban affirming care for minors. Based on the American Counseling Association *Code of Ethics* (2014), competencies for working with transgender clients (Burnes et al., 2010), and social justice competencies (Toporek, Lewis, & Ratts, 2010), counselors need to advocate for the rights of transgender people to exist, use public facilities, and receive medical care while we also advocate for the protections of medical providers who in some states could be prosecuted for providing care to trans patients. Now is the time to step forward and engage in the fight. The dominance of cisgender privilege is quite literally crushing the transgender community, and although therapists tend to work on a small individual/family scale, this is a moment that calls for more public engagement.

When working with families, being outspoken about your support for trans rights is paramount. Being explicit about my understanding that transgender people have always existed and will continue to exist, that the identity is not a question or something to poke and prod for veracity is foundational to my approach with Alex. To join with the parents, Charlie especially, I had to demonstrate my ability to hear nuance, engage with his specific experience, and see the best in him. In my work with families, it has served me well to treat each member of the family as a person doing their best with the information they have. This is the foundation from which families can successfully navigate questions about if (and when) the young person needs to access medical care to support their identity. Conversations about puberty blockers, hormone therapy, and surgeries come after this primary work is firmly in place.

It is not the job of the therapist to talk anyone into (or out of) accessing medical care to support their transgender identity. Rather, it is the job of the therapist to help families function at the highest level possible, access information, be connected to communities and resources, and make informed decisions. A family with a 12-year-old will need personalized support navigating these questions, and a therapist can be a great help in connecting them to other families living through these same issues. By meeting other trans families and seeing examples of adolescents thriving in their trans and nonbinary identities, with some accessing puberty blockers and hormones, Alex and their family can feel less isolated and on the edge of their social world. In this way, gender identity development can exist in the same matrix as other aspects of identity—things we as parents expect to evolve and develop over time. Therapists can help parents remain open and engaged to the unfolding process of witnessing their child become more and more themselves, thereby providing that crucial ingredient of support and engagement that deeply impacts child well-being.

Conclusion

Alex benefited greatly from having a space for their parents to explore, make mistakes, and learn about transgender and nonbinary identities. Meeting other families with trans children and teens created a network of mirroring and alliances for all three family members and a rich resource where they could bring specific questions as they arose. The issues they faced when Alex was 12 were different than when they were 15, and having a deep and broad community was paramount. Alex continues to identify as a nonbinary transgender person, and now at age 15 has added understanding of other aspects of their identity as well. They have recently become more interested in learning more about their heritage as a person of Korean descent and have enlisted Lisa and Charlie to take Korean classes with them. The family continues to prioritize "being in it together" above all else and ensuring that they are relating with one another in real and authentic ways that fit for their family as opposed to letting That Monster Feeling take over and make decisions for them. They continue to meet with me as needed, mostly to process continuing anxiety about Alex's future as a trans person in a violently oppressive anti-trans culture.

Sample Case Notes

Session 3

Subjective: Charlie expressed his perception that Alex's gender was the result of "peer pressure" and an "attempt to be cool" and brought up a resource he found on the internet about Rapid-Onset Gender Dysphoria.

Objective: Charlie's speech was tense and pressured at times, and he interrupted and talked over Lisa when she questioned his assessment. After therapist validated and joined Charlie in his fear and concern for Alex, Charlie reported feeling calmer, spoke more slowly, and allowed Lisa to participate in the conversation.

Assessment: From a narrative perspective, Charlie is currently under the influence of dominant discourses that invalidate trans and nonbinary identities, and position gender nonconformity as ahistorical and a product of internet culture. Throughout the session, Charlie appeared to become more open to the idea that his panic and fear (externalized by the clients as That Monster Feeling) was limiting his ability to learn and connect with Alex.

Plan: Continue identifying the role oppressive anti-trans discourses (The Monster Feeling) are playing in individual emotional experience and family interactions; begin to invite alternative re-storying by providing clients with resources to learn the history of transgender people (see resource list).

Resources

For Adolescents

The Gender Quest Workbook by Rylan Jay Testa, Jayme Peta, & Deborah Coolhart. Instant Help Books.

It's Perfectly Normal: Changing Bodies, Growing Up, Sex, and Sexual Health by Robie H. Harris. Family Library.

Some Assembly Required: The Not-So-Secret Life of a Transgender Teen by Arin Andrews. Simon & Schuster.

Current Resources for Therapists and Adult Clients to Better Understand Gender Identity

Beyond the Gender Binary (book) by Alok Vaid-Menon. Pocket Change Collective.

The Bold World: A Memoir of Family and Transformation (book) by Jodie Patterson. Random House.

Gender Queer: A Memoir (graphic novel) by Maia Kobabe. Lion Forge Comics Oni Press.

Serano, J. (2018). *Everything you need to know about Rapid Onset Gender Dysphoria.* https://juliaserano.medium.com/everything-you-need-to-know-about-rapid-onset-gender-dysphoria-1940b8afdeba (article)

Trans* Ally Workbook: Getting Pronouns Right (booklet) by Davey Shlasko. Think Again Training and Consultation.

Historical Resources for Therapists and Adult Clients to Learn the History of Transgender and Gender-Diverse People

Before We Were Trans: A New History of Gender (book) by Kit Heyam. Seal Press.

Disclosure (film) by Sam Feder.

Female Husbands (book) by Jen Manion. Cambridge University Press.

Transgender History (book) by Susan Stryker. Seal Press.

Transgender Warriors (book) by Leslie Feinberg. Beacon Press.

Discussion Questions

1. What is the main role of the therapist in working with transgender adolescents and their parents? Does this case challenge any of your notions about the role of assessment in this work?
2. How does narrative inquiry invite therapists to challenge dominant cultural discourses? Does this bring up any misgivings or confusion about your role?
3. As a therapist, what might you need to learn about transgender history as well as the current political landscape to work effectively with Alex and their family?

4. What professional community might you need to find to work with transgender families? How would you respond if you received a request from a client who wanted to be connected to more community?

References

American Counseling Association. (2014). *2014 ACA code of ethics*. https://www .counseling.org/docs/default-source/default-document-library/2014-code-of -ethics-finaladdress.pdf

Andrzejewski, J., Pampati, S., Steiner, R. J., Boyce, L., & Johns, M. M. (2021). Perspectives of transgender youth on parental support: Qualitative findings from the resilience and transgender youth study. *Health Education & Behavior, 48*(1), 74–81. https://doi.org/10.1177/1090198120965504

Burnes, T. R., Singh, A. A., Harper, A. J., Harper, B., Maxon-Kann, W., Pickering, D. L., Moundas, S., Scofield, T. R., Roan, A., Hosea, J., & ALGBTIC Transgender Committee. (2010). American Counseling Association: Competencies for counseling with transgender clients. *Journal of LGBT Issues in Counseling, 4*(3–4), 135–159.

Chang, S., Singh, A., & Dickey, L. M. (2018). *A clinician's guide to gender affirming care: Working with transgender and gender non-conforming clients*. New Harbinger Publications.

Johns, M. M., Lowry, R., Andrzejewski, J., Barrios, L. C., Demissie, Z., McManus, T., Rasberry, C. N., Robin, L., & Underwood, J. M. (2019). Transgender identity and experiences of violence victimization, substance use, suicide risk, and sexual risk behaviors among high school students—19 states and large urban school districts, 2017. *Morbidity and Mortality Weekly Report, 68*(3), 67–71. https://doi.org/10.15585/mmwr.mm6803a3

Kuvalanka, K. A., Weiner, J. L., Munroe, C., Goldberg, A. E., & Gardner, M. (2017). Trans and gender-nonconforming children and their caregivers: Gender presentations, peer relations, and well-being at baseline. Journal of Family Psychology, 31(7), 889–899. https://doi.org/10.1037/fam0000338

Lefevor, G. T., Boyd-Rogers, C. C., Sprague, B. M., & Janis, R. A. (2019). Health disparities between genderqueer, transgender, and cisgender individuals: An extension of minority stress theory. *Journal of Counseling Psychology, 66*(4), 385–395. https://doi.org/10.1037/ cou0000339

Olson, K. R., Durwood, L., DeMeules, M., & McLaughlin, K. A. (2016). Mental health of transgender children who are supported in their identities. *Pediatrics, 137*(3), Article e20153223. https://doi.org/10.1542/peds.2015-3223

Ryan, C. (2010). Engaging families to support lesbian, gay, bisexual, and transgender youth: The family acceptance project. *Prevention Researcher, 17*(4), 11–13. https://doi.org/10.1037/e509042011-003

Ryan, C., Russell, S. T., Huebner, D., Diaz, R., & Sanchez, J. (2010). Family acceptance in adolescence and the health of LGBT young adults. *Journal*

of Child and Adolescent Psychiatric Nursing, 23(4), 205–213. https://doi
.org/10.1111/j.1744-6171.2010.00246.x

Serano, J. (2018). *Everything you need to know about Rapid Onset Gender Dys-phoria.* https://juliaserano.medium.com/everything-you-need-to-know-about
-rapid-onset-gender-dysphoria-1940b8afdeba

Toporek, R. L., Lewis, J. A., & Ratts, M. J. (2010). The ACA advocacy com-petencies: An overview. In M. J. Ratts, R. L. Toporek, & J. A. Lewis (Eds.),
ACA advocacy competencies: A social justice framework for counselors (pp.
11–20). American Counseling Association.

White, M., & Epston, D. (1990). *Narrative means to therapeutic ends.* Norton.

Winslade, J., & Monk, G. (2008). *Narrative mediation: Loosening the grip of conflict.* Jossey-Bass, Wiley Imprint.

Index

About the Editors

Jennifer N. Baggerly, PhD, LPC-S, RPT-S, is professor of counseling and play therapy at the University of North Texas at Dallas. She is a licensed professional counselor supervisor and a registered play therapist supervisor with more than 25 years of play therapy experience. Dr. Baggerly also provides counseling and play therapy at Kaleidoscope Behavioral Health in Flower Mound, Texas. She is an award-winning counselor educator and distinguished leader in the field of counseling and play therapy.

Some of her notable awards across the decades include UNT Dallas Graduate School Outstanding Faculty Award (2022), Texas Counseling Association Outstanding Supervisor Award (2021), Viola Brody Outstanding Play Therapist Award (2005), and Post-Secondary Counselor of the Year for Hillsborough Counseling Association (2004). She served as chair of the board of directors for the Association for Play Therapy from 2013 to 2014 and was a member of the board from 2009 to 2015. Having published in more than 75 publications, Dr. Baggerly is recognized as a prominent expert in children's crisis intervention and play therapy. She has provided Disaster Response Play Therapy throughout the world including Hurricane Maria in Puerto Rico, tsunami in Sri Lanka, Hurricane Katrina in Louisiana, hurricanes in Florida, and tornadoes in Texas and Oklahoma. She has demonstrated her play therapy skills through several training videos such as *Disaster Mental Health and Crisis Stabilization for Children* and *Trauma Informed Child Centered Play Therapy*.

Athena A. Drewes, PsyD, MA, MS Ed, RPT-S, is a licensed psychologist, certified school psychologist, registered play therapist and play therapist supervisor, and noted author and coeditor of more than 13 books on play therapy including *The Therapeutic Powers of Play: 20 Core Agents of Change* (with Charles Schaefer, 2014) and *Cultural Issues in Play Therapy*, 2nd ed. (with Eliana Gil, 2021). She has produced a video demonstrating her Prescriptive Integrative Play Therapy approach through the American Psychological Association Children and Adolescents Series IX. She has had a long and prestigious career as a passionate play therapist with more than 45 years of clinical experience in working with children and adolescents with complex trauma and sexual abuse in schools, residential treatment, and foster care settings.

She is currently semiretired in Ocala, Florida, is a guardian ad litem (court-appointed special advocate for foster care children), and has a private practice focusing on supervision on the national and international level, consultation, and national and international training. She is founder and president emeritus of the New York Association for Play Therapy and past director of the Association for Play Therapy.

About the Contributors

Samuel Bore, PhD, LPC-S, is associate professor and chair of counseling programs at the University of North Texas at Dallas in the School of Behavioral Health and Human Services. Dr. Bore is also a certified school counselor and licensed professional counselor in Texas, with expertise in school counseling, marriage, and family counseling. He has more than 20 peer-reviewed publications in research areas such as group work in schools, school counselor and administrators' collaboration, ethics in school counseling, self-injury among teenagers, cultural straddling among immigrants and refugees, and spirituality.

Brooks Bull, PhD, LMFT, is adjunct instructor at Antioch University in New England, a licensed marriage and family therapist, and owner of Collaborative Therapy and Coaching. They provide trauma-informed, socially just therapy to people of all genders. They offer therapy to individuals, couples, and polycules as well as nontherapeutic coaching. They also provide short-term therapy for transgender and nonbinary people to access medical services. Dr. Bull has published numerous articles and chapters on families with trans children, sex therapy with queer clients, and collaborative and narrative therapies.

Sara Cantu, PhD, LPC-S, LMFT-S, RPT-S, CEDS-C, counsels children and adolescents in private practice in Frisco, Texas. She is also director of curriculum and certification for the International Association for Eating Disorder Professionals. Sara has worked with children, adolescents, and adults affected by eating disorders and their families at all levels of care. She is a certified eating disorder specialist approved consultant.

Peggy L. Ceballos, PhD, NCC, is associate professor in the Department of Counseling and Higher Education at the University of North Texas. She is a national certified counselor, certified child centered play therapy-supervisor, and a certified child parent relationship therapy-supervisor. Her research and numerous publications focus on play therapy and counseling for Latinx populations. She has received several major grants related to play therapy research.

Allison Crowe, PhD, LCMHCS, NCC, is professor in the counselor education program and interim department chair in the Department of Interdisciplinary Professions at East Carolina University. She is a licensed clinical mental health counselor and supervisor in North Carolina and a past president of the North Carolina Counseling Association. She has published more than 60 peer-reviewed scholarly journal articles, many of which focus on topics related to mental health concerns and the stigma that surrounds these.

Dalena Dillman Taylor, PhD, LMHC, RPT-S, is associate professor at the University of North Texas in the Department of Counseling and Higher Education. She earned her doctoral degree in counseling and completed her master's degree in counseling from the University of North Texas. Dr. Dillman Taylor's primary research interests include advancement of Adlerian Play Therapy field toward evidence-based practice, counseling and educational services for high-need children and families, and counselor development and supervision.

Anelie Etienne, LMSW, dedicates her career to improving systems and serving youth impacted by poverty, mental illness, substance abuse, housing instability, and other contributing factors to child neglect and maltreatment. She has worked with the local department of social services for nearly a decade as a child protective services investigator, project manager for families involved with the child welfare system, and currently as grants coordinator, she accesses federal, state, and local funding to create housing opportunities.

Tracie Faa-Thompson, MA, AASW, PGdipNDPT, CAEBC-I, is a social worker, certified animal ethology and behavior consultant-instructor, certified filial therapist, and is cofounder of Animal Assisted Play Therapy. She is the founder of Turn About Pegasus, an equine-assisted program for at-risk youth and families with a variety of difficulties. She is EAGALA approved for both mental health and equine specialist roles. She is also a practice teacher of social work students and a trainer in life story work and attachment theory. She specializes in adoption, working with traumatized children and their adoptive and foster families in the United Kingdom.

Caitlin Frawley, PhD, LMHC, earned her doctorate degree in counselor education from the University of Central Florida. She completed her master's degree in mental health counseling at Teachers College, Columbia University, in New York City. She is a licensed mental health counselor. Her clinical experiences include providing play therapy and counseling to children in the foster care system and youth survivors of sexual abuse.

Robert Jason Grant, EdD, LPC, RPT-S, is the creator of AutPlay® Therapy. He is a therapist, supervisor, and consultant, and uses several years of advanced training and his own lived neurodivergent experience to provide affirming services to children and their families. He is an international trainer and keynote presenter and multi-published author of several articles and books. He is currently serving as past chair on the board of directors for the Association for Play Therapy.

Chi-Sing "Denny" Li, PhD, LPC-S, LMFT, is professor in the Counselor Education Department of Sam Houston State University. He has been a licensed professional counselor (LPC) and a licensed marriage and family therapist (LMFT) in Texas for 30 years. His research and numerous publications are focused on cross-cultural issues in counseling, group counseling, and crisis and trauma counseling. Dr. Li was awarded the Outstanding Counselor Educator of the Year in 2023 by the Texas Association for Counselor Education and Supervision.

Yu-Fen Lin, PhD, LPC-S, is associate professor of counseling at the University of North Texas at Dallas. She serves as internship coordinator in her counseling program. She is the 2023 president elect of the Texas Association of Counselor Education and Supervision. Dr. Lin has numerous publications on multicultural counseling and gender wellness. In her private practice, she enjoys supervising many LPC associates and working with Asian American clients across all ages.

Kristin K. Meany-Walen, PhD, LMHC, RPT-S, is adjunct professor at University of Northern Iowa and a counselor in private practice. Her areas of expertise include Adlerian Play Therapy, school-based counseling, and wellness. Kristin frequently presents, publishes, and conducts research on these topics. She coauthored *Doing Play Therapy: From Building the Relationship to Facilitating Change and Partners in Play: An Adlerian Approach to Play Therapy* (3rd ed.).

Domonique Messing, LCSW, RPT, MBA, is a clinical social worker and registered play therapist. She currently serves clients in private practice and specializes in working with children, adolescents, young adults, parents, and expectant mothers. Domonique has extensive experience in various evidence-based treatments, practicing from a person-centered approach.

Felicia R. Neubauer, MSW, LCSW, currently works in private practice in Medford, New Jersey, as a therapist, as well as a TF-CBT trainer and consultant. Her work passion is helping children, adults, and families to heal from trauma and mental health issues.

Jason O. Perry, PhD, LCMHC, is teaching assistant professor and director of the McClammy Counseling and Research Laboratory at East Carolina University. He has a passion for serving the needs of the people from his home of Eastern North Carolina. He has nearly 23 years of combined experience in the areas of child and family mental health, adolescent substance abuse, career counseling, and corrections.

Keith I. Raymond, MA, CMHC, NCC, is a doctoral counseling student at Montclair State University. He holds a master of arts in clinical mental health counseling from New Jersey City University. Keith is a national certified counselor (NCC), licensed professional counselor (LPC), and psychotherapist working in private practice providing counseling services to children, adolescents, adults, families, and couples. His counseling specialty areas are providing play therapy services in various clinical settings and social justice advocacy for Black, indigenous, and people of color (BIPOC).

Lisa Remey, MEd, LPC-S, RPT-S™, Certified FirstPlay® Practitioner, and private practice owner, Bluebonnet Center for Play Therapy in New Braunfels, Texas. She has specialized in play therapy for 20 years and has worked with children, families, and the military community, supporting them from infancy to adolescence and is passionate about training play therapists through speaking and supervision.

Ana Guadalupe Reyes, PhD, LPC, NCC, CHST (elle/le/they/them), is assistant professor in the Department of Counseling at California State University, Fullerton. They are a national certified counselor, licensed professional counselor in the state of Texas, and certified humanistic sand tray therapist. Dr. Reyes is also a Usui Reiki master/teacher who practices various forms of energy healing. With more than 13 years of experience working with marginalized and racialized communities in multiple settings, Dr. Reyes integrates somatic, liberatory, and holistic approaches into their work as a scholar, educator, advocate, and counselor.

Marium Sadiq, MA, LPC, RPT, is a third-year counseling doctoral student at the University of North Texas. She is a licensed professional counselor and a registered play therapist who practices using Child-Centered Play Therapy. Throughout her time as a therapist, she has continuously noticed the impact of CCPT as a culturally aware approach to help support children with depression.

Clarissa L. Salinas, PhD, LPC-S, RPT-S, is assistant professor of counseling at the University of Texas Rio Grande Valley. She teaches a variety of courses to include Introduction to Counseling, Internship, and Child and Adolescent Counseling. She also works in private practice, where she provides play therapy to children in the community. Her scholarly contributions include publications on the topics of creative interventions, play therapy, and teaching and learning at a Hispanic Serving Institution (HSI).

Angela I. Sheely-Moore, PhD, is associate professor in the Counseling Department at Montclair State University. With eight years of clinical experience counseling children and families from diverse populations in school and agency settings, Dr. Sheely-Moore specializes in researching counseling services to marginalized communities from a social justice lens. She has published in the areas of multicultural competencies, play-based counseling services, and counselor education andragogy.

Risë VanFleet, PhD, RPT-S, CDBC, CAEBI, is a licensed psychologist (PA), registered play therapist-supervisor, certified dog behavior consultant, and certified animal ethology and behavior instructor with 48 years of clinical, supervisory, administrative, and teaching experience. She is well known internationally for her decades of work training mental health professionals in Play Therapy and Filial Therapy. She is president of the Family Enhancement & Play Therapy Center, Inc., in Boiling Springs, Pennsylvania. She is the founder and president of the International Institute for Animal Assisted Play Therapy®.